Board Review Series

Biochemistry
3rd edition

Board Review Series

Biochemistry

3rd edition

Dawn B. Marks, Ph.D.
Professor of Biochemistry
Department of Biochemistry
Temple University School of Medicine
Philadelphia, Pennsylvania

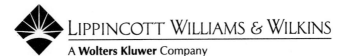

LIPPINCOTT WILLIAMS & WILKINS
A **Wolters Kluwer** Company

Philadelphia • Baltimore • New York • London
Buenos Aires • Hong Kong • Sydney • Tokyo

Editor: Elizabeth A. Nieginski
Managing Editor: Marette D. Magargle-Smith
Marketing Manager: Jennifer Conrad
Development Editor: Marjory I. Fraser

Copyright © 1999 Lippincott Williams & Wilkins

351 West Camden Street
Baltimore, Maryland 21201-2436 USA

Printed in the United States of America
First Edition,

Library of Congress Cataloging-in-Publication Data

Marks, Dawn B.,
        Biochemistry / Dawn B. Marks. — 3rd ed.
            p.   cm. — (Board review series)
        Includes index.
        ISBN 0–683–30491–7
        1. Biochemistry—Outlines, syllabi, etc. 2. Biochemistry—Examinations,
questions, etc. I. Title. II. Series.
        QP518.3.M37   1998
        572—dc21
        DNLM/DLC
        for Library of Congress   98–34102
                                                                                                        CIP

The publishers have made every effort to trace the copyright holders for borrowed material. If they have inadvertently overlooked any, they will be pleased to make the necessary arrangements at the first opportunity.

To purchase additional copies of this book, call our customer service department at **(800) 638-3030** or fax orders to **(301) 824-7390.** For other book services, including chapter reprints and large quantity sales, ask for the Special Sales Department. International customers should call **(301) 714-2324.**

Visit Lippincott Williams & Wilkins on the Internet: http://www.lww.com. Lippincott Williams & Wilkins customer service representatives are available from 8:30 am to 6:00 pm. EST.

04
7 8 9 10

Contents

Preface

This book is intended to aid students in preparing for examinations, particularly the United States Medical Licensing Examination (USMLE) Step 1. The basic material of biochemistry is presented in an integrative fashion in the conviction, based on 30 years of teaching, that details are easier to remember if they are presented within the context of the physiologic functioning of the human body. Changes in this edition include an update of information, more clinically-slanted questions (to match the changing format of the USMLE), and the addition of a chapter on the biochemical functions of tissues and the problems that result when a tissue malfunctions.

I hope that this edition will aid students not only with their immediate task of passing a set of examinations, but also with the more long-term objective of fitting the subject of biochemistry into the framework of basic and clinical sciences, so essential to understanding their future patients' problems.

How to Use This Book

Anyone who has been teaching for a number of years knows that students, particularly those in medical school or in other programs within the health sciences, do not have an infinite amount of time to study or to review any given course. Therefore, this book was designed to make it easier for you to review biochemistry only at the depth you require, depending on the purpose for your review and the amount of time you have available.

Each chapter is divided into topics; each topic begins with a comprehensive summary in a shaded box. As you read each summary, if you remember the details, skip to the shaded box that contains the summary of the next topic. If you do not remember the details, review the more in-depth presentations of the topic under the subheadings that follow each summary.

If you are really pressed for time, read only the material that begins at the left margin. If you have more time, read material that is indented toward the right. The farther toward the right you read, the more detail you get.

After you finish a chapter, try the questions and compare your answers to those in the explanations. If you have difficulty with the questions, review the chapter again.

By following the process outlined above, you can save time by reviewing only the topics you need to review and by concentrating only on the details you have forgotten.

Dawn B. Marks

Acknowledgments

I would like to thank Rosanne Hallowell of Williams & Wilkins for her support and for her flexibility in adapting to my hectic schedule.

I am especially indebted to Matthew Chansky, the artist who revamped the drawings from the previous edition into a much livelier format.

Dawn B. Marks

1

Fuel Metabolism

Overview

- The major fuels of the body, carbohydrates, fats, and proteins, are obtained from the diet and stored in the body's fuel depots.
- In the fed state (after a meal), ingested fuel is used to meet the immediate energy needs of the body and excess fuel is stored.
- During fasting (e.g., between meals or overnight), stored fuels are used to derive the energy needed to survive until the next meal.
- In prolonged fasting (starvation), changes occur in the use of fuel stores that permit survival for extended periods of time.
- The level of insulin in the blood increases in the fed state and promotes the storage of fuel, while the level of glucagon increases in the fasting state and promotes the release of stored fuel.

I. Metabolic Fuels and Dietary Components

- Carbohydrates, fats, and proteins serve as the major fuels of the body and are obtained from the diet. After digestion and absorption, these fuels can be oxidized for energy.
- Fuel consumed in excess of the body's immediate energy needs is stored, mainly as fat, but also as glycogen. To some extent, body protein can also be used as fuel.
- The daily energy expenditure of an individual includes the energy required for the basal metabolic rate (BMR) and the energy required for physical activity.
- In addition to providing energy, the diet also produces precursors for the synthesis of structural components of the body and supplies essential compounds which the body cannot synthesize (e.g., the essential fatty acids and amino acids, and the vitamins and minerals which often serve as cofactors for enzymes).

A. Fuels

- When **fuels** are metabolized in the body, **heat** is generated and adenosine triphosphate (**ATP**) is synthesized.

1. **Energy produced by oxidizing fuels to CO_2 and H_2O**

   a. **Carbohydrates** produce about **4 kcal/g.**

    b. Proteins produce about **4 kcal/g.**

    c. Fats produce more than twice as much energy **(9 kcal/g).**

    d. Alcohol, present in many diets, produces about **7 kcal/g.**

  2. Physicians and nutritionists often use the term **"calorie"** in place of **kilocalorie.**

  3. Heat generated by fuel oxidation is used to maintain **body temperature.**

  4. ATP generated by fuel metabolism is used for biochemical reactions, muscle contraction, and other energy-requiring processes.

B. Composition of body fuel stores (Figure 1-1)

  1. Triacylglycerol (triglyceride)

    a. Adipose triacylglycerol is the major fuel store of the body.

    b. Adipose tissue stores fuel very efficiently. It has more stored calories per gram and less water (15%) than other fuel stores. (Muscle tissue is about 80% water.)

  2. Glycogen stores, although small, are extremely important.

    a. Liver glycogen is used to maintain blood glucose during the early stages of fasting.

    b. Muscle glycogen is oxidized for muscle contraction.

  3. Protein does not serve solely as a source of fuel and can be degraded only to a limited extent.

    a. Approximately one-third of total body protein can be degraded.

    b. If too much protein is oxidized for energy, body functions can be severely compromised.

C. Daily energy expenditure is the amount of energy required each day.

  1. BMR is the energy used by a person who has fasted for at least 12 hours and is awake but at rest.
    – A rough estimate is: BMR = 24 kcal/kg body weight per day.

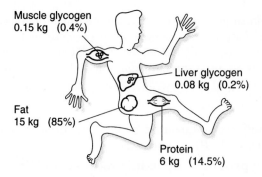

Muscle glycogen
0.15 kg (0.4%)

Liver glycogen
0.08 kg (0.2%)

Fat
15 kg (85%)

Protein
6 kg (14.5%)

Figure 1-1. **Fuel composition of the average 70-kg man after an overnight fast** (in kg and as a percentage of total calories).

2. **Specific dynamic action (SDA),** also called diet-induced thermogenesis (DIT), is the elevation in metabolic rate that occurs during digestion and absorption of foods. It is often ignored in calculations because its value is usually unknown and probably small (less than 10% of the total energy).

3. **Physical activity**

   a. The number of calories that physical activity adds to the daily energy expenditure varies considerably. A person can expend about 5 calories (kcal) each minute while walking but 20 calories while running.

   b. The daily energy requirement for an extremely sedentary person is about 30% of the BMR. For a more active person, it may be 50% or more of the BMR.

D. **Other dietary requirements and recommendations**

1. **Lipids**

   a. **Fat** should constitute 30% or less of the total calories—10% each of polyunsaturated, monounsaturated, and saturated fatty acids.

   b. **Cholesterol** intake should be no more than 300 mg/day.

   c. **Essential fatty acids** are the precursors of the polyunsaturated fatty acids required for the **synthesis of** prostaglandins and other **eicosanoids. Linoleic** and **α-linolenic acids** are the major dietary sources.

2. **Protein**

   – **The recommended protein** intake is **0.8 g/kg body weight** per day.

   a. **Essential amino acids**

      (1) **Nine** amino acids cannot be synthesized in the body and, therefore, must be present in the diet in order for protein synthesis to occur. The essential amino acids are **histidine, isoleucine, leucine, lysine, methionine, phenylalanine, threonine, tryptophan,** and **valine.**

      (2) Only a small amount of **histidine** is required in the diet; however, **larger amounts** are required for **growth** (e.g., children, pregnant women, people recovering from injuries).

      (3) Because **arginine** can be synthesized only in limited amounts, it is required in the diet for **growth.**

   b. **Nitrogen balance**

      (1) **Dietary protein**, which contains about 16% nitrogen, is the body's primary source of nitrogen.

      (2) **Proteins** are constantly being synthesized and degraded in the body.

      (3) As amino acids are oxidized, the nitrogen is converted to **urea** and excreted by the kidneys. Other nitrogen-containing compounds produced from amino acids are also excreted in the urine (**uric acid, creatinine,** and **NH_4^+**).

(4) Nitrogen balance (the normal state in the adult) occurs when **degradation** of body protein **equals synthesis**. The amount of nitrogen excreted in the urine each day equals the amount of nitrogen ingested daily.

(5) Negative nitrogen balance occurs when **degradation** of body protein **exceeds synthesis**. More nitrogen is excreted than ingested. It results from an inadequate amount of protein in the diet or from the absence of one or more essential amino acids.

(6) Positive nitrogen balance occurs when **degradation** of body protein is **less than synthesis**. Less nitrogen is excreted than ingested. It occurs during growth and synthesis of new tissue.

3. Vitamins and minerals

a. Vitamins and minerals are required in the diet. Many serve as **cofactors for enzymes.**

b. Minerals required in large amounts include **calcium and phosphate,** which serve as structural components of bone. Minerals required in trace amounts include **iron**, which is a component of heme.

II. The Fed or Absorptive State (Figure 1-2)

- Dietary carbohydrates are cleaved during digestion, forming monosaccharides (mainly glucose) that enter the blood. Glucose is oxidized by various tissues for energy or is stored as glycogen in the liver and in muscle. In the liver, glucose is also converted to triacylglycerols, which are packaged in very low density lipoproteins (VLDL) and released into the blood. The fatty acids of the VLDL are stored in adipose tissue.

- Dietary fats (triacylglycerols) are digested to fatty acids and 2-monoacylglycerols (2-monoglycerides). These digestive products are resynthesized to triacylglycerols by intestinal epithelial cells, packaged in chylomicrons, and secreted via the lymph into the blood. The fatty acids of chylomicrons are stored in adipose triacylglycerols.

- Dietary proteins are digested to amino acids and absorbed into the blood. The amino acids are used by various tissues to synthesize proteins and to produce nitrogen-containing compounds (e.g., purines, heme, creatine, epinephrine), or they are oxidized to produce energy.

A. Digestion and absorption

1. Carbohydrates

a. Starch, the storage form of carbohydrate in plants, is the major dietary carbohydrate.

(1) Salivary α-amylase (in the mouth) and **pancreatic α-amylase** (in the intestine) cleave starch to disaccharides and oligosaccharides.

(2) Enzymes with **maltase** and **isomaltase** activity are found in complexes located on the surface of the brush border of intestinal epithelial cells. They complete the conversion of starch to glucose.

b. Sucrose and lactose (ingested disaccharides) are cleaved by enzymes that are part of the complexes on the surface of intestinal epithelial cells.

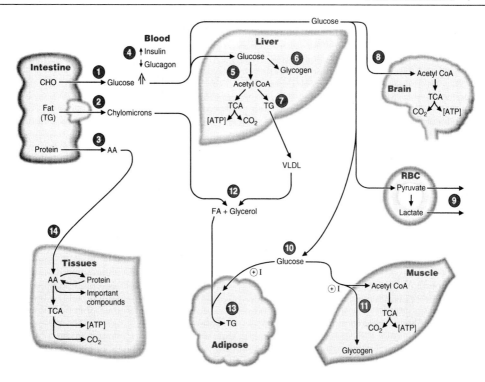

Figure 1-2. The fed state. The circled numbers serve as a guide, indicating the approximate order in which the processes begin to occur. AA = amino acid; FA = fatty acid; I = insulin; RBC = red blood cells; TG = triacylglycerols; VLDL = very low density lipoprotein; $\oplus$ = stimulated by.

(1) **Sucrase** converts sucrose to **fructose** and **glucose.**

(2) **Lactase** converts lactose to **glucose** and **galactose.**

c. **Monosaccharides** (mainly **glucose** and some **fructose** and **galactose**) are absorbed by the intestinal epithelial cells and pass into the blood.

2. **Fats**

a. **Triacylglycerol** is the primary dietary fat. It is obtained from the fat stores of the plants and animals that serve as food.

– The triacylglycerols are **emulsified** in the intestine by **bile salts** and **digested** by **pancreatic lipase** to **2-monoacylglycerols** and **fatty acids** which are packaged into **micelles** (solubilized by bile salts) and absorbed into intestinal epithelial cells, where they are reconverted to **triacylglycerols.**

b. After digestion and resynthesis, the triacylglycerols are packaged in **chylomicrons** that first enter the lymph and then the blood.

3. **Proteins**

a. Proteins are **digested** first by **pepsin** in the stomach and then by a series of enzymes in the intestine.

(1) The pancreas produces **trypsin, chymotrypsin, elastase,** and the **carboxypeptidases,** which act in the lumen of the intestine.

(2) **Aminopeptidases, dipeptidases,** and **tripeptidases** are associated with the intestinal epithelial cells.

    b. Proteins are ultimately **degraded** to a mixture of **amino acids,** which then enter intestinal epithelial cells, where some amino acids are metabolized. The remainder pass into the blood.

B. Digestive products in the blood

    1. Hormone levels change when the products of digestion enter the blood.

        a. Insulin levels rise principally as a result of **increased blood glucose levels,** and, to a lesser extent, increased blood levels of amino acids.

        b. Glucagon levels fall in response to glucose but rise in response to amino acids. Overall, after a mixed meal (containing carbohydrate, fat, and protein), glucagon levels remain fairly constant in the blood.

    2. Glucose and **amino acids** leave the intestinal epithelial cells and travel through the hepatic portal vein to the **liver.**

C. The fate of glucose in the fed (absorptive) state

    1. The fate of glucose in the liver

      – Liver cells either oxidize glucose or convert it to glycogen and triacylglycerols.

        a. Glucose is **oxidized** to CO_2 and H_2O to meet the immediate energy needs of the liver.

        b. Excess glucose is **stored** in the liver as **glycogen,** which is used during periods of fasting to maintain blood glucose.

        c. Excess glucose can be **converted to fatty acids** and a **glycerol** moiety, which combine to form **triacylglycerols,** which are released from the liver into the blood as **VLDL.**

    2. The fate of glucose in other tissues

        a. The **brain,** which depends on glucose for its energy, **oxidizes glucose to CO_2 and H_2O,** producing ATP.

        b. Red blood cells, lacking mitochondria, oxidize glucose to **pyruvate** and **lactate,** which are released into the blood.

        c. Muscle cells take up glucose by a **transport** process that is **stimulated by insulin.** They **oxidize glucose** to CO_2 and H_2O to generate ATP for contraction, and they also **store** glucose as **glycogen** for use during contraction.

        d. Adipose cells take up glucose by a **transport** process that is **stimulated by insulin.** These cells oxidize glucose to produce energy and convert it to the glycerol moiety used to produce triacylglycerol stores.

D. The fate of lipoproteins in the fed state

    1. The triacylglycerols of **chylomicrons** (produced from dietary fat) and **VLDL** (produced from glucose by the liver) are **digested** in capillaries by **lipoprotein lipase** to form fatty acids and glycerol.

    2. The **fatty acids** are taken up by **adipose tissue,** converted to **triacylglycerols,** and stored.

E. The fate of amino acids in the fed state

    – Amino acids from dietary proteins enter cells and are:

1. Used for **protein synthesis** (which occurs on ribosomes and requires mRNA). Proteins are constantly being synthesized and degraded.

2. Used to make **nitrogenous compounds** such as heme, creatine phosphate, epinephrine, and the bases of DNA and RNA.

3. Oxidized to generate **ATP**.

III. Fasting (Figure 1-3)

- As blood glucose levels decrease after a meal, insulin levels decrease and glucagon levels increase, stimulating the release of stored fuels into the blood.
- The liver supplies glucose and ketone bodies to the blood. The liver maintains blood glucose levels by glycogenolysis and gluconeogenesis and synthesizes ketone bodies from fatty acids supplied by adipose tissue.
- Adipose tissue releases fatty acids and glycerol from its triacylglycerol stores. The fatty acids are oxidized to CO_2 and H_2O by tissues. In liver, they are converted to ketone bodies. The glycerol is used for gluconeogenesis.
- Muscle releases amino acids. The carbons are used by the liver for gluconeogenesis, and the nitrogen is converted to urea.

A. The liver during fasting

– The liver produces **glucose** and **ketone bodies** that are released into the blood and serve as sources of energy for other tissues.

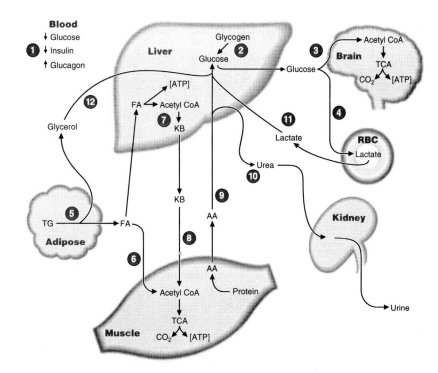

Figure 1-3. The fasting (basal) state. This state occurs after an overnight (12-hour) fast. The circled numbers serve as a guide, indicating the approximate order in which the processes begin to occur. KB = ketone bodies. For other abbreviations, see Figure 1-2.

1. **Production of glucose by the liver**
   – The liver has the major responsibility for **maintaining blood glucose levels.** Glucose is required particularly by tissues such as the brain and red blood cells. The brain oxidizes glucose to CO_2 and H_2O, while red blood cells oxidize glucose to pyruvate and lactate.

   a. **Glycogenolysis**
      – About 2-3 hours after a meal, the liver begins to break down its glycogen stores by the process of glycogenolysis, and glucose is released into the blood. Glucose is taken up by tissues and oxidized.

   b. **Gluconeogenesis**
      (1) After about 4-6 hours of fasting, the **liver** begins the process of gluconeogenesis. Within 30 hours, liver glycogen stores are depleted, leaving gluconeogenesis as the major process responsible for maintaining blood glucose.

      (2) **Carbon sources** for gluconeogenesis are:
         (a) **Lactate** produced by tissues like red blood cells or exercising muscle
         (b) **Glycerol** from breakdown of triacylglycerols in adipose tissue
         (c) **Amino acids,** particularly alanine, from muscle protein
         (d) **Propionate** from oxidation of odd-chain fatty acids (minor source)

2. **Production of ketone bodies by the liver**

   a. As glucagon levels rise, adipose tissue breaks down its **triacylglycerol stores** into fatty acids and glycerol, which are released into the blood.

   b. Through the process of **β-oxidation**, the liver converts the fatty acids to acetyl CoA.

   c. **Acetyl CoA** is used by the liver for the synthesis of the ketone bodies, **acetoacetate and β-hydroxybutyrate**. The liver cannot oxidize ketone bodies and releases them into the blood.

B. **Adipose tissue during fasting**

   1. As glucagon levels rise, adipose **triacylglycerol stores** are **mobilized.** The liver converts the fatty acids to ketone bodies and the glycerol to glucose.

   2. Tissues such as muscle oxidize the fatty acids to CO_2 and H_2O.

C. **Muscle during fasting**

   1. **Degradation of muscle protein**

      a. During fasting, muscle protein is degraded, producing amino acids, which are partially metabolized by muscle and released into the blood, mainly as **alanine** and **glutamine.**

      b. Tissues, such as **gut** and **kidney**, metabolize the glutamine.

      c. The products (mainly **alanine**) travel to the **liver** where the carbons are converted to glucose or ketone bodies and the nitrogen is converted to urea.

2. Oxidation of fatty acids and ketone bodies

    a. During **fasting**, muscle oxidizes fatty acids released from adipose tissue and ketone bodies produced by the liver.

    b. During **exercise**, muscle can also use its own glycogen stores as well as glucose, fatty acids, and ketone bodies from the blood.

IV. Prolonged Fasting (Starvation)

- In starvation (prolonged fasting), muscle decreases its use of ketone bodies. As a result, ketone body levels rise in the blood, and the brain uses them for energy. Consequently, the brain needs less glucose, and gluconeogenesis slows, sparing muscle protein.
- These changes in the fuel utilization patterns of various tissues enable us to survive for extended periods of time without food.

A. Metabolic changes in starvation (Figure 1-4)

    – When the body enters the **starved state,** after **3-5 days of fasting,** changes occur in the use of fuel stores.

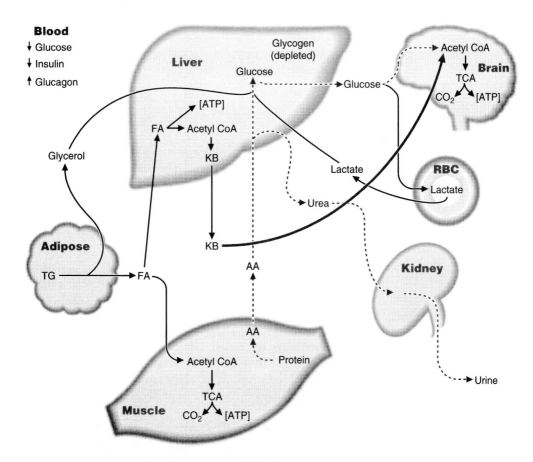

Figure 1-4. The starved state. This state occurs after 3-5 days of fasting. Dashed lines indicate processes that have decreased, and the heavy solid line indicates a process that has increased relative to the fasting state. For abbreviations, see Figures 1-2 and 1-3.

1. Muscle decreases its use of ketone bodies and oxidizes fatty acids as its primary energy source.

2. Because of decreased use by muscle, **blood ketone body levels rise.**

3. The **brain** then takes up and **oxidizes ketone bodies** to derive energy. Consequently, the brain decreases its use of glucose, although glucose is still a major fuel for the brain.

4. Liver **gluconeogenesis decreases.**

5. **Muscle protein is spared** (i.e., less muscle protein is degraded to provide amino acids for gluconeogenesis).

6. Because of decreased conversion of amino acids to glucose, **less urea is produced** from amino acid nitrogen in starvation than after an overnight fast.

B. Fat: the primary fuel

– The body uses its fat stores as its primary source of energy during starvation, conserving functional protein.

1. Overall, fats are quantitatively the most important fuel in the body.

2. The length of time that a person can survive without food depends mainly on the amount of fat stored in adipose tissue.

V. Clinical Correlations

A. Obesity

Obesity is associated with problems such as **hypertension, cardiovascular disease, and Type 2 diabetes mellitus** [formerly called non–insulin-dependent diabetes mellitus (NIDDM)]. Treatment involves altering lifestyle, particularly by decreasing food intake and increasing exercise.

B. Type 1 diabetes mellitus [formerly called insulin-dependent diabetes mellitus (IDDM)]

In untreated Type 1 diabetes mellitus (DM), insulin levels are low because of destruction of β cells of the pancreas, usually by an autoimmune process. Before insulin became widely available, individuals with Type 1 DM behaved metabolically as if they were in a constant state of starvation. Ingestion of food did not result in a rise in insulin, so fuel was not stored. Muscle protein and adipose triacylglycerol were degraded. Glucose and ketone bodies were produced by the liver in amounts that led to excretion by the kidneys. Severe weight loss ensued, and death occurred at an early age. Since insulin became available, these metabolic derangements have been treated.

C. Anorexia nervosa

Anorexia nervosa is characterized by **self-induced weight loss**. Those frequently affected include young, affluent, white women, who in spite of an emaciated appearance, often claim to be "fat." It is partially a behavioral problem; those afflicted are obsessed with losing weight.

D. Bulimia

People with bulimia suffer from binges of **overeating** followed by **self-induced vomiting** to avoid gaining weight.

E. Cystic fibrosis

Cystic fibrosis is the most common lethal **genetic disease** among the white population of the United States. Proteins of **chloride ion channels** are **defective**, and both eccrine and exocrine **gland** function are affected. Pulmonary disease and pancreatic insufficiency frequently occur. Food, particularly fats and proteins, are only partially digested, and **nutritional deficiencies** result.

F. Nontropical sprue

Nontropical sprue (adult celiac disease) results from a **reaction to gluten**, a protein found in grains. Intestinal epithelial cells are damaged, and **malabsorption** results. Common symptoms are steatorrhea, diarrhea, and weight loss.

G. Kwashiorkor

Kwashiorkor commonly occurs in children in third world countries where the **diet**, which is **adequate in calories**, is **low in protein**. A deficiency of dietary protein causes a decrease in protein synthesis that eventually affects the regeneration of intestinal epithelial cells and, thus, the problem is further compounded by **malabsorption**. Hepatomegaly and a **distended abdomen** are often observed.

H. Marasmus

Marasmus results from a **diet deficient** in both **protein and calories**. Persistent starvation ultimately results in death.

I. High-protein diets

When high-protein diets are very low in calories and the protein is of **low biologic value** (i.e., lacking in essential amino acids), **negative nitrogen balance** results. Body protein is degraded as amino acids are converted to glucose. A decrease in heart muscle can lead to death. Even if the protein is of high quality, ammonia and urea levels rise, putting increased stress on the kidneys. Vitamin deficiencies may occur due to a lack of fruits and vegetables.

J. Intravenous feeding

Solutions containing **5 g/dL glucose** are frequently infused into the veins of hospitalized patients. These solutions should be administered only for brief periods of time, because they lack the essential fatty and amino acids and because a high enough volume cannot be given each day to provide an adequate number of calories. More nutritionally complete solutions are available for long-term parenteral administration.

K. Hyperthyroidism

One of the most common forms of hyperthyroidism is Graves' disease. In this disease, the body produces antibodies that stimulate the thyroid gland to produce **excess thyroid hormone**. It is characterized by an **elevated BMR**,

an enlarged thyroid (goiter), protruding eyes, nervousness, tremors, palpitations, excessive perspiration, and weight loss.

L. Hypothyroidism

Hypothyroidism results from a **deficiency of thyroid hormone**. The **BMR is decreased**, and mucopolysaccharides accumulate on the vocal cords and in subcutaneous tissue. Common symptoms are lethargy, dry skin, a husky voice, decreased memory, and weight gain.

Review Test

Directions: Each of the numbered items or incomplete statements in this section is followed by answers or by completions of the statement. Select the **one** lettered answer or completion that is **best** in each case.

Questions 1–3

A young woman who has a sedentary job and does not exercise consulted a physician about her weight, which was 110 lb. A dietary history indicates that she eats approximately 100 g of carbohydrate, 20 g of protein, and 40 g of fat daily.

1. How many calories (kcal) does this woman consume each day?

(A) 1440
(B) 1340
(C) 940
(D) 840
(E) 640

2. What is the woman's approximate daily energy expenditure in calories (kcal) per day at this weight?

(A) 1200
(B) 1560
(C) 1800
(D) 2640
(E) 3432

3. Based on the woman's current weight, diet, and sedentary lifestyle, the physician correctly concludes that she should

(A) increase her exercise level
(B) decrease her protein intake
(C) increase her caloric intake
(D) decrease her fat intake to less than 30% of her total calories

4. In the normal adult, the fuel store that contains the fewest calories is

(A) adipose triacylglycerol
(B) liver glycogen
(C) muscle glycogen
(D) muscle protein

5. It is more advantageous for the human body to store fuel as triacylglycerol in adipose tissue than as protein in muscle because adipose triacylglycerol stores contain

(A) more calories and more water
(B) less calories and less water
(C) less calories and more water
(D) more calories and less water

6. Which one of the following amino acids is essential in the human diet?

(A) Serine
(B) Lysine
(C) Glutamate
(D) Tyrosine
(E) Cysteine

7. Which of the following statements concerning fuel metabolism is correct?

(A) Muscle protein cannot be used as a source of fuel for the body
(B) Negative nitrogen balance occurs when the amount of nitrogen excreted in the urine is less than the amount of nitrogen ingested in the diet
(C) Dietary protein is not required because amino acids can be synthesized from glucose
(D) A person who ingests 100 g of protein/day will excrete about 16 g of nitrogen in the urine

8. After fasting for 12 hours, a student consumes a large bag of pretzels. This meal will

(A) replenish liver glycogen stores
(B) increase the rate of gluconeogenesis
(C) reduce the rate at which fatty acids are converted to adipose triacylglycerols
(D) increase blood glucagon levels
(E) result in glucose being oxidized to lactate by the brain and to CO_2 and H_2O by red blood cells

9. Which of the following would be observed in a person who is resting after an overnight fast?

(A) Liver glycogen stores are completely depleted
(B) Liver gluconeogenesis is not an important process
(C) Muscle glycogen stores are used to maintain blood glucose
(D) Fatty acids are released from adipose triacylglycerol stores
(E) The liver is oxidizing ketone bodies to CO_2 and H_2O

10. Which of the following would be observed in a person after 1 week of starvation?

(A) The brain uses glucose and ketone bodies as fuel sources
(B) Liver glycogen stores are only partially depleted, owing to an increase in gluconeogenesis
(C) Nitrogen balance is maintained because muscle protein releases amino acids to compensate for the lack of dietary protein
(D) Fatty acids from adipose stores are the major source of fuel for red blood cells

11. When compared with his state after an overnight fast, a person who fasts for 1 week will have

(A) higher levels of blood glucose
(B) less muscle protein
(C) more adipose tissue
(D) lower levels of ketone bodies in the blood

12. Patients with anorexia nervosa, untreated Type 1 diabetes mellitus, hyperthyroidism, and nontropical sprue all will

(A) have a high BMR
(B) have high insulin levels in the blood
(C) experience weight loss
(D) suffer from malabsorption
(E) have low levels of ketone bodies in the blood

Directions: Each group of items in this section consists of lettered options followed by a set of numbered items. For each item, select the **one** lettered option that is most closely associated with it. Each lettered option may be selected once, more than once, or not at all.

Questions 13–16

(A) Protein
(B) Triacylglycerols
(C) Liver glycogen
(D) Muscle glycogen

Match each of the characteristics below with the source of stored energy that it best describes.

13. The largest form of stored energy in the body

14. The energy source reserved for strenuous muscular activity

15. The primary source of carbon for maintaining blood glucose during an overnight fast

16. The major precursor of urea in the urine

Questions 17–21

(A) Liver
(B) Brain
(C) Skeletal muscle
(D) Red blood cells

Match each of the characteristics below with the tissue it best describes.

17. After a fast of a few days, ketone bodies become an important fuel

18. Ketone bodies are used as a fuel after an overnight fast

19. Fatty acids are not a significant fuel source at any time

20. During starvation, this tissue uses amino acids to maintain blood glucose levels

21. This tissue converts lactate from muscle to a fuel for other tissues

Answers and Explanations

1-D. The woman consumes 400 calories (kcal) of carbohydrate (100 g × 4 kcal/g), 80 calories of protein (20 × 4), and 360 calories of fat (40 × 9) for a total of 840 calories daily.

2–B. This woman's daily energy expenditure is 1560 calories (kcal). Daily energy expenditure equals BMR plus activity. Her weight is 110 lb/2.2 = 50 kg. Her BMR (about 24 kcal/kg) is 50 kg × 24 = 1200 kcal/day. She is sedentary and needs only 360 additional kcal (30% of her BMR) to support her physical activity. Therefore, she needs 1200 + 360 = 1560 kcal each day.

3–C. Because her caloric intake (840 kcal/day) is less than her expenditure (1560 kcal/day), the woman is losing weight. She needs to increase her caloric intake. Exercise would cause her to lose more weight. She is probably in negative nitrogen balance because her protein intake is low (0.8 g/kg/day is recommended). Although her fat intake is 43% of her total calories and recommended levels are less than 30%, she should increase her total calories by increasing her carbohydrate and protein intake rather than decreasing her fat intake.

4–B. In the average (70-kg) man, adipose tissue contains 15 kg of fat or 135,000 calories (kcal). Liver glycogen contains about 0.08 kg of carbohydrate (320 calories), and muscle glycogen contains about 0.15 kg of carbohydrate (600 calories). In addition, about 6 kg of muscle protein (24,000 calories) can be used as fuel. Therefore, liver glycogen contains the fewest available calories.

5–D. Adipose tissue contains more calories (kcal) and less water than muscle protein. Triacylglycerol stored in adipose tissue contains 9 kcal/g, and adipose tissue has about 15% water. Muscle protein contains 4 kcal/g and has about 80% water.

6–B. Lysine cannot be synthesized and must be obtained in the diet. Serine and glutamate can be synthesized from glucose. Cysteine can be synthesized from serine, obtaining its sulfur from methionine. Tyrosine is produced from phenylalanine.

7–D. Muscle protein provides amino acids for gluconeogenesis, which produces glucose that is oxidized during fasting. Protein contains about 16% nitrogen; therefore, a person in nitrogen balance will excrete about 16 g of nitrogen for every 100 g of protein ingested. A person in negative nitrogen balance excretes more nitrogen in the urine than is ingested in dietary protein per day. Nine amino acids must be provided in the diet because they cannot be synthesized by the body.

8–A. After a meal of carbohydrates, glycogen is stored in the liver and in muscle, and triacylglycerols are stored in adipose tissue. The level of glucagon in the blood decreases, and gluconeogenesis decreases. The brain oxidizes glucose to CO_2 and H_2O while the red blood cells produce lactate.

9–D. During fasting, fatty acids are released from adipose tissue and oxidized by other cells. Liver glycogen is not depleted until about 30 hours of fasting. After an overnight fast, both glycogenolysis and gluconeogenesis by the liver help maintain blood glucose. Muscle glycogen stores are not used to maintain blood glucose. The liver produces ketone bodies but does not oxidize them.

10–A. After 3–5 days of starvation, the brain begins to use ketone bodies, in addition to glucose, as a fuel source. Glycogen stores in the liver are depleted during the first 30 hours of fasting. Inadequate protein in the diet results in negative nitrogen balance. Red blood cells cannot oxidize fatty acids, because they do not have mitochondria.

11–B. If a person who has fasted overnight continues to fast for 1 week, muscle protein will continue to decrease because it is being converted to blood glucose. However, it will not decrease at as rapid a rate as with a briefer fast, because the brain is using ketone bodies and, therefore, less glucose. His blood glucose levels will decrease only slightly, because initially glycogenolysis and then gluconeogenesis by the liver act to maintain blood glucose levels. Adipose tissue will decrease as triacylglycerol is mobilized. Fatty acids from adipose tissue will be converted to ketone bodies in the liver. Blood ketone body levels will rise, and ketone bodies will be used by the brain.

12–C. All of these patients will lose weight—the anorexic patients because of insufficient calories in the diet, the patients with Type 1 diabetes mellitus because of low insulin levels that result in the excretion of glucose and ketone bodies in the urine, those with hyperthyroidism because of an increased BMR, and those with nontropical sprue because of decreased absorption of food from the gut. The untreated diabetic patients will have high ketone levels because of low insulin. Ketone levels may be elevated in anorexia and also in sprue.

13–B. Adipose triacylglycerols contain the largest amount of stored energy.

14–D. Muscle glycogen is used for energy during exercise.

15–C. Liver glycogenolysis is the major process for maintaining blood glucose after an overnight fast.

16–A. The nitrogen in amino acids derived from protein is converted to urea and excreted in the urine.

17–B. The brain begins to use ketone bodies when levels start to rise after 3–5 days of fasting.

18–C. Skeletal muscle oxidizes ketone bodies, which are synthesized in the liver from fatty acids derived from adipose tissue.

19–D. Oxidation of fatty acids occurs in mitochondria. Red blood cells lack mitochondria and therefore cannot use fatty acids.

20–A. The liver converts amino acids to blood glucose by gluconeogenesis.

21–A. Exercising muscle produces lactate, which the liver can convert to glucose by gluconeogenesis. Blood glucose is oxidized by red blood cells and other tissues.

2

Basic Aspects of Biochemistry

Overview

- Acids dissociate, releasing protons and producing their conjugate bases.
- Bases accept protons, producing their conjugate acids.
- Buffers consist of acid-base conjugate pairs that can donate and accept protons, thereby maintaining the pH of a solution.
- Proteins, which are composed of amino acids, serve in many roles in the body (e.g., as enzymes, structural components, hormones, and antibodies).
- Interactions between amino acid residues produce the three-dimensional conformation of a protein.
- Enzymes are proteins that catalyze biochemical reactions.

I. Brief Review of Organic Chemistry

- Biochemical reactions involve the functional groups of molecules.

A. Identification of carbon atoms (Figure 2-1)
- Carbon atoms are either **numbered** or given **Greek letters.**

B. Functional groups in biochemistry
Types of groups
- Alcohols, aldehydes, ketones, carboxyl groups, anhydrides, sulfhydryl groups, amines, esters and amides are all important components of biochemical compounds (Figure 2-2).

C. Biochemical reactions
1. Reactions are classified according to the functional groups that react (e.g., **esterifications, hydroxylations, carboxylations, and decarboxylations**).

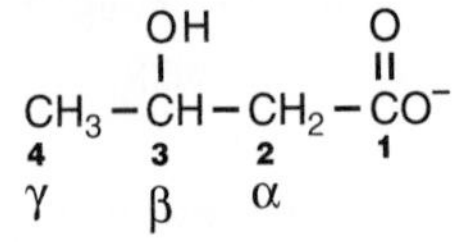

$$
\begin{array}{ccccc}
& \overset{\displaystyle OH}{|} & & \overset{\displaystyle O}{\|} & \\
CH_3 & - CH & - CH_2 & - CO^- & \\
\underset{\gamma}{4} & \underset{\beta}{3} & \underset{\alpha}{2} & 1 &
\end{array}
$$

Figure 2-1. Identification of carbon atoms in an organic compound. Carbons are numbered starting from the most oxidized carbon-containing group, or they are assigned Greek letters, with the carbon next to the most oxidized group designated as the α-carbon. This compound is 3-hydroxybutyrate or β-hydroxybutyrate. It is a ketone body.

17

Carbon–Oxygen groups

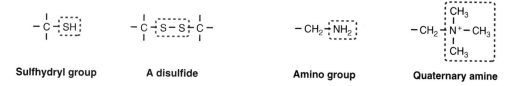

| Alcohol | Aldehyde | Ketone | Carboxylic acid | Ether | Acid anhydride |

Carbon–Sulfur groups

Carbon–Nitrogen groups

| Sulfhydryl group | A disulfide | Amino group | Quaternary amine |

Esters and Amides

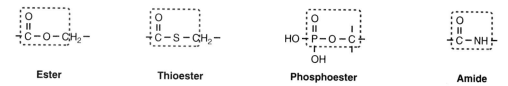

| Ester | Thioester | Phosphoester | Amide |

Figure 2-2. A brief review of organic chemistry.

2. **Oxidations** of sulfhydryl groups to disulfides, of alcohols to aldehydes and ketones, and of aldehydes to carboxylic acids frequently occur.

   a. Many of these oxidations are reversed by **reductions**.

   b. In **oxidation** reactions, electrons are lost. In **reduction** reactions, electrons are gained.

   c. As **foods are oxidized**, electrons are released and passed through the electron transport chain. Adenosine triphosphate (**ATP**) is generated and supplies the energy to drive various functions of the body.

II. Acids, Bases, and Buffers

- Many biochemical compounds, ranging from small molecules to large polymers, are capable of releasing or accepting protons at physiologic pH, and as a consequence, may carry a charge.
- Most biochemical reactions occur in aqueous solutions.
- The pH of a solution is the negative $\log_{10}$ of its hydrogen ion concentration $[H^+]$.
- Acids are proton donors, and bases are proton acceptors.
- The Henderson-Hasselbalch equation describes the relationship between pH, pK (the negative log of the dissociation constant), and the concentrations of an acid and its conjugate base.

- Buffers consist of solutions of acid-base conjugate pairs that resist changes in pH when H^+ or OH^- are added.
- Acids that are ingested or produced by the body are buffered by bicarbonate and by proteins, particularly hemoglobin. These buffers help to maintain the pH in the body within the range compatible with life.

A. Water

1. Water is the **solvent of life**. It dissociates

$$H_2O \rightleftharpoons H^+ + OH^-$$

with an equilibrium constant

$$K = \frac{[H^+][OH^-]}{[H_2O]}$$

2. Because the extent of dissociation is not appreciable, H_2O remains constant at 55.5 M, and the ion product of H_2O is

$$K_w = [H^+][OH^-] = 1 \times 10^{-14}$$

3. The **pH** of a solution is the negative $\log_{10}$ of its hydrogen ion concentration $[H^+]$:

$$pH = -\log_{10}[H^+]$$

– For pure water,

$$[H^+] = [OH^-] = 1 \times 10^{-7}$$

Therefore, **the pH of pure water is 7.**

B. Acids and bases

– Acids are compounds that donate protons, and bases are compounds that accept protons.

1. **Acids dissociate.**

   a. **Strong acids**, such as hydrochloric acid (HCl), dissociate completely.

   b. **Weak acids**, such as **acetic acid, dissociate only to a limited extent:**

$$HA \rightleftharpoons H^+ + A^-$$

   where HA is the acid and A^- its conjugate base.

   c. The **dissociation constant** for a weak acid is

$$K = \frac{[H^+][A^-]}{[HA]}$$

2. The **Henderson-Hasselbalch equation** was derived from the equation for the dissociation constant:

$$pH = pK + \log_{10}\frac{[A^-]}{[HA]}$$

where pK is the negative $\log_{10}$ of K, the dissociation constant.

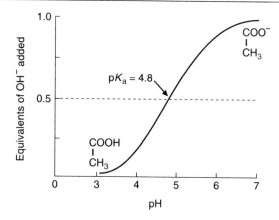

Figure 2-3. The titration curve of acetic acid. The molecular species that predominate at low (acetic acid) and high pH (acetate) are shown. At low pH (high [H⁺]), the molecule is protonated and has zero charge. As alkali is added, [H⁺] decreases (H⁺ + OH⁻ → H₂O), acetic acid dissociates, and the carboxyl group becomes negatively charged.

3. The **major acids** produced by the body include **phosphoric acid, sulfuric acid, lactic acid,** and the ketone bodies, **acetoacetic acid** and **β-hydroxybutyric acid.** CO_2 is also produced, which combines with H_2O to form **carbonic acid** in a reaction catalyzed by carbonic anhydrase:

$$CO_2 + H_2O \;\rightleftharpoons\; H_2CO_3 \rightleftharpoons H^+ + HCO_3^-$$
$$\text{carbonic}$$
$$\text{anhydrase}$$

C. Buffers

1. Buffers consist of **solutions of acid-base conjugate pairs,** such as acetic acid and acetate.

   a. Near its pK, a buffer maintains the pH of a solution, resisting changes due to addition of acids or bases (Figure 2-3). For a weak acid, the pK is often designated pK_a.

   b. At the pK_a, [A⁻] and [HA] are equal, and the buffer has its maximal capacity.

2. **Buffering mechanisms in the body**

   – The **normal pH range** of arterial blood is **7.37 to 7.43.**

   a. The major buffers of blood are **bicarbonate** (HCO_3^-/H_2CO_3) and **hemoglobin** (Hb/HHb).

   b. These buffers act in conjunction with mechanisms in the kidneys for excreting protons and mechanisms in the lungs for exhaling CO_2 to maintain the pH within the normal range.

III. Amino Acids and Peptide Bonds

- An amino acid usually contains a carboxyl group, an amino group, and a side chain, all bonded to the α-carbon atom.
- Amino acids are usually of the L-configuration.
- At physiologic pH, amino acids carry a positive charge on their amino groups and a negative charge on their carboxyl groups.

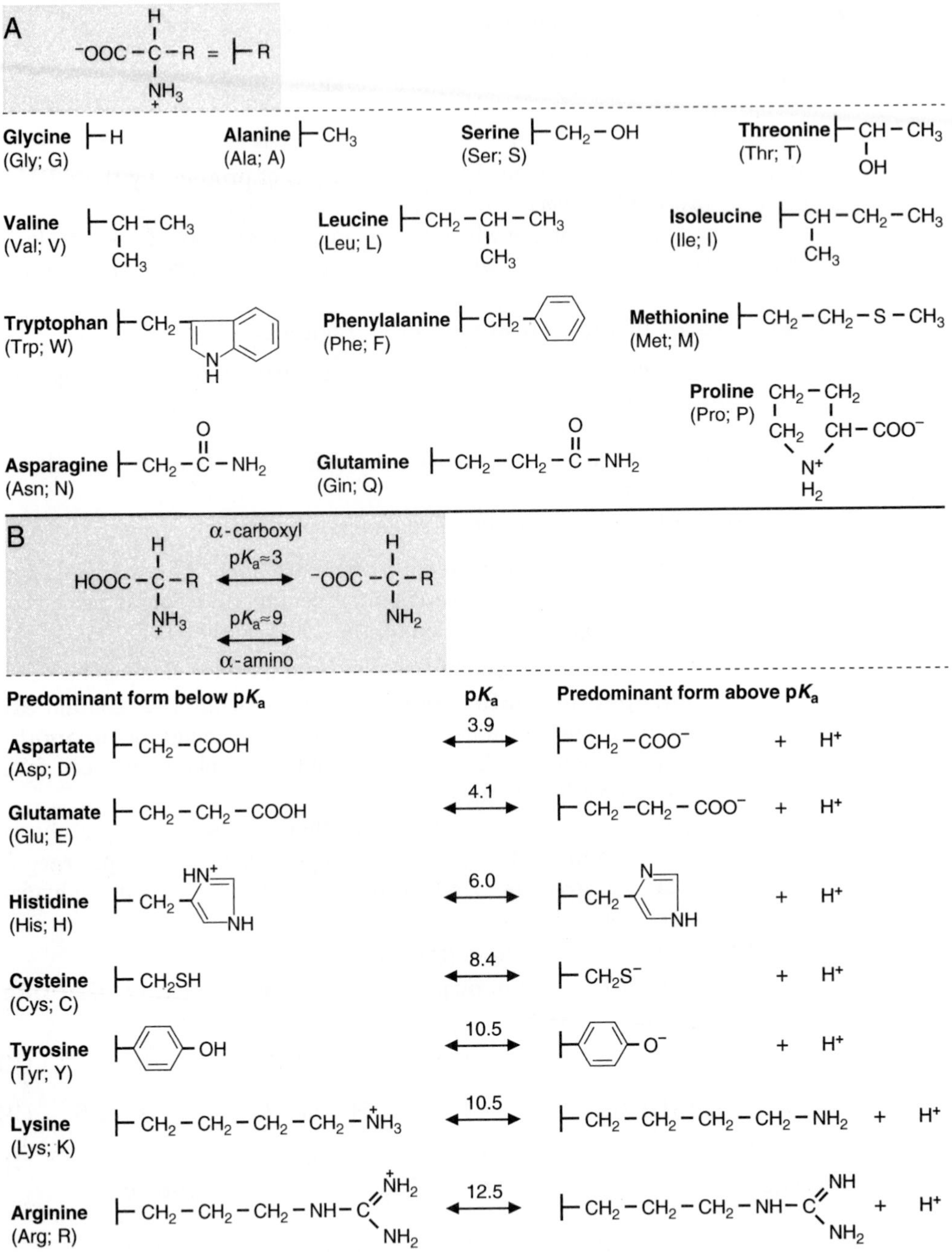

A

$$^-OOC - \underset{\underset{\overset{+}{NH_3}}{|}}{\overset{\overset{H}{|}}{C}} - R \;=\; {\vdash}R$$

Glycine ${\vdash}H$
(Gly; G)

Alanine ${\vdash}CH_3$
(Ala; A)

Serine ${\vdash}CH_2-OH$
(Ser; S)

Threonine ${\vdash}CH-CH_3$
(Thr; T) $\quad\;\; |$
$\qquad\qquad\; OH$

Valine ${\vdash}CH-CH_3$
(Val; V) $\quad\; |$
$\qquad\; CH_3$

Leucine ${\vdash}CH_2-CH-CH_3$
(Leu; L) $\qquad\qquad |$
$\qquad\qquad\quad\; CH_3$

Isoleucine ${\vdash}CH-CH_2-CH_3$
(Ile; I) $\qquad |$
$\qquad\quad CH_3$

Tryptophan ${\vdash}CH_2$
(Trp; W)

Phenylalanine ${\vdash}CH_2$
(Phe; F)

Methionine ${\vdash}CH_2-CH_2-S-CH_3$
(Met; M)

Proline CH_2-CH_2
(Pro; P) $\;\; | \qquad\quad |$
$\qquad\; CH_2 \quad CH-COO^-$
$\qquad\qquad\;\; \underset{H_2}{N^+}$

Asparagine ${\vdash}CH_2-\overset{\overset{O}{\|}}{C}-NH_2$
(Asn; N)

Glutamine ${\vdash}CH_2-CH_2-\overset{\overset{O}{\|}}{C}-NH_2$
(Gln; Q)

B

$$HOOC-\underset{\underset{\overset{+}{NH_3}}{|}}{\overset{\overset{H}{|}}{C}}-R \;\; \underset{\underset{\alpha\text{-amino}}{pK_a\approx 9}}{\overset{\overset{\alpha\text{-carboxyl}}{pK_a\approx 3}}{\longleftrightarrow}} \;\; ^-OOC-\underset{\underset{NH_2}{|}}{\overset{\overset{H}{|}}{C}}-R$$

Predominant form below pK_a	pK_a	Predominant form above pK_a
Aspartate ${\vdash}CH_2-COOH$ (Asp; D)	3.9	${\vdash}CH_2-COO^-$ $\quad+\quad H^+$
Glutamate ${\vdash}CH_2-CH_2-COOH$ (Glu; E)	4.1	${\vdash}CH_2-CH_2-COO^-$ $\quad+\quad H^+$
Histidine ${\vdash}CH_2$ (His; H)	6.0	${\vdash}CH_2$ $\quad+\quad H^+$
Cysteine ${\vdash}CH_2SH$ (Cys; C)	8.4	${\vdash}CH_2S^-$ $\quad+\quad H^+$
Tyrosine ${\vdash}$⬡$-OH$ (Tyr; Y)	10.5	${\vdash}$⬡$-O^-$ $\quad+\quad H^+$
Lysine ${\vdash}CH_2-CH_2-CH_2-CH_2-\overset{+}{N}H_3$ (Lys; K)	10.5	${\vdash}CH_2-CH_2-CH_2-CH_2-NH_2$ $\quad+\quad H^+$
Arginine ${\vdash}CH_2-CH_2-CH_2-NH-C\overset{\overset{+}{N}H_2}{\underset{NH_2}{}}$ (Arg; R)	12.5	${\vdash}CH_2-CH_2-CH_2-NH-C\overset{NH}{\underset{NH_2}{}}$ $\quad+\quad H^+$

Figure 2-4. Structures of the amino acids. Abbreviations are given for all amino acids. (A) Amino acids that do not have ionizable side chains. (B) Side chains that are ionizable. In B, for each amino acid, the species that predominates at a pH below the pK_a is shown on the left; the species that predominates at a pH above the pK_a is shown on the right. Note that the charge changes from 0 to - or from + to 0. At the pK_a, equal amounts of both species are present.

- The side chains of the amino acids contain different chemical groups. Some side chains carry a charge.
- Peptide bonds link adjacent amino acid residues in a protein chain.

A. Amino acids (Figure 2-4)

- There are 20 amino acids used for the synthesis of proteins by the mRNA-directed process that occurs on ribosomes (see Chapter 3).
- Other amino acids exist for which there is no genetic code; for example, in the urea cycle or in proteins where they are generated by post-translational modifications.

1. Structures of the amino acids (see Figure 2-4)

a. Most amino acids contain a **carboxyl group,** an **amino group,** and a **side chain** (R group), all attached to the α-carbon. Exceptions are:

(1) **Glycine,** which does not have a side chain. Its α-carbon contains two hydrogens.

(2) **Proline,** in which the nitrogen is part of a ring.

b. All of the 20 amino acids except glycine are of the **L-configuration** (Figure 2-5). Because glycine does not contain an asymmetric carbon atom, it is not optically active and, thus, it is neither D nor L.

c. The **classification** of amino acids is based on their side chains.

(1) **Hydrophobic amino acids** have side chains that contain **aliphatic** groups (valine, leucine, and isoleucine) or **aromatic groups** (phenylalanine, tyrosine, and tryptophan) that can form hydrophobic interactions.

- **Tyrosine** has a phenolic group that carries a negative charge above its pK_a ($\approx$10.5), so it is not hydrophobic in this pH range.

(2) **Hydroxyl groups** found on serine and threonine can form hydrogen bonds.

(3) **Sulfur** is present in cysteine and methionine.

- The **sulfhydryl groups** of two cysteines can form a **disulfide,** producing cystine:

$$
\underset{\textbf{Cysteine}}{\overset{\overset{\displaystyle COO^-}{|}}{\underset{\underset{\displaystyle NH_3^+}{|}}{H - C}} - CH_2 - SH} + \underset{\textbf{Cysteine}}{HS - CH_2 - \overset{\overset{\displaystyle COO^-}{|}}{\underset{\underset{\displaystyle NH_3^+}{|}}{CH}}} \rightleftharpoons \underset{}{\overset{\overset{\displaystyle COO^-}{|}}{\underset{\underset{\displaystyle NH_3^+}{|}}{H - C}} - CH_2 - S - S - CH_2 - \underset{\textbf{Cystine}}{\overset{\overset{\displaystyle COO^-}{|}}{\underset{\underset{\displaystyle NH_3^+}{|}}{CH}}}}
$$

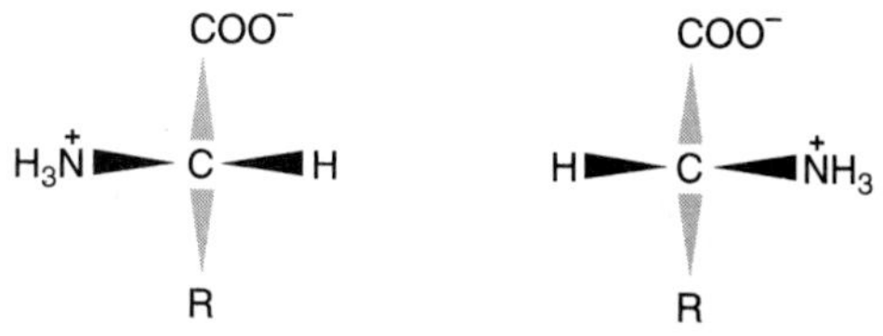

L-Amino acid   D-Amino acid

Figure 2-5. L- and D-amino acids. Groups at the broad parts of the arrows are closer to the viewer than groups at the narrow parts. R is the side chain. These forms are mirror images. They cannot be superimposed.

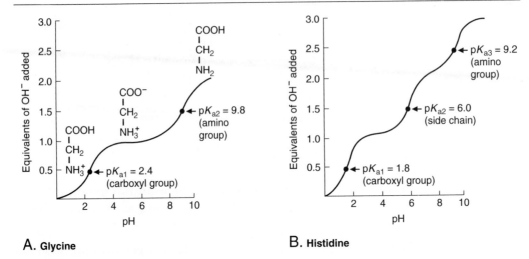

Figure 2-6. Titration curves for glycine (A) and histidine (B). The molecular species of glycine present at various pHs are indicated by the molecules above the curve. For histidine, pK_{a2} is the dissociation constant of the imidazole (side chain) group.

(4) Ionizable groups are present on the side chains of seven amino acids. They can **carry a charge,** depending on the pH. When charged, they can form **electrostatic interactions.**

(5) Amides are present on the side chains of **asparagine and glutamine.**

(6) The side chain of **proline forms a ring** with the nitrogen attached to the α-carbon.

2. Charges on amino acids (see Figure 2-4*B*)

    a. Charges on α-amino and α-carboxyl groups

       -At physiologic pH, the **α-amino group** is protonated ($pK_a{\approx}9$) and carries a **positive charge,** and the **carboxyl group** is dissociated ($pK_a{\approx}2$) and carries a **negative charge.**

    b. Charges on side chains

       (1) Positive charges are present on the side chains of the basic amino acids, **arginine, lysine,** and **histidine** at pH 7.

       (2) Negative charges are present on the side chains of the acidic amino acids, **aspartate and glutamate** at pH 7.

       (3) The **isoelectric point (pI)** is the pH at which the number of **positive charges equals** the number of **negative charges.**

3. Titration of amino acids

   – Ionizable groups on amino acids carry protons at low pH (high [H⁺]) that dissociate as the pH increases.

   a. For an amino acid that does not have an ionizable side chain, two pK_as are observed during titration (Figure 2-6*A*).

       (1) The first **(pK_{a1})** corresponds to the **α-carboxyl group** ($pK_{a1}{\approx}2$). As the proton dissociates, the carboxyl group goes from a zero to a minus charge.

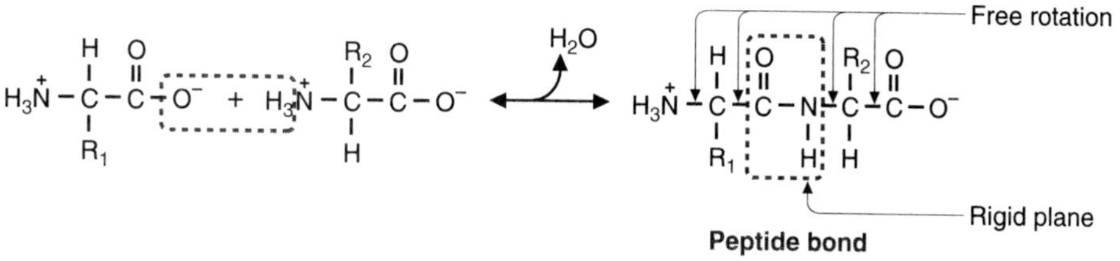

Figure 2-7. The peptide bond.

    (2) The second (**pK$_{a2}$**) corresponds to the **α-amino group** (pK$_{a2}$≈9). As the proton dissociates, the amino group goes from a positive to a zero charge.

  b. For an amino acid with an ionizable side chain, **three pK$_a$s** are observed during titration (see Figure 2-6*B*).

    (1) The α-carboxyl and α-amino groups have pK$_a$s of about 2 and 9, respectively.

    (2) The **third pK$_a$** varies with the amino acid and depends on the pK$_a$ of the side chain (see Figure 2-4*B*).

B. Peptide bonds

– Peptide bonds covalently join the α-carboxyl group of each amino acid to the α-amino group of the next amino acid in the protein chain (Figure 2-7).

  1. Characteristics

    a. The **atoms** involved in the peptide bond form a **rigid, planar unit.**

    b. Because of its **partial double-bond character**, the peptide bond has **no freedom of rotation**.

    c. However, the bonds involving the **α-carbon** can **rotate freely.**

  2. Peptide bonds are extremely stable. Cleavage generally involves the action of proteolytic enzymes.

IV. Protein Structure

- The primary structure of a protein consists of the amino acid sequence along the chain.

- Secondary structure involves α-helices, β-sheets, and other types of folding patterns.

- Tertiary structure (the three-dimensional conformation of a protein) involves electrostatic and hydrophobic interactions and hydrogen and disulfide bonds.

- Quaternary structure refers to the interaction of one or more subunits to form a protein.

- Proteins serve in many roles (e.g., as enzymes, hormones, receptors, antibodies, structural components, transporters of other compounds, and contractile elements in muscle).

A. General aspects of protein structure (Figure 2-8)

– The **linear sequence** of amino acid residues in a polypeptide chain determines the three-dimensional configuration of a protein, and the **structure** of a protein determines its function.

1. The **primary structure** is the sequence of amino acids along the polypeptide chain.

   a. By convention, the **sequence** is written from left to right, starting with the **N-terminal** amino acid.

   b. Because there are no dissociable protons in peptide bonds, the **charges** on a polypeptide chain are due only to the N-terminal amino group, the C-terminal carboxyl group, and the side chains on amino acid residues (see Figure 2-4*B*).

      – A protein will **migrate** in an **electric field**, depending on the sum of its charges at a given pH (the net charge).

      (1) Positively charged proteins are cations and migrate toward the **cathode (-).**

      (2) Negatively charged proteins are anions and migrate toward the **anode (+).**

      (3) At the **isoelectric pH** (the pI), the net charge is zero, and the protein does not migrate.

2. **Secondary structure** includes various types of local conformations in which the atoms of the side chains are not involved.

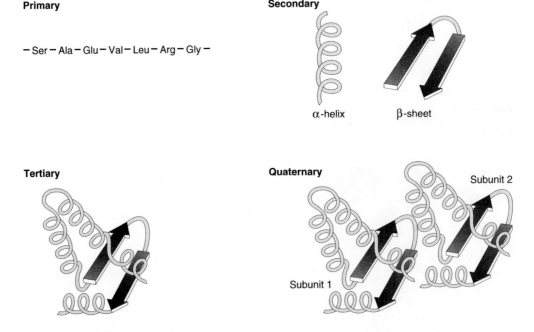

Figure 2-8. Schematic diagram of the primary, secondary, tertiary, and quaternary structure of a protein.

a. An **α-helix** is generated when each carbonyl of a peptide bond forms a **hydrogen bond** with the -NH of a peptide bond four amino acid residues further along the chain (Figure 2-9).

  (1) The side chains of the amino acid residues extend outward from the central axis of the rod-like structure.

  (2) The α-helix is disrupted by proline residues, in which the ring imposes geometric constraints, and by regions in which numerous amino acid residues have charged groups or large, bulky side chains.

b. **β-Sheets** are formed by **hydrogen bonds** between two extended polypeptide chains or between two regions of a single chain that folds back on itself (Figure 2-10).

  (1) These **interactions** are between the **carbonyl** of one peptide bond and the **-NH** of another.

  (2) The chains may run in the same direction or in opposite directions.

c. **Supersecondary structures**

  (1) Certain folding patterns involving α-helices and β-sheets are frequently found and include the **helix-turn-helix**, the **leucine zipper**, and the **zinc finger**.

  (2) Other types of **helices** or **loops** and **turns** can occur that differ from one protein to another (random coils).

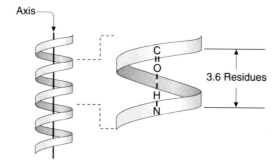

Figure 2-9. An α-helix. The enlarged segment shows the hydrogen bonding that occurs between the carbonyl (C = O) of one peptide bond and the -NH of another peptide bond that is four amino acid residues further along the chain.

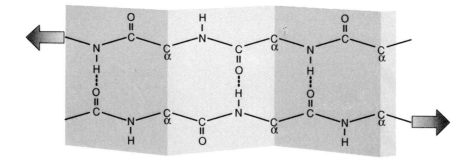

Figure 2-10. The structure of an antiparallel β-sheet. The orientation is indicated by *arrows*.

3. The **tertiary structure** of a protein refers to its overall **three-dimensional conformation.** It is produced by interactions between amino acid residues that may be located at a considerable distance from each other in the primary sequence of the polypeptide chain (Figure 2-11).

   a. **Hydrophobic amino acid residues** tend to collect in the **interior** of globular proteins, where they exclude water, while **hydrophilic residues** are usually found on the **surface,** where they interact with water.

   b. The types of interactions between amino acid residues that produce the **three-dimensional shape** of a protein include **hydrophobic** interactions, **electrostatic** interactions, and **hydrogen bonds**, all of which are **noncovalent. Covalent disulfide bonds** also occur.

4. **Quaternary structure** refers to the spatial arrangement of **subunits** in a protein that consists of more than one polypeptide chain (see Figure 2-8).

   – The subunits are joined together by the same types of **noncovalent interactions** that join various segments of a single chain to form its tertiary structure.

5. **Denaturation and renaturation**

   a. Proteins can be **denatured** by agents such as **heat** and **urea** that cause **unfolding** of polypeptide chains without causing hydrolysis of peptide bonds.

   b. If a denatured protein returns to its native state after the denaturing agent is removed, the process is called **renaturation**.

6. **Post-translational modifications** of proteins occur after the protein has been synthesized on the ribosome.

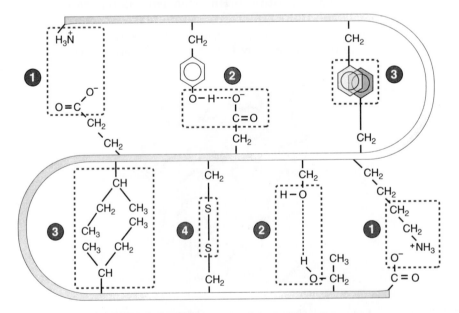

Figure 2-11. Interactions between amino acid residues in a polypeptide chain. ❶ Electrostatic interactions; ❷ hydrogen bonds; ❸ hydrophobic interactions; ❹ a disulfide bond.

– Phosphorylation, glycosylation, ADP-ribosylation, methylation, hydroxylation, and acetylation affect the charge and the interactions between amino acid residues, **altering the three-dimensional configuration** and, thus, the function of the protein.

B. Hemoglobin (Figure 2-12)

1. Structure of hemoglobin

– Adult hemoglobin (HbA) consists of **four polypeptide chains** (two α and two β chains), each containing a molecule of **heme.**

a. The α **and** β **chains** of HbA are **similar** in three-dimensional configuration to each other and to the single chain of muscle myoglobin although their amino acid sequences differ.

b. Eight regions of α-helix occur in each chain.

c. Heme fits into a crevice in each globin chain and interacts with two histidine residues.

2. Function of hemoglobin

a. The **oxygen saturation curve** for hemoglobin is **sigmoidal** (Figure 2-13).

   (1) Each heme binds **one O_2** molecule, for a total of four O_2 molecules per HbA molecule. HbA changes from the taut or tense **(T) form** to the relaxed **(R) form** when oxygen binds.

   (2) Binding of O_2 to one heme group in hemoglobin increases the affinity for O_2 of its other heme groups. This effect produces the sigmoidal oxygen saturation curve.

b. The binding of **protons** to HbA stimulates the release of O_2, a manifestation of **the Bohr effect** (see Figure 2-13).

   (1) Thus, O_2 is readily released in the tissues where [H^+] is high due to the production of CO_2 by metabolic processes:

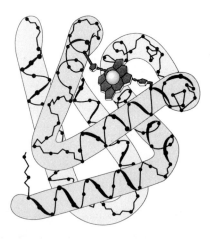

Figure 2-12. The structure of the β-chain of hemoglobin. Cylindrical regions contain α-helices. The planar structure near the top center of the polypeptide chain is heme. (From: ENZYME STRUCTURE AND MECHANISM by Fersht © 1977 by W.H. Freeman and Company. Used with permission.)

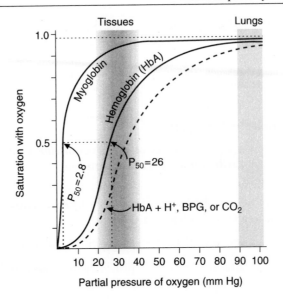

Figure 2-13. Oxygen saturation curves for myoglobin and adult hemoglobin (HbA). Myoglobin has a hyperbolic saturation curve. HbA has a sigmoidal curve. The HbA curve shifts to the right at lower pH, with higher concentrations of 2,3-biphosphoglycerate (BPG), or as CO_2 binds to HbA in the tissues. Under these conditions, O_2 is released more readily. P_{50} is the partial pressure of O_2 at which half-saturation with O_2 occurs.

$$CO_2 + H_2O \rightleftharpoons H_2CO_3 \rightleftharpoons H^+ + HCO_3^-$$

Tissues $\rightarrow$ $\quad\quad\quad H^+ + HbAO_2 \rightleftharpoons HHbA + O_2$ $\quad \leftarrow$ **Lung**

  (2) These reactions are reversed in the lung. O_2 binds to HbA, and CO_2 is exhaled.

 c. Covalent binding of **CO_2** to HbA in the tissues also causes the release of O_2.

 d. Binding of **2,3-bisphosphoglycerate (BPG)** (formerly known as 2,3-diphosphoglycerate [DPG]), a side product of glycolysis in red blood cells, decreases the affinity of HbA for O_2. Consequently, O_2 is more readily released in tissues when BPG is bound to HbA.

  – **Fetal hemoglobin (HbF),** composed of 2 α subunits and and 2 γ subunits, has a lower affinity for BPG than does HbA and, therefore, HbF has a higher affinity for O_2.

C. Collagen refers to a group of very similar structural proteins that are found, for example, in the **extracellular matrix,** the **vitreous humor** of the eye, and in **bone and cartilage.**

 1. Structure of collagen

  a. Collagen consists of **three chains** that wind around each other to form a **triple helix** (Figure 2-14).

  b. Collagen contains approximately 1000 amino acids, one-third of which are **glycine.** The sequence Gly-X-Y frequently occurs, in which X is often **proline** and Y is **hydroxyproline** or **hydroxylysine.**

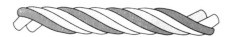

Figure 2-14. The triple helix of collagen. Three polypeptide chains wrap around each other as indicated by the shading. Cross-links hold the chains together.

2. Synthesis of collagen

a. The polypeptide chains of **preprocollagen** are synthesized on the **rough endoplasmic reticulum**, and the signal (pre) sequence is cleaved.

b. Proline and **lysine** residues are **hydroxylated** by a reaction that requires O_2 and **vitamin C.**

c. Galactose and **glucose** are added to hydroxylysine residues.

d. The **triple helix** forms, procollagen is secreted from the cell, and cleaved to form collagen.

e. Cross-links are produced. The side chains of lysine and hydroxylysine residues are oxidized to form aldehydes, which can undergo aldol condensation or form Schiff bases with the amino groups of lysine residues.

D. Insulin

1. Structure of insulin (Figure 2-15)

– Insulin is a polypeptide hormone that is produced by the **β cells** of the **pancreas**. It has 51 amino acids in **two polypeptide chains**, which are linked by two **disulfide bridges**.

2. Synthesis of insulin

a. Preproinsulin is synthesized on the rough endoplasmic reticulum and the pre- (signal) sequence is removed to form proinsulin.

b. In secretory granules, **proinsulin** is cleaved, and the **C-peptide** is released. The remainder of the molecule forms the active hormone.

V. Enzymes

- A major role of proteins is to serve as enzymes, catalysts of biochemical reactions.
- The active sites of enzymes are the regions where substrates bind and are converted to products, which are released.
- The rate (v) of many enzyme-catalyzed reactions can be described by the Michaelis-Menten equation. For enzymes that exhibit Michaelis-Menten kinetics, plots of velocity versus substrate concentration are hyperbolic.
- The Michaelis-Menten equation can be rearranged to give the Lineweaver-Burk equation.
- Competitive inhibitors compete with the substrate for binding at the active site of the enzyme.
- Noncompetitive inhibitors bind to the enzyme or the enzyme-substrate complex at a site different from the active site.

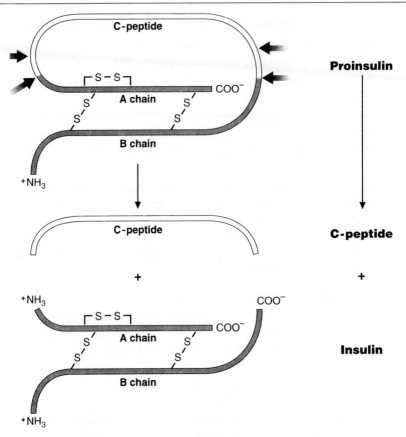

Figure 2-15. The cleavage of proinsulin to form insulin. Heavy arrows indicate the sites of cleavage, which release the C-peptide. The A and B chains of insulin are joined by disulfide bonds.

- Allosteric enzymes bind activators or inhibitors at sites other than the active site. Plots of the velocity versus substrate concentration for allosteric enzymes produce curves that are sigmoidal.

A. General properties of enzymes

1. The reactions of the cell would not occur rapidly enough to sustain life if enzyme catalysts were not present.

2. **Substrates** bind at the **active sites** of enzymes, where they are converted to products and released.

3. Enzymes are usually **highly specific** for their substrates and products.

   a. Many enzymes recognize only a single compound as a substrate.

   b. Some enzymes, such as those involved in digestion, are less specific.

4. Many enzymes require **cofactors** that frequently are **metal ions** or derivatives of **vitamins.**

5. Enzymes **decrease** the **energy of activation** for a reaction. They do not affect the equilibrium concentrations of the substrates and products.

B. Dependence of velocity on [E], [S], temperature, and pH

1. The **velocity** of a reaction, **v, increases with the enzyme concentration, [E]**, if the substrate concentration, **[S]**, is constant.

2. If [E] is constant, v increases with [S] until the **maximum velocity, V_{max}**, is attained.
   – At **V_{max}**, all the **active sites** of the enzyme are **saturated** with substrate.

3. The **velocity** of a reaction **increases with temperature** until a maximum is reached, after which the velocity decreases due to denaturation of the enzyme.

4. Each enzyme-catalyzed reaction has an **optimal pH** at which appropriate charges are present on both the enzyme and the substrate, and the velocity is at a maximum.
   – Changes in the pH can alter these charges so that the reaction proceeds at a slower rate. If the pH is too high or too low, the enzyme can also undergo **denaturation**.

C. The Michaelis-Menten equation

1. If, during a reaction, an **enzyme-substrate complex** is formed that **dissociates** (to re-form the free enzyme and the substrate) or **reacts** (to release the product and regenerate the free enzyme):

$$E + S \underset{k_2}{\overset{k_1}{\rightleftharpoons}} ES \overset{k_3}{\longrightarrow} E + P$$

where E is the enzyme, S the substrate, ES the enzyme-substrate complex, P the product, and k_1, k_2, and k_3 are rate constants.

2. From this concept, the **Michaelis-Menten** equation was derived:

$$v = \frac{V_m \, [S]}{K_m + [S]}$$

where $K_m = (k_2 + k_3)/k_1$ and V_{max} is the maximum velocity.

A

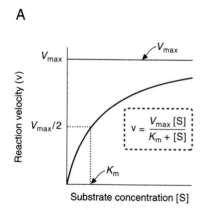

B

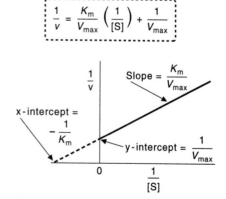

Figure 2-16. The velocity of an enzyme-catalyzed reaction that exhibits Michaelis-Menten kinetics. (A) Velocity (v) versus substrate concentration ([S]); (B) Lineweaver-Burk plot. Note the points on each plot from which V_{max} and K_m can be determined. V_{max} = maximum velocity, and K_m = the substrate concentration at $\frac{1}{2}$ V_{max}.

3. The rate of formation of products (the velocity of the reaction) is related to the **concentration of the enzyme-substrate complex:**

$$v = k_3[ES]$$

V_{max} is reached when all of the enzyme is in the enzyme-substrate complex.

4. **K_m** is the **substrate concentration** at which **$v = \frac{1}{2} V_{max}$.**
   – When $[S] = K_m$, substitution of K_m for $[S]$ in the Michaelis-Menten equation yields $v = \frac{1}{2} V_{max}$.

5. When the velocity is plotted versus $[S]$, a **hyperbolic curve** is produced (Figure 2-16*A*).

D. The **Lineweaver-Burk equation** (see Figure 2-16*B*)
   – Because of the difficulty in determining V_{max} from a hyperbolic curve, the Michaelis-Menten equation was transformed by Lineweaver and Burk into an equation for a straight line.

E. **Inhibitors** of enzymes decrease the rate of enzymatic reactions.

1. **Competitive inhibitors** compete with the substrate for the active site of the enzyme and form an enzyme-substrate complex, EI (see Figure 2-17*A*).
   a. Competitive inhibition is reversed by increasing $[S]$.
   b. **V_{max}** remains the same, but the **apparent K_m (K'_m) is increased.**
   c. For Lineweaver-Burk plots, **lines** for the inhibited reaction **intersect** on the **Y-axis** with those for the uninhibited reaction.

2. **Noncompetitive inhibitors** bind to the enzyme or the enzyme-substrate complex at a site different from the active site, decreasing the activity of the enzyme (see Figure 2-17*B*). Thus, **V_{max} is decreased.**

A. **Competitive inhibition**
   • V_{max} does not change
   • K_m increases

B. **Pure noncompetitive inhibition**
   • V_{max} decreases
   • K_m changes under some conditions

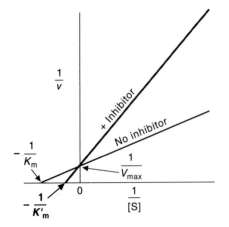
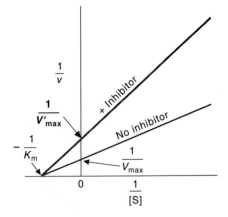

Figure 2-17. Effect of inhibitors on Lineweaver-Burk plots. (A) Competitive inhibition. (B) Pure noncompetitive inhibition (in which the inhibitor binds to E and ES with the same affinity). If the affinities differ, the lines will not intersect on the x-axis and the apparent K_m (K'_m) will differ from K_m. V'_{max} = the apparent V_{max}.

3. Irreversible inhibitors bind tightly to the enzyme and **inactivate** it.

F. Allosteric enzymes

1. Allosteric enzymes **bind activators or inhibitors** at sites other than the active site (Figure 2-18).

2. **Sigmoidal curves** are generated by plots of v versus [S].

   a. An allosteric enzyme has two or more subunits each with **substrate binding sites** that exhibit **cooperativity**. Binding of a substrate molecule at one site facilitates binding of other substrate molecules at other sites.

      (1) Allosteric activators cause the enzyme to bind substrate more readily.

      (2) Allosteric inhibitors cause the enzyme to bind substrate less readily.

   b. Similar effects occur during O_2 binding to **hemoglobin** (see Figure 2-13).

G. Regulation of enzyme activity by covalent modification

   – Enzyme activity may increase or decrease after the covalent addition of a chemical group.

1. Phosphorylation affects many enzymes.

   – Pyruvate dehydrogenase and glycogen synthase are inhibited by phosphorylation, while glycogen phosphorylase is activated.

2. Phosphatases that remove the phosphate groups alter the activities of these enzymes.

H. Regulation by protein-protein interactions

   – Proteins can bind to enzymes, altering their activity. For example, regulatory subunits inhibit the activity of protein kinase A. When these regulatory subunits bind cyclic AMP (cAMP) and are released from the enzyme, the catalytic subunits become active.

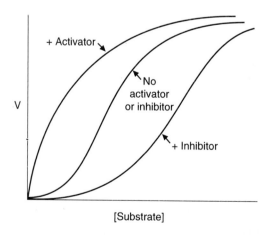

Figure 2-18. Effect of activators and inhibitors on an allosteric enzyme.

I. Isoenzymes

1. Isoenzymes (or isozymes) are enzymes that catalyze the same reaction but differ in their amino acid sequence and, therefore, in many of their properties.

2. Tissues contain **characteristic isozymes** or mixtures of isozymes. Enzymes such as lactate dehydrogenase and creatine kinase differ from one tissue to another.

   a. **Lactate dehydrogenase** contains four subunits. Each subunit may be either of the heart (H) or the muscle (M) type. Five isozymes exist (HHHH, HHHM, HHMM, HMMM, and MMMM).

   b. **Creatine kinase**, contains two subunits. Each subunit may be either of the muscle (M) or the brain (B) type. Three isozymes exist (MM, MB, and BB). The MB fraction is most prevalent in heart muscle.

VI. Clinical Correlations

A. Acid-base disturbances

Hypoventilation causes retention of CO_2 by the lungs, which can lead to a **respiratory acidosis**. Hyperventilation can cause a **respiratory alkalosis**. **Metabolic acidosis** can result from accumulation of metabolic acids (lactic acid or the ketone bodies, β-hydroxybutyric acid and acetoacetic acid), or ingestion of acids or compounds that are metabolized to acids (e.g., methanol, ethylene glycol). **Metabolic alkalosis** is due to increased HCO_3^-, which is accompanied by an increased pH. Acid-base disturbances lead to compensatory responses that attempt to restore normal pH. For example, a metabolic acidosis causes hyperventilation and the release of CO_2, which tends to lower the pH. During metabolic acidosis, the kidneys excrete NH_4^+, which contains H^+ buffered by ammonia:

$$H^+ + NH_3 \rightleftharpoons NH_4^+$$

B. Hemoglobinopathies

Many types of **mutations** produce alterations in the structure of hemoglobin. One common mutation results in **sickle cell anemia**, in which the β chain of hemoglobin contains a valine rather than a glutamate at position 6. Thus, in the mutant hemoglobin (HbS), a hydrophobic amino acid replaces an amino acid with a negative charge. This change allows deoxygenated molecules of HbS to polymerize. Red blood cells that contain large complexes of HbS molecules can assume a sickle shape. These cells undergo **hemolysis** and an **anemia** results. Painful **vaso-occlusive crises** also occur, and **end-organ damage** may result.

C. Problems associated with connective tissue

Mutations in the synthesis and processing of **collagen** occur in **Ehlers-Danlos syndrome**, which is characterized by abnormalities of skin, ligaments, and internal organs. The skin is fragile and often stretches easily. Joint laxity occurs. Abnormalities in type I **collagen** genes have been found in **osteogenesis imperfecta**. In this condition, bones are fragile and are readily fractured. In **scurvy**, which is due to **vitamin C deficiency**, hydroxylation of proline residues is decreased, and an unstable form of **collagen** is produced.

Bones, teeth, blood vessels, and other structures rich in collagen develop abnormally. Bleeding gums and poor wound healing are often observed. **Marfan's syndrome** results from a defect in the protein **fibrillin**. Clinical manifestations are variable but often include tall stature with arachnodactyly (long, thin fingers and toes), mitral valve prolapse, and lens dislocation.

D. Diabetes mellitus

Diabetes mellitus, which is due to a **deficiency of insulin** (Type 1 or insulin-dependent diabetes mellitus, **IDDM**) or to decreased secretion of insulin or **resistance** of tissues to insulin action (Type 2 or noninsulin-dependent diabetes mellitus, **NIDDM**), results in **hyperglycemia**. Autoimmunity plays a role in the etiology of IDDM. In this condition, the plasma usually contains antibodies to islet cells of the pancreas, including those that produce insulin.

E. Deficient or defective enzymes

Thousands of diseases related to deficient or defective enzymes occur. Many of them are **rare**. For example, in **phenylketonuria** (which has an incidence of 1 in 10,000 births in whites and Asians), the enzyme **phenylalanine hydroxylase,** which converts phenylalanine to tyrosine, is deficient. Phenylalanine accumulates, and tyrosine becomes an essential amino acid that is required in the diet. **Mental retardation** is a result of metabolic derangement. A more **common problem** is **lactase deficiency**, which occurs in more than 80% of Native-, African-, and Asian-Americans. Lactose is not digested at a normal rate and accumulates in the gut where it is metabolized by bacteria. **Bloating, abdominal cramps,** and **watery diarrhea** result.

F. Therapeutic uses of enzyme kinetics

Drugs are frequently used therapeutically to **inhibit enzymes**; for example 5-fluorouracil (5-FU) is used to inhibit the enzyme thymidylate synthetase. This enzyme converts dUMP to dTMP, which ultimately provides the thymine for DNA synthesis. **5-FU** is used as a **chemotherapeutic agent** to inhibit the proliferation of cancer cells.

G. Monitoring tissue damage by measuring enzyme levels in the blood

Enzymes, which are normally produced in cells, are released into the blood when cells are injured. For example, after a **heart attack**, there is an increase in blood levels of **creatine kinase (CK)**, particularly the **MB isozyme**. The extent of damage and the rate of recovery can be estimated by periodically measuring the levels of CK and its MB isozyme.

Review Test

Directions: Each of the numbered items or incomplete statements in this section is followed by answers or by completions of the statement. Select the **one** lettered answer or completion that is **best** in each case.

$$
\begin{array}{c}
H - C = O \\
| \\
H - C - OH \\
| \\
HO - C - H \\
| \\
H - C - OH \\
| \\
H - C - OH \\
| \\
CH_2OH
\end{array}
$$

1. The most oxidized group in the compound shown above is

(A) an acid
(B) an aldehyde
(C) a ketone
(D) an alcohol

Questions 2 and 3

Use the following structure for questions 2 and 3.

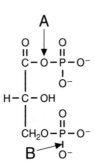

2. The bond labeled A in the compound shown is

(A) an anhydride
(B) an ether
(C) an ester
(D) a phosphodiester

3. The bond labeled B in the compound shown is

(A) an anhydride
(B) an ether
(C) an ester
(D) a phosphodiester

4. The conversion of β-hydroxybutyrate to acetoacetate occurs by what type of reaction?

$$
\underset{CH_3-CH-CH_2-COO^-}{\overset{OH}{|}} \rightleftharpoons \underset{CH_3-C-CH_2-COO^-}{\overset{O}{\parallel}}
$$

(A) Oxidation
(B) Reduction
(C) Dehydration
(D) Dehydroxylation

5. Physiologic pH is 7.4. What is the $[H^+]$ of a solution at physiologic pH?

(A) -7.4
(B) 0.6
(C) 0.6×10^{-8}
(D) 1.0×10^{-8}
(E) 4.0×10^{-8}

Questions 6 and 7

6. The ionization of a weak acid, expressed as

$$HA \rightleftharpoons H^+ + A^-$$

has an equilibrium constant (K_a) equal to

(A) log $[A^-]/[HA]$
(B) $[HA]/[A^-]$
(C) $[H^+][A^-]/[HA]$
(D) $[A^-]/[HA]$
(E) $[HA]/[H^+][A^-]$

7. When the pH for a solution of this acid is equal to the pK$_a$, the ratio of the concentrations of the salt and the acid ([A$^-$]/[HA]) is

(A) 0
(B) 1
(C) 2
(D) 3
(E) 4

8. Proteins are effective buffers because they contain

(A) a large number of amino acids
(B) amino acid residues with different pK$_a$s
(C) N-terminal and C-terminal residues that can donate and accept protons
(D) peptide bonds that readily hydrolyze, consuming hydrogen and hydroxyl ions
(E) a large number of hydrogen bonds in α-helices

Questions 9 and 10

Use the structure below to answer questions 9 and 10.

Asp-Ala-Ser-Glu-Val-Arg

9. The C-terminal amino acid of the hexapeptide shown is

(A) alanine
(B) asparagine
(C) aspartate
(D) arginine

10. At physiologic pH (7.4), this hexapeptide will contain a net charge of

(A) –2
(B) –1
(C) 0
(D) +1
(E) +2

11. Which one of the following types of bonds is covalent?

(A) Hydrophobic
(B) Hydrogen
(C) Disulfide
(D) Electrostatic

12. In sickle cell anemia, the hemoglobin molecule (HbS) is abnormal. If the β chains of normal hemoglobin (HbA) and HbS have the N-terminal sequences shown below and the chains otherwise are the same, which of the following statements is TRUE?
HbA Val-His-Leu-Thr-Pro-Glu-Glu-Lys-Ser-Ala-Val-Thr . . .
HbS Val-His-Leu-Thr-Pro-Val-Glu-Lys-Ser-Ala-Val-Thr . . .

(A) HbS contains one more hydrophobic amino acid than HbA
(B) HbS contains one more negative charge than HbA
(C) Neither HbS nor HbA contains an amino acid that has a side chain with a pK$_a$ of 6
(D) The entire sequences shown for both HbA and HbS can form α-helices

13. Which one of the following conditions causes hemoglobin to release oxygen more readily?

(A) Metabolic alkalosis
(B) Increased production of 2,3-bisphosphoglycerate (BPG)
(C) Hyperventilation, leading to decreased levels of CO$_2$ in the blood
(D) Replacement of the β subunits with γ subunits

14. Production of which of the following proteins would be most directly affected in scurvy?

(A) Myoglobin
(B) Collagen
(C) Insulin
(D) Hemoglobin

15. The active site of an enzyme

(A) is formed only after addition of a specific substrate
(B) is directly involved in binding of allosteric inhibitors
(C) resides in a few adjacent amino acid residues in the primary sequence of the polypeptide chain
(D) binds competitive inhibitors

16. An enzyme catalyzing the reaction

$$E + A \rightleftharpoons EA \rightarrow E + P$$

was mixed with 4 mM substrate. The initial rate of product formation was 25% of V_{max}. The K_m for the enzyme is

(A) 2 mM
(B) 4 mM
(C) 9 mM
(D) 12 mM
(E) 25 mM

17. The velocity (v) of an enzyme-catalyzed reaction

(A) decreases as the substrate concentration increases
(B) is lowest when the enzyme is saturated with substrate
(C) is related to the substrate concentration at $\frac{1}{2} V_{max}$
(D) is independent of the pH of the solution

Questions 18 and 19

Refer to the following reaction when answering questions 18 and 19:

$$Fumarate + H_2O \underset{fumarase}{\rightleftharpoons} malate$$

18. Fumarase catalyzes the conversion of fumarate to malate. It has a K_m of 5 μM for fumarate and a V_{max} of 50 μmol/min/mg of protein when measured in the direction of malate formation. The concentration of fumarate required to give a velocity of 25 μmol/min/mg protein is

(A) 2 μM
(B) 5 μM
(C) 10 μM
(D) 20 μM
(E) 50 μM

19. The K_m for fumarase is approximately 5 μM for fumarate. The fumarate concentration in mitochondria is approximately 2 mM. If the fumarate concentration dropped to 1 mM, the reaction rate would

(A) increase slightly
(B) decrease slightly
(C) decrease by one half
(D) stay exactly the same

20. The liver enzyme glucokinase catalyzes the phosphorylation of glucose to glucose 6-phosphate. The value of K_m for glucose is about 7 mM. Blood glucose is 5 mM under fasting conditions and can rise in the liver to 20 mM after a high-carbohydrate meal. Therefore, if a person who is fasting eats a high-carbohydrate meal, the velocity of the glucokinase reaction will

(A) remain at less than 50% V_{max}
(B) remain above 90% V_{max}
(C) increase from less than 50% V_{max} to more than 50% V_{max}
(D) decrease from more than 50% V_{max} to less than 50% V_{max}

21. A drug that is a competitive inhibitor of an enzyme

(A) increases the apparent K_m but does not affect V_{max}
(B) decreases the apparent K_m but does not affect V_{max}
(C) increases V_{max} but does not affect the apparent K_m
(D) decreases V_{max} but does not affect the apparent K_m
(E) decreases both V_{max} and K_m

Questions 22–25

Refer to the graph when answering questions 22-25:

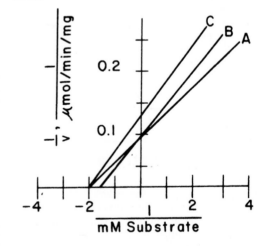

22. The value of K_m for the enzyme depicted by curve A is

(A) 0.5 mM
(B) 1 mM
(C) 2 mM
(D) 1 μmol/min/mg
(E) 10 μmol/min/mg

23. The value of V_{max} for the enzyme depicted by curve A is

(A) 0.1 μmol/min/mg
(B) 1 μmol/min/mg
(C) 10 μmol/min/mg
(D) 0.5 mM
(E) 2 mM

24. Curve B depicts the effect of an inhibitor on the system described by curve A. This inhibitor

(A) is a competitive inhibitor
(B) is a noncompetitive inhibitor
(C) increases the V_{max}
(D) decreases the K_m

25. Curve C depicts the effect of a different inhibitor of the system described by curve A. This second inhibitor

(A) is a competitive inhibitor
(B) is a noncompetitive inhibitor
(C) increases the V_{max}
(D) decreases the K_m

Questions 26 and 27

Refer to the graph when answering questions 26 and 27:

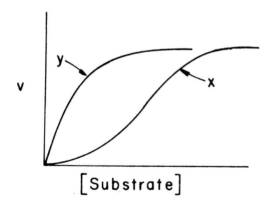

$$[\text{Substrate}]$$

The plot represents the relationship between substrate concentration and velocity for a single enzyme in the absence (curve x) and presence (curve y) of a compound that binds allosterically to the enzyme.

26. In the presence of the allosteric compound

(A) K_m and V_{max} both increase
(B) K_m and V_{max} both decrease
(C) K_m increases and V_{max} decreases
(D) K_m decreases and V_{max} increases
(E) K_m decreases and V_{max} stays the same

27. The allosteric compound is

(A) a competitive inhibitor
(B) a noncompetitive inhibitor
(C) an irreversible inhibitor
(D) an activator

28. Isocitrate dehydrogenase catalyzes the reaction

Isocitrate + $NAD^+ \rightarrow$ α-ketoglutarate + CO_2 + NADH + H^+

The curves illustrated below are obtained when the initial velocity (v) of the reaction is plotted against isocitrate concentration in the presence of various levels of ADP and excess NAD^+. Which of the following statements about this system is correct?

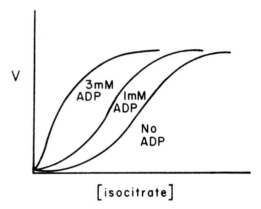

$$[\text{isocitrate}]$$

(A) Isocitrate dehydrogenase exhibits simple Michaelis-Menten kinetics in the absence of ADP
(B) ADP increases the K_m of the enzyme for isocitrate
(C) ADP increases the V_{max} of the enzyme
(D) ADP activates the enzyme

Directions: Each group of items in this section consists of lettered options followed by a set of numbered items. For each item, select the **one** lettered option that is most closely associated with it. Each lettered option may be selected once, more than once, or not at all.

Questions 29–32

(A) $^-OOC - CH_2 - CH_2 - CH - COO^-$
           |
          $^+NH_3$

(B) 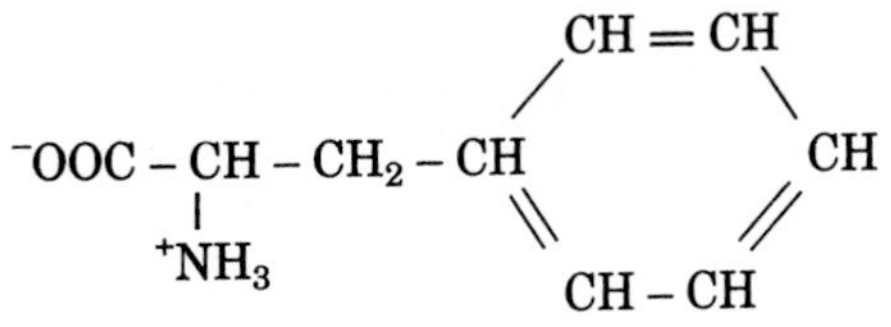 $^-OOC - CH - CH_2 - CH$ ⟨ring structure⟩ CH
           |
          $^+NH_3$

(C) $^-OOC - CH - CH_2 - S - S - CH_2 - CH - COO^-$
           | |
          $^+NH_3$ $^+NH_3$

(D) $CH_3 - S - CH_2 - CH_2 - CH - COO^-$
                                       |
                                     $^+NH_3$

Match each statement below with the compound above that it best describes.

29. Produced from two amino acids by an oxidation reaction

30. Contains an aromatic side chain

31. Contains a side chain that participates in electrostatic interactions

32. Migrates toward the anode in an electric field

Questions 33–37

(A) Hemoglobin
(B) Myoglobin
(C) Collagen
(D) Insulin

Match each characteristic below with the protein it best describes.

33. Requires vitamin C for its synthesis

34. Has one oxygen binding site and one polypeptide chain

35. Contains four molecules of heme per molecule of protein

36. Is converted into a triple helix during its synthesis

37. Is composed of two polypeptide chains joined by disulfide bonds

Answers and Explanations

1–B. The most oxidized group in this molecule of glucose is an aldehyde (see carbon 1). The other functional groups are alcohols.

2–A. Bond A, an anhydride, is formed when a carboxylic acid and a phosphoric acid react, splitting out H_2O.

3–C. Bond B, a phosphate ester, is formed when phosphoric acid reacts with an alcohol, splitting out H_2O.

4–A. An alcohol is oxidized to a ketone when β-hydroxybutyrate is converted to acetoacetate. These compounds are ketone bodies.

5–E. If the pH is 7.4, [H⁺] is $10^{-7.4}$, or $10^{0.6} \times 10^{-8}$, or 4×10^{-8}.

6–C. The equilibrium constant is equal to the product of the concentrations of the products divided by the product of the concentrations of the reactants, or in this case, $K_a = [H^+][A^-]/[HA]$.

7–B. The Henderson-Hasselbalch equation, $pH = pK_a + \log_{10} [A^-]/[HA]$, gives the relationship between these parameters. If $pH = pK_a$, $\log_{10} [A^-]/[HA] = 0$, and $[A^-]/[HA] = 1$.

8–B. The side chains of the amino acid residues in proteins contain functional groups with different pK_as. Therefore, they can donate and accept protons at various pH values and act as buffers over a broad pH spectrum. There is only one N-terminal amino group ($pK_a \approx 9$) and one C-terminal carboxyl group ($pK_a \approx 3$) per polypeptide chain. Peptide bonds are not readily hydrolyzed, and such hydrolysis would not provide buffering action. Hydrogen bonds have no buffering capacity.

9–D. By convention, peptides are drawn with the N-terminal amino acid on the left and the C-terminal amino acid on the right. Therefore, this peptide contains arginine at its C-terminus.

10–B. The N-terminal aspartate contains a positive charge on its N-terminal amino group and a negative charge on the carboxyl group of its side chain. Glutamate contains a negative charge on the carboxyl group of its side chain. The C-terminal arginine contains a negative charge on its C-terminal carboxyl group and a positive charge on its side chain. Thus, the overall charges are +2 and ⁻3, which gives a net charge of ⁻1.

11–C. Disulfide bonds are covalent.

12–A. The glutamate at position 6 in HbA is replaced by valine in HbS. Therefore, HbS has one more hydrophobic amino acid and one less negative charge than HbA. Both HbA and HbS contain histidine, which has a side chain with a pK_a of 6. Both sequences contain proline, which is cyclic and interrupts formation of an α-helix.

13–B. Increased [H⁺], BPG, and CO_2 decrease the affinity of HbA for O_2. Fetal hemoglobin (HbF = $\alpha_2\gamma_2$) has a greater affinity for O_2 than HbA ($\alpha_2\beta_2$). Increased BPG would cause O_2 to be more readily released.

14–B. Scurvy is caused by a deficiency of vitamin C. The hydroxylation of proline and lysine residues in collagen requires vitamin C and oxygen. Globin synthesis might be indirectly affected because absorption of iron from the intestine is stimulated by vitamin C. Iron is involved in heme synthesis, which regulates globin synthesis.

15–D. The active site is formed when the enzyme folds into its three-dimensional configuration and may involve amino acid residues that are far apart in the primary sequence. Substrate molecules bind at the active site. Competitive inhibitors compete with the substrate. (Both bind at the active site.) Allosteric inhibitors bind at a site other than the active site.

16–D. In the Michaelis-Menten equation, $v = (V_{max} \times [S])/(K_m + [S])$. In this case, $\frac{1}{4} V_{max} = (V_{max} \times 4)/(K_m + 4)$, or $K_m = 12$ mM.

17–C. The velocity of an enzyme-catalyzed reaction increases as the substrate concentration increases. It is highest when the enzyme is saturated with substrate. Then, v equals V_{max}, the maximum velocity. The velocity depends on K_m. Enzymes have an optimal pH at which their activity is maximal.

18–B. A velocity of 25 is $\frac{1}{2} V_{max}$ ($V_{max} = 50$). $K_m = [S]$ at $\frac{1}{2} V_{max}$. $K_m = 5$ μM.

19–B. The velocity decreases slightly when the concentration of the substrate drops from 2 mM to 1 mM. At 2 mM, $v = (V_{max} \times 2000$ μM$)/(5$ μM $+ 2000$ μM$) = 99.8\% V_{max}$. At 1 mM, $v = (V_{max} \times 1000$ μM$)/(5$ μM $+ 1000$ μM$) = 99.5\% V_{max}$.

20–C. During fasting, $v = (5 \times V_{max})/(7 + 5) = 42\% V_{max}$. In the fed state, $v = (20 \times V_{max})/(7 + 20) = 74\% V_{max}$. Glucokinase is more active in the fed than in the fasting state.

21–A. A competitive inhibitor competes with the substrate for the active site of the enzyme, in effect increasing the apparent K_m. As the substrate concentration is increased, the substrate, by competing with the inhibitor, can overcome its inhibitory effects, and eventually the normal V_{max} is reached.

22–A. The intercept on the x axis is $-1/K_m = -2$. Therefore, $K_m = 0.5$ mM.

23–C. The intercept on the y axis is $1/V_{max} = 0.1$. Therefore, $V_{max} = 10$ μmol/min/mg.

24–A. With this inhibitor, V_{max} is the same (the y intercept is the same), but the apparent K_m is larger (the x intercept is less negative). Therefore, this is a competitive inhibitor.

25–B. With this inhibitor, V_{max} is lower but K_m is the same. It is a pure noncompetitive inhibitor.

26–E. K_m, the substrate concentration at $\frac{1}{2} V_{max}$, is lower for curve y than for curve x. As the substrate concentration increases, both curves approach a plateau (V_{max}) that has the same velocity.

27–D. The allosteric compound increases the rate of the reaction at lower substrate concentrations, so it is an activator of the reaction.

28–D. Without ADP, the curve is sigmoidal, thus Michaelis-Menten kinetics are not exhibited. V_{max} is the same at all ADP concentrations shown. The substrate concentration at $\frac{1}{2} V_{max}$ decreases as the ADP concentration increases; therefore, ADP decreases the K_m, activating the enzyme. (The velocity is higher at lower substrate concentrations in the presence of ADP.)

29–C. The sulfhydryl (-SH) groups of two cysteines react to form the disulfide bond (-S-S-) of cystine (compound C).

30–B. Phenylalanine (compound B) contains an aromatic phenyl ring.

31–A. The side chain of glutamate (compound A) contains a carboxyl group that carries a negative charge and participates in electrostatic interactions.

32–A. Glutamate is the only one of these amino acids that carries a net charge. It migrates toward the positive electrode (the anode).

33–C. Proline and lysine residues in collagen are hydroxylated in a reaction that requires vitamin C.

34–B. Each myoglobin molecule contains one polypeptide chain and one heme molecule that binds one O_2 molecule. Each hemoglobin molecule contains four polypeptide chains, four molecules of heme, and four molecules of oxygen.

35–A. Each molecule of hemoglobin contains four molecules of heme. Each myoglobin molecule contains one molecule of heme.

36–C. Collagen forms a triple helix during its synthesis.

37–D. Insulin is composed of an A chain and a B chain, which are linked by disulfide bonds.

3

Gene Expression and the Synthesis of Proteins

Overview

- Genetic information is encoded in DNA, which, in eukaryotes, is located mainly in nuclei with small amounts in mitochondria.
- Genetic information is inherited and expressed. Inheritance occurs by the process of replication. The strands of parental DNA serve as templates for synthesis of copies that are passed to daughter cells.
- Mutations that result from damage to DNA can lead to genetic alterations, including abnormal cell growth and cancer. Repair mechanisms can correct damaged DNA.
- Recombination of genes promotes genetic diversity.
- Expression of genes requires two steps, transcription and translation. DNA is transcribed to produce messenger RNA (mRNA), which is translated to produce proteins. Ribosomal RNA (rRNA) and transfer RNA (tRNA) participate in the process of translation.
- Proteins are involved in cell structure, and they function as enzymes, determining the reactions that occur in cells. Thus, proteins, the products of genes, determine what cells look like and how they behave.
- Gene expression is regulated. Only a small fraction of the genome is expressed in any one cell.
- Recombinant DNA technology was developed to study and manipulate genes.

I. Nucleic Acid Structure

- The monomeric units of nucleic acids are nucleotides; each nucleotide contains a heterocyclic nitrogenous base, a sugar, and phosphate.
- DNA contains the bases adenine (A), guanine (G), cytosine (C), and thymine (T). RNA contains A, G, and C, but has uracil (U) instead of thymine.
- Deoxyribose is present in DNA, whereas RNA contains ribose.
- Polynucleotides consist of nucleosides joined by 3′,5′-phosphodiester bridges. The genetic message resides in the sequence of bases along the polynucleotide chain.
- In DNA, two polynucleotide chains are joined by pairing between their bases (adenine with thymine and guanine with cytosine), and they form a double helix. One chain runs in a 5′ to 3′ direction and the other runs 3′ to 5′.
- DNA molecules interact with histones to form strands of nucleosomes, which wind into more tightly coiled structures.

Purines

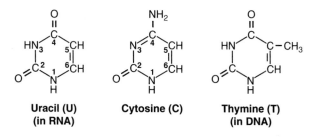

Adenine (A)   Guanine (G)

Pyrimidines

Uracil (U)   Cytosine (C)   Thymine (T)
(in RNA)   (in DNA)

Figure 3-1. The nitrogenous bases of the nucleic acids.

- RNA is single-stranded, but the strands loop back on themselves and the bases pair: guanine with cytosine and adenine with uracil.
- Messenger RNA (mRNA) has a cap at the 5′ end and a poly(A) tail at the 3′ end.
- Ribosomal RNA (rRNA) has extensive base-pairing.
- Transfer RNA (tRNA) forms a cloverleaf structure that contains many unusual nucleotides and an anticodon.

A. The structure of DNA

1. Chemical components of DNA

- Each polynucleotide chain of DNA contains nucleotides, which consist of a **nitrogenous base** (A, G, C, or T), **deoxyribose,** and **phosphate** (Figures 3-1, 3-2, and 3-3).

   a. The bases are the **purines** adenine (A) and guanine (G), and the **pyrimidines** cytosine (C) and thymine (T).

   b. Phosphodiester bonds join the 3′-carbon of one sugar to the 5′-carbon of the next (Figure 3-4).

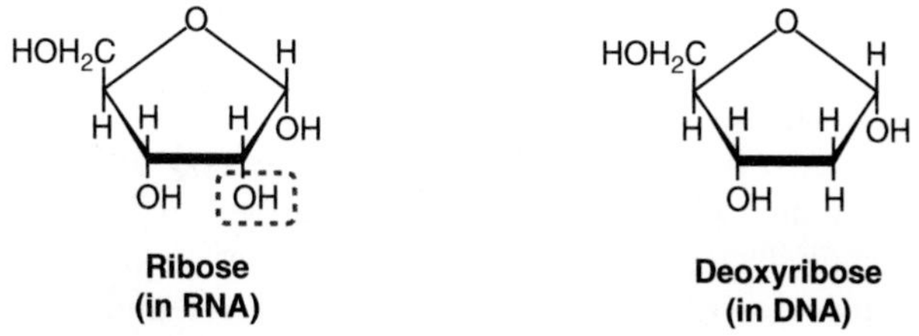

Ribose   Deoxyribose
(in RNA)   (in DNA)

Figure 3-2. The sugars of the nucleic acids. Ribose has a hydroxyl group on carbon 2 (dotted box); deoxyribose does not.

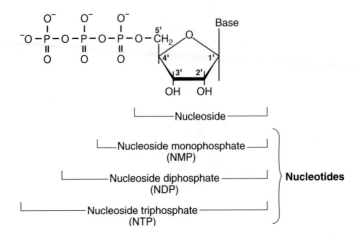

Figure 3-3. Nucleoside and nucleotide structures.

2. DNA double helix

a. Each DNA molecule is composed of two **polynucleotide chains** joined by hydrogen bonds between the bases (Figure 3-5).

(1) Adenine on one chain forms a base pair with **thymine** on the other chain.

(2) Guanine base-pairs with **cytosine.**

(3) The **base sequences** of the two strands are **complementary**. Adenine on one strand is matched by thymine on the other, and guanine is matched by cytosine.

b. The **chains are antiparallel.** One chain runs in a **5′ to 3′** direction; the other chain runs **3′ to 5′** (Figure 3-6).

c. The double-stranded molecule is twisted to form a **helix** with major and minor grooves (Figure 3-7).

(1) The **base pairs** that join the two strands are **stacked** like a spiral staircase in the interior of the molecule.

(2) The **phosphate groups** are on the outside of the double helix. Two acidic groups of each phosphate are involved in phosphodiester bonds. The third is free and dissociates its proton at physiologic pH, giving the molecule a **negative charge** (see Figure 3-4).

(3) The **B form of DNA,** first described by Watson and Crick, is right-handed and contains **10 base pairs per turn.**

– Other forms of DNA include the A form, which is similar to the B form but more compact, and the Z form, which is left-handed and has its bases positioned more toward the periphery of the helix.

3. Denaturation, renaturation, and hybridization

a. Denaturation: Alkali or **heat** cause the **strands** of DNA to **separate** but do not break phosphodiester bonds.

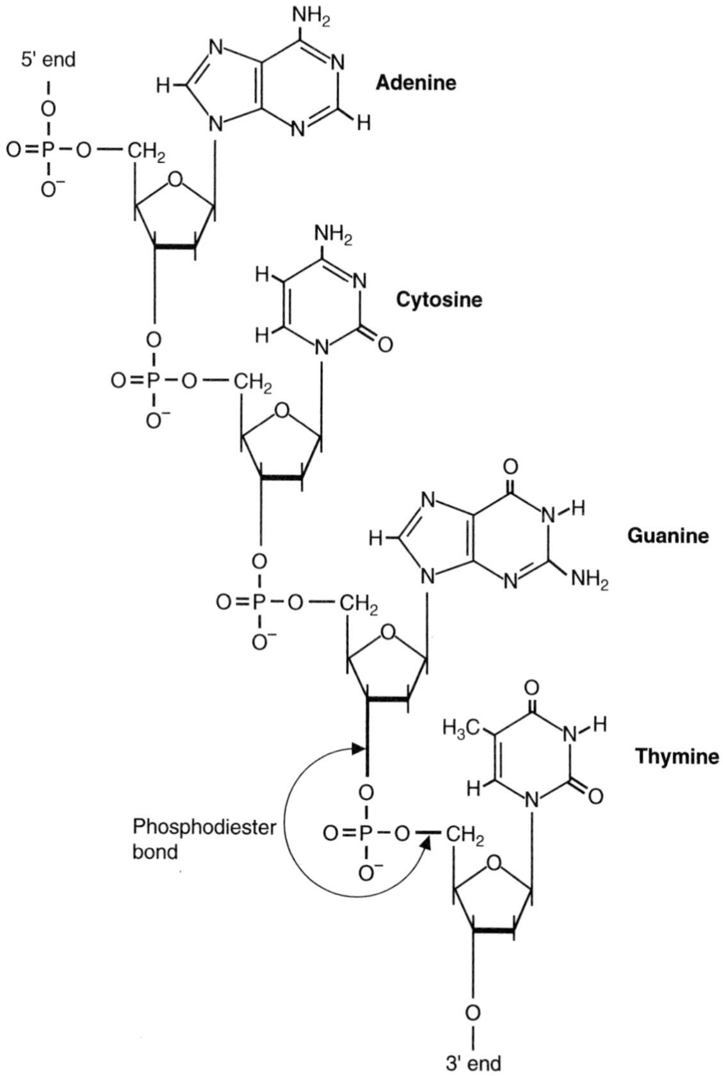

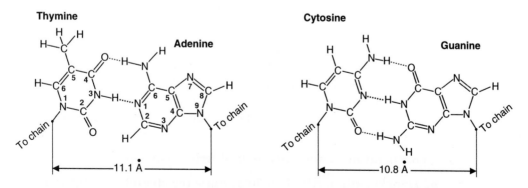

Figure 3-4. A segment of a polynucleotide strand. This strand contains thymine and deoxyribose, so it is a segment of DNA.

Figure 3-5. The base pairs of DNA.

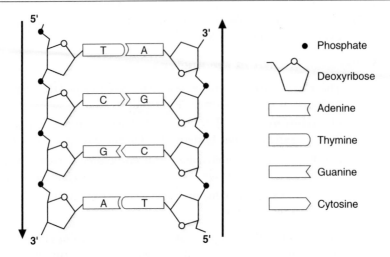

Figure 3-6. Antiparallel strands of DNA. Note that the strands run in opposite directions.

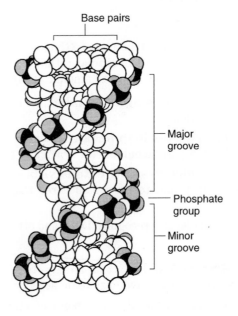

Figure 3-7. The DNA double helix.

b. **Renaturation:** If strands of DNA are separated by heat and then the **temperature** is slowly **decreased** under the appropriate conditions, **base pairs re-form** and complementary strands of DNA come back together.

c. **Hybridization:** A single strand of DNA pairs with complementary base sequences on another strand of DNA or RNA.

4. **DNA molecules are extremely large.**

a. The entire chromosome of the bacterium *Escherichia coli* is circular and contains more than 4×10^6 base pairs.

b. The DNA molecule in the longest human chromosome is linear and is over 7.2 cm long.

5. Packing of DNA in the nucleus

a. The **chromatin** of eukaryotic cells consists of DNA complexed with histones in **nucleosomes** (Figure 3-8).

   (1) Histones are relatively small, basic proteins with a high content of **arginine** and **lysine**. (Prokaryotes do not have histones.)

   (2) Eight histone molecules form an octamer around which approximately 140 base pairs of DNA are wound to form a nucleosome core.

   (3) The DNA that joins one nucleosome core to the next is complexed with histone H1.

b. The "beads on a string" nucleosomal structure of chromatin is further compacted to form solenoid structures (helical, tubular coils).

B. The structure of RNA

1. RNA differs from DNA

a. The polynucleotide structure of **RNA** is similar to DNA except that RNA contains the sugar **ribose** rather than deoxyribose and **uracil** rather than thymine. (A small amount of thymine is present in tRNA.)

b. **RNA** is generally **single-stranded** (in contrast to DNA, which is double-stranded).

   (1) When **strands loop back** on themselves, the bases on opposite sides can pair: adenine with uracil and guanine with cytosine.

   (2) RNA molecules have extensive base-pairing, which produces secondary and tertiary structures that are important for RNA function.

   (3) RNA molecules recognize DNA and other RNA molecules by base-pairing.

c. Some **RNA molecules** act as **catalysts** of reactions; thus, RNA, as well as protein, can have enzymatic activity.

   (1) Ribozymes, usually precursors of rRNA, remove internal segments of themselves, splicing the ends together.

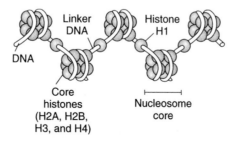

Figure 3-8. A polynucleosome. (Adapted from Olins DE, Olins AL: Nucleosomes: The structural quantum in chromosomes. *American Scientist* 66:708, 1978.)

(2) RNAs also act as **ribonucleases,** cleaving other RNA molecules (e.g., RNaseP cleaves tRNA precursors).

(3) Peptidyl transferase, an enzyme in protein synthesis, consists of RNA.

2. **Messenger RNA (mRNA)** contains a cap structure and a poly(A) tail.

   a. The **cap** consists of **methylated guanine triphosphate** attached to the hydroxyl group on the ribose at the 5′ end of the mRNA.
   – The N7 in the guanine is methylated.
   – The 2′-hydroxyl groups of the first and second ribose moieties of the mRNA also may be methylated (Figure 3-9).

   b. The **poly(A) tail** contains up to 200 adenine (A) nucleotides attached to the hydroxyl group at the 3′ end of the mRNA.

3. **Ribosomal RNA (rRNA)** contains many loops and extensive base-pairing.
   – rRNA molecules differ in their sedimentation coefficients (S). They associate with proteins to form **ribosomes** (Figure 3-10).

   a. Prokaryotes have three types of rRNA: 16S, 23S, and 5S rRNA.

   b. Eukaryotes have four types of cytosolic rRNA: 18S, 28S, 5S, and 5.8S rRNA. Mitochondrial ribosomes are similar to prokaryotic ribosomes.

4. **Transfer RNA (tRNA)** has a cloverleaf structure and contains modified nucleotides. Transfer RNA molecules are relatively small, containing about 80 nucleotides.

   a. In eukaryotic cells, many nucleotides in tRNA are modified.

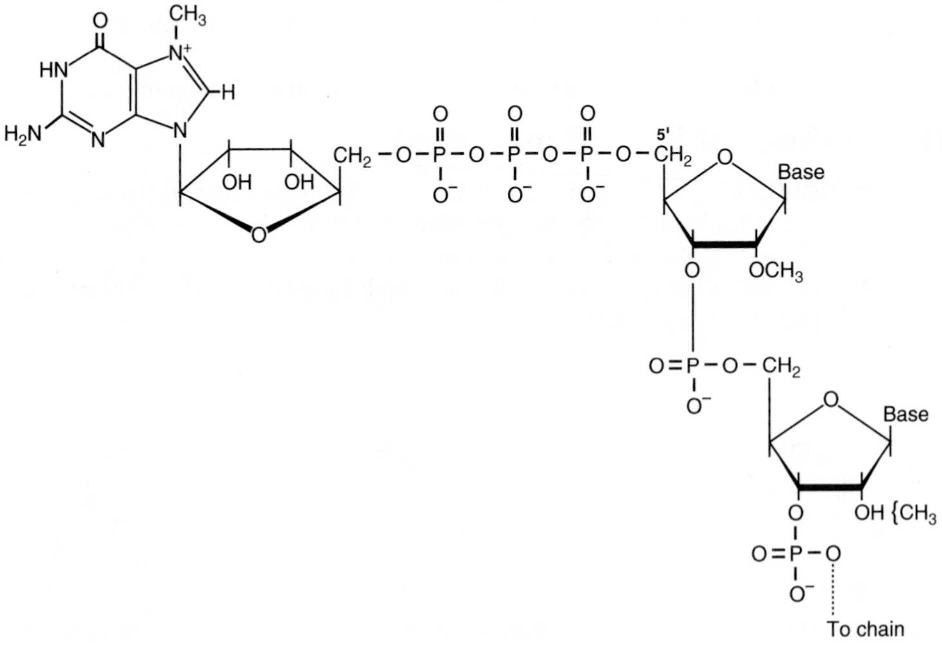

Figure 3-9. The cap structure of mRNA.

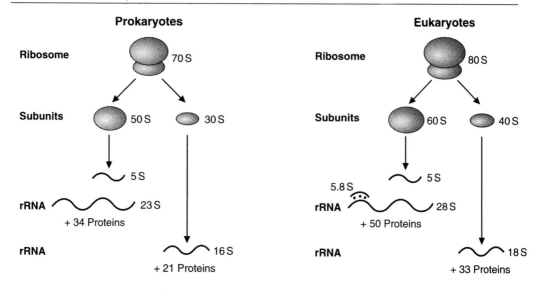

Figure 3-10. The composition of ribosomes.

  – Modified nucleotides containing **pseudouridine (ψ), dihydrouridine (D),** and **ribothymidine (T)** are present in most tRNAs (Figure 3-11).

  b. All tRNA molecules have a similar **cloverleaf structure** even though their base sequences differ (Figure 3-12).

   (1) The first loop from the 5′ end, the **D loop,** contains dihydrouridine.
   (2) The middle loop contains the **anticodon,** which base-pairs with the codon in mRNA.
   (3) The third loop, the **TψC loop,** contains both ribothymidine and pseudouridine.
   (4) The **CCA sequence** at the 3′ end carries the amino acid.

II. Synthesis of DNA (Replication)

  ● Replication, the process of DNA synthesis, occurs during the S phase of the cell cycle in eukaryotes and is catalyzed by a complex of proteins that includes the enzyme DNA polymerase.
  ● Each strand of the parent DNA acts as a template for the synthesis of its complementary strand.

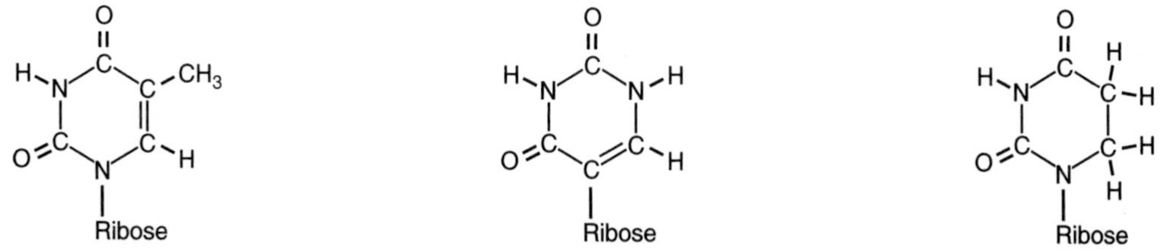

Ribothymidine (T)   **Pseudouridine (ψ)**   **Dihydrouridine (D)**

Figure 3-11. Three modified nucleosides found in most tRNAs.

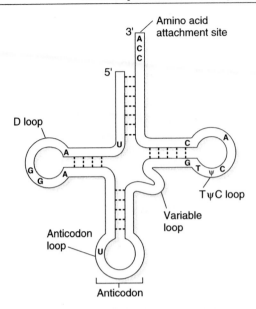

Figure 3-12. The cloverleaf structure of tRNA. Bases that commonly occur in a particular position are indicated by *letters.* Base-pairing in stem regions is indicated by *dashed lines* between strands. ψ = pseudouridine; *T* = ribothymidine; *D* = dihydrouridine.

- DNA polymerase copies the template strand in the 3′ to 5′ direction and synthesizes the new strand in the 5′ to 3′ direction. Deoxyribonucleoside triphosphates serve as the precursors.
- DNA polymerase cannot initiate the synthesis of a new strand. A short stretch of RNA serves as a primer.
- Other proteins and enzymes are required to unwind the parental strands and allow both strands to be copied simultaneously.
- Errors that occur during replication are corrected by enzymes associated with the replication complex.
- Damage that occurs to DNA molecules can be corrected by repair mechanisms, which usually involve removal and replacement of the damaged region with the intact undamaged strand serving as a template.
- DNA molecules can recombine. A portion of a strand from one molecule can be exchanged for a portion of a strand from another molecule.
- Genes can be transposed (moved from one chromosomal site to another).

A. **The cell cycle of eukaryotic cells** (Figure 3-13)

   1. During the G_1 (first gap) phase, cells **prepare to duplicate** their chromosomes.

   2. During the **S** (synthesis) phase, **synthesis of DNA** (replication) occurs.

   3. During the G_2 (second gap) phase, cells **prepare to divide.**

   4. During the **M** (mitosis) phase, **cell division** occurs.

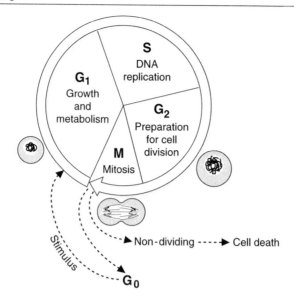

Figure 3-13. The cell cycle of eukaryotes.

5. Cells can traverse the cell cycle many times.

– They can leave the cycle never to divide again, or they can enter a phase (sometimes called G_0) in which they remain for extended periods. In response to an appropriate stimulus, these cells reenter the cell cycle and divide again.

B. Mechanism of replication

1. Replication is bidirectional and semiconservative (Figure 3-14).

a. Bidirectional means that replication begins at a site of origin and simultaneously moves out in both directions from this point.
– Prokaryotes have one site of origin on each chromosome.
– Eukaryotes have multiple sites of origin on each chromosome.

b. Semiconservative means that, following replication, each daughter molecule of DNA contains one intact parental strand and one newly synthesized strand joined by base pairs.

2. Replication forks are the sites at which DNA synthesis is occurring.

– The **parental strands** of DNA separate and the helix unwinds ahead of a replication fork (Figure 3-15).

a. Helicases unwind the helix, and **single-strand binding proteins** hold it in a single-stranded conformation.

b. Topoisomerases act to prevent the extreme supercoiling of the parental helix that would result as a consequence of unwinding at a replication fork.

– Topoisomerases break and rejoin DNA chains.
– **DNA gyrase,** a topoisomerase inhibited by quinolones, is found only in prokaryotes.

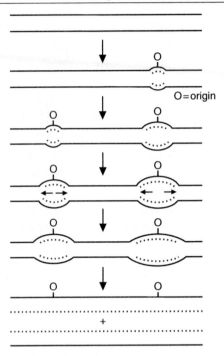

O = origin

Figure 3-14. Replication of a eukaryotic chromosome. *Solid lines* are parental strands. *Dotted lines* are newly synthesized strands. Synthesis is bidirectional from each point of origin *(O)*.

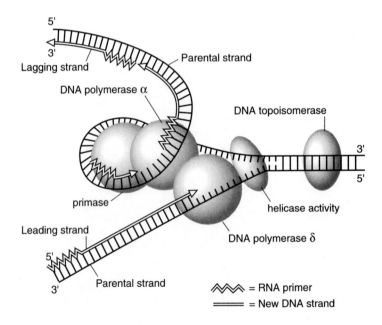

Figure 3-15. The eukaryotic replication complex located at a replication fork. The lagging strand loops around the complex. Single-strand binding proteins (not shown) are attached to the regions of single-stranded DNA.

3. **DNA polymerases** catalyze the synthesis of DNA.

   a. **Prokaryotes** have three DNA polymerases: **pol I, pol II, and pol III.** Pol III is the replicative enzyme, and pol I is involved in repair.

   b. **Eukaryotes** have five DNA polymerases: α, β, γ, δ, and ε. DNA polymerase α is involved in replication of nuclear DNA. Polymerase δ acts in conjunction with α during replication. Polymerases β and ε are involved in repair of nuclear DNA, and γ functions in mitochondria.

   c. **DNA polymerases** can only copy a DNA template in the 3′ to 5′ direction and produce the newly synthesized strand in the 5′ to 3′ direction.

   d. **Deoxyribonucleoside triphosphates** (dATP, dGTP, dTTP, and dCTP) are the precursors for DNA synthesis.

   (1) Each precursor pairs with the corresponding base on the template strand and forms a phosphodiester bond with the hydroxyl group on the 3′-carbon of the sugar at the end of the growing chain (Figure 3-16).

   (2) Pyrophosphate is produced and cleaved to two inorganic phosphates.

4. **DNA polymerase** requires a **primer** (Figure 3-17).

   a. DNA polymerases **cannot initiate** synthesis of new strands.

   b. **RNA serves as the primer** for DNA polymerase in vivo.

   – The RNA primer, which contains about 10 nucleotides, is formed by copying of the parental strand in a reaction catalyzed by **primase.**

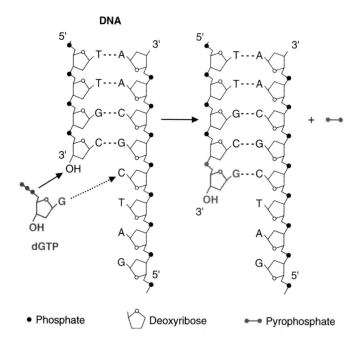

Figure 3-16. The action of DNA polymerase.

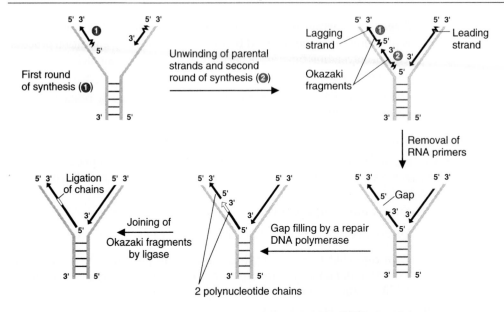

Figure 3-17. Mechanism of DNA synthesis at the replication fork. Two rounds of polymerase action are shown (❶ and ❷). The number of nucleotides added in each round is much larger than shown; in eukaryotes, about 10 ribonucleotides and 200 deoxyribonucleotides are polymerized on the lagging strand. Synthesis on the leading strand is continuous. The unshaded regions of the arrows indicate the nucleotides added by the repair action of a DNA polymerase.

   c. DNA polymerase adds deoxyribonucleotides to the 3′-hydroxyls of the RNA primers and subsequently to the ends of the growing DNA strands.

   d. DNA parental (template) strands are copied simultaneously at replication forks, although they run in opposite directions.

      (1) The **leading strand** is formed by continuous copying of the parental strand that runs 3′ to 5′ **toward** the replication fork.

      (2) The **lagging strand** is formed by discontinuous copying of the parental strand that runs 3′ to 5′ **away from** the replication fork.

        – As more of the helix is unwound, synthesis of the lagging strand begins from another primer. The short fragments formed by this process are known as **Okazaki fragments.**

        – The RNA **primers are removed by nucleases** (e.g., RNase H); then the resulting **gaps are filled** with the appropriate deoxyribonucleotides by another DNA polymerase.

        – Finally, the **Okazaki fragments are joined by DNA ligase,** an enzyme that catalyzes formation of phosphodiester bonds between two polynucleotide chains.

   e. In eukaryotic cells, about 200 deoxyribonucleotides are added to the lagging strand in each round of synthesis, whereas in prokaryotes 1000 to 2000 are added.

  5. The **fidelity of replication** is very high with an overall error rate of 10^{-9} to 10^{-10}.

   a. Errors (insertion of an inappropriate nucleotide) that occur during replication can be **corrected by editing** during the replication process. This proofreading function is performed by a 3′ to 5′ exonuclease activity associated with the polymerase complex.

   b. Postreplication repair processes (e.g., mismatch repair) also increase the fidelity of replication.

C. Mutations

– **Changes in DNA** molecules cause mutations. After replication, these changes result in a permanent alteration of the base sequence in the daughter DNA.

1. **Changes causing mutations** include:

   a. Uncorrected errors made during replication

   b. Damage that occurs to replicating or nonreplicating DNA caused by oxidative deamination, radiation, or chemicals, resulting in cleavage of DNA strands or chemical alteration or removal of bases

2. **Types of mutations** include:

   a. Point mutations (substitution of one base for another)

   b. Insertions (addition of one or more nucleotides within a DNA sequence)

   c. Deletions (removal of one or more nucleotides from a DNA sequence)

D. DNA repair (Figure 3-18)

– In general, repair involves **removal** of the segment of DNA that contains a damaged region or mismatched bases, **filling in the gap** by action of a DNA polymerase that uses the undamaged sister strand as a template, and **ligation** of the newly synthesized segment to the remainder of the chain.
– **Endonucleases, exonucleases,** a **DNA polymerase,** and a **ligase** are required for repair.

1. **Nucleotide excision repair** involves the removal of a group of **nucleotides** (including the damaged nucleotide) from a DNA strand.

2. **Base excision repair** involves a specific **glycosylase** that removes a **damaged base** by hydrolyzing an N-glycosidic bond, producing an apurinic or apyrimidinic site, which is cleaved and, subsequently, repaired.

3. **Mismatch repair** involves the removal of the portion of the **newly-synthesized strand** of recently replicated DNA that contains a pair of mismatched bases. Bacteria recognize the newly synthesized strand because, in contrast to the parental strand, it has not yet been methylated. The recognition mechanism in eukaryotes is not known.

E. Rearrangements of genes

– Several processes produce new combinations of genes, thus promoting genetic diversity.

1. **Recombination** occurs between homologous DNA segments, that is, those that have very similar sequences.

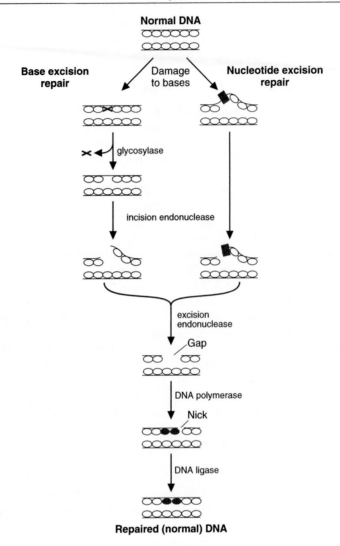

Figure 3-18. Base excision and nucleotide excision repair of DNA. Circles indicate normal bases; x's and ∎, damaged bases. The actual number of nucleotides removed (the size of the gap) is larger than that shown.

   2. Transposition involves movement of a DNA segment from one site to a nonhomologous site.

   – Transposons ("jumping genes") are mobile genetic elements that facilitate the movement of genes.

F. Reverse transcription

   1. Synthesis of DNA from an **RNA template** is catalyzed by **reverse transcriptase**.

   2. Retroviruses contain RNA as their genetic material.

   a. The retroviral RNA serves as a template for synthesis of DNA by reverse transcriptase.

b. The DNA that is generated can be inserted into the genome (chromosomes) of the host cell and be expressed.

3. Reverse transcriptase also may play a role in normal development.

III. Synthesis of RNA (Transcription)

- Transcription, the synthesis of RNA from a DNA template, is catalyzed by RNA polymerase. RNA polymerase copies a DNA template in the 3' to 5' direction and synthesizes a single-stranded RNA molecule in a 5' to 3' direction. Unlike DNA polymerase, RNA polymerase can initiate the synthesis of new strands.
- In eukaryotes, the primary product of transcription is modified and trimmed before it participates in protein synthesis.
- Eukaryotic messenger RNA, produced by RNA polymerase II, is capped at the 5' end and has a poly(A) tail added at the 3' end. Introns (segments that do not code for protein) are removed, and exons (segments that produce the mature mRNA) are spliced together.
- Eukaryotic ribosomal RNA is produced by RNA polymerase I as a 45S precursor that is methylated and cleaved to form three of the rRNAs (18S, 28S, and 5.8S) that appear in ribosomes. The 5S rRNA is produced from a separate gene by RNA polymerase III.
- Eukaryotic transfer RNA is produced by RNA polymerase III as a precursor that is trimmed at the 5' and 3' ends. Introns are removed and exons are spliced together.
  - Unusual nucleotides are produced in mature tRNA by posttranscriptional modification of normal nucleotides, and a CCA sequence is added at the 3' end.
- Eukaryotic RNA must travel from the nucleus to the cytoplasm for translation.
- Bacteria do not contain nuclei, so transcription and translation occur simultaneously. A single RNA polymerase produces mRNA, rRNA, and tRNA in bacteria. Bacterial transcripts (e.g., those from *E. coli*) do not contain introns.

A. RNA polymerase

1. RNA polymerase can **initiate** the synthesis of **new chains.** A primer is not required.

2. The DNA template is copied in the 3' to 5' direction, and the RNA chain grows in the 5' to 3' direction.

3. **Ribonucleoside triphosphates** (ATP, GTP, UTP, and CTP) serve as the **precursors** for the RNA chain. The process is similar to that for DNA synthesis (see Figure 3-16).

B. Synthesis of RNA in bacteria

1. The RNA polymerase of *E. coli* contains **four subunits,** $\alpha_2\beta\beta'$, which form the core enzyme, and a fifth subunit, the **sigma factor (σ),** which is required for initiation of RNA synthesis.

2. Genes contain a **promoter region** to which RNA polymerase binds.

   a. Promoters contain the consensus sequence **TATAAT** (called the Pribnow or TATA box) about 10 bases upstream from (before) the start point of transcription.

– A **consensus sequence** consists of the most commonly found sequence of bases in a given region of all DNAs tested.

  b. A **second consensus sequence** (TTGACA) is usually located upstream from the Pribnow box, about 35 nucleotides (-35) from the start point of transcription.

3. When RNA polymerase binds to a **promoter,** local unwinding of the DNA helix occurs, so that the DNA strands partially separate. The polymerase then begins transcription, copying the **template strand.**

  a. As the polymerase moves along the DNA, the next region of the double helix unwinds while the single-stranded region that has already been transcribed rejoins its partner.

  b. Termination occurs in a region in which the transcript forms a hairpin loop that precedes four U residues.

  c. The ρ (rho) factor aids in the termination of some transcripts.

4. **mRNA** is often produced as a **polycistronic transcript** that is translated as it is being transcribed.

  a. A polycistronic mRNA produces several different proteins during translation, one from each cistron.

  b. *E. coli* mRNA has a short half-life. It is degraded in minutes.

5. **rRNA** is produced as a **large transcript** that is cleaved, producing the 16S rRNA that appears in the 30S ribosomal subunit and the 23S and 5S rRNAs that appear in the 50S ribosomal subunit.
  – The 30S and 50S ribosomal subunits combine to form the 70S ribosome.

6. **tRNA** usually is produced from **larger transcripts** that are cleaved. One of the cleavage enzymes, RNaseP, contains an RNA molecule that acts as a catalyst.

C. Synthesis of RNA in nuclei of eukaryotes

  1. mRNA synthesis (Figure 3-19)

  a. Eukaryotic genes that produce mRNA contain a **basal promoter region.** This region binds transcription factors, proteins that bind RNA polymerase II. Promoters contain a number of conserved sequences.

  (1) A **TATA** (Hogness) **box,** containing the consensus sequence TATA-TAA, is located about 25 base pairs upstream (-25) from the transcription start site.

  (2) A **CAAT box** is frequently found about 70 base pairs upstream from the start site.

  (3) **GC-rich regions** (GC boxes) often occur between -40 and -110.

  b. **Enhancers** are DNA sequences that function in the **stimulation** of the transcription rate. They can be located thousands of base pairs upstream or downstream from the start site. Other sequences called **silencers** function in the **inhibition** of transcription.

  c. **RNA polymerase II** initially produces a large primary transcript called heterogeneous nuclear RNA (**hnRNA**), which contains exons and introns.

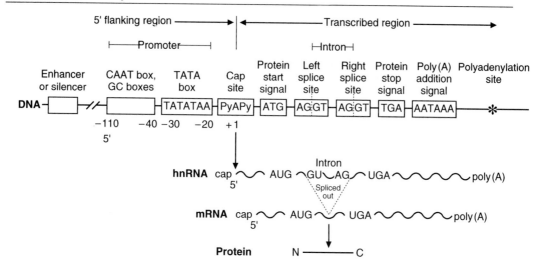

Figure 3-19. The structure of a eukaryotic gene and its products. As is customary, DNA sequences are given for the non-template strand. The DNA template strand, of course, is present. Its sequence is complementary and antiparallel to that of the non-template strand. The sequence of the RNA transcript is identical to that of the corresponding region of the non-template strand of the DNA, except that, in RNA, U replaces T. *Py* = pyrimidine.

   (1) Exons are sequences within a transcript that appear in the mature **mRNA.**

   (2) Introns are sequences within the primary transcript that are **removed** and do not appear in the mature mRNA.

  d. Processing of hnRNA yields mature mRNA, which enters the cytoplasm through nuclear pores (Figure 3-20).

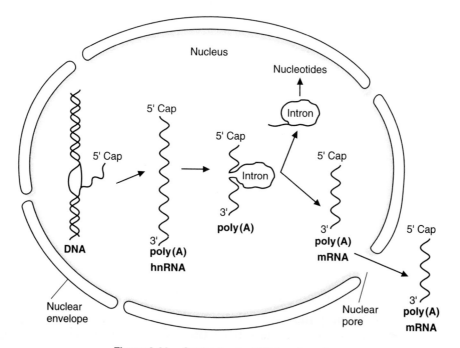

Figure 3-20. Synthesis of mRNA in eukaryotes.

(1) The **primary transcript** (hnRNA) is capped at its 5′ end as it is being transcribed.

(2) A **poly(A) tail,** 20 to 200 nucleotides in length, is added to the 3′ end of the transcript.

    – The sequence AAUAAA in hnRNA serves as a signal for cleavage of the hnRNA and addition of the poly(A) tail by poly(A) polymerase. ATP serves as the precursor.

(3) **Splicing** reactions remove introns and connect the exons.

    – The **splice point** at the **left** flank of an intron usually has the sequence AG followed by an **invariant GU**. At the **right** flank, an **invariant AG** is frequently followed by GU (see Figure 3-19).

    – Small nuclear RNAs complexed with protein (**snRNPs**) [e.g., U1 and U2] are involved in the cleavage and splicing process. A **lariat** structure is generated during the splicing reaction (see Figure 3-20).

(4) Some hnRNAs contain 50 or more exons that must be spliced correctly to produce functional mRNA. Other hnRNAs have no introns.

2. rRNA synthesis and assembly of ribosomes (Figure 3-21)

    a. A **45S precursor** is produced by RNA polymerase I from rRNA genes located in the fibrous region of the nucleolus. Many copies of the genes are present, linked together by spacer regions.

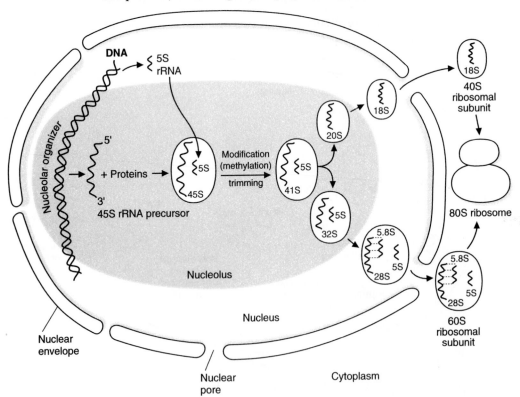

Figure 3-21. Synthesis of rRNA and assembly of ribosomes.

b. The **45S precursor** is modified by methylation and undergoes a number of cleavages that ultimately produce 18S rRNA and 28S rRNA; the latter is hydrogen-bonded to a 5.8S rRNA.

c. **18S rRNA** complexes with proteins and forms the 40S ribosomal subunit.

d. The **28S, 5.8S, and 5S rRNAs** complex with proteins and form the 60S ribosomal subunit. 5S rRNA is produced by RNA polymerase III outside of the nucleolus.

e. The **ribosomal subunits migrate** through the nuclear pores into the cytoplasm where they complex with mRNA, forming 80S ribosomes. (Because sedimentation coefficients reflect both shape and particle weight, they are not additive.)

f. rRNA precursors can contain **introns** that are removed during maturation. In some organisms, the enzymatic activity that removes rRNA introns resides in the rRNA precursor. No proteins are required. These autocatalytic RNAs are known as **ribozymes**.

3. tRNA synthesis (Figure 3-22)

a. **RNA polymerase III** is the enzyme that produces tRNA. The promoter is located within the coding region of the gene.

b. **Primary transcripts** for tRNA are cleaved at the 5′ and 3′ ends.

c. Some precursors contain **introns** that are removed.

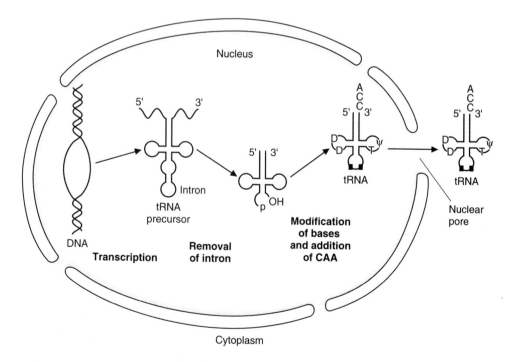

Figure 3-22. Synthesis of tRNA. D, T, ψ, and ∎ are unusual nucleotides produced by posttranscriptional modifications.

    d. During processing of tRNA precursors, **nucleotides** are **modified**. Posttranscriptional modification includes the conversion of uridine to pseudouridine (ψ), ribothymidine (T), and dihydrouridine (D). Other unusual nucleotides are also produced.

    e. Addition of the sequence **CCA** to the **3′ end** is catalyzed by nucleotidyl transferase.

IV. Protein Synthesis (Translation of mRNA)

- During translation, messenger RNA (mRNA) determines the sequence of the amino acids in the protein that is produced.
- mRNA combines with ribosomes, which contain rRNA. Many ribosomes can be attached simultaneously to a single molecule of mRNA, forming a polysome.
- tRNA carries amino acids to the ribosomal site of protein synthesis. The anticodon in each aminoacyl-tRNA combines with the complementary codon in mRNA. A codon is the sequence of three nucleotides in mRNA that specifies a particular amino acid.
- Initiation of a polypeptide chain begins with the amino acid methionine (codon = AUG).
- Subsequently, amino acids are added to the growing polypeptide chain according to the codon sequence in the mRNA. Aminoacyl-tRNAs and GTP provide the energy for chain elongation.
- A protein is synthesized from its N- to its C-terminus, following the codons in the mRNA in a 5′ to 3′ direction.
- When synthesis of the polypeptide is complete, a termination codon (UGA, UAG, or UAA) causes the polypeptide chain to be released.

A. The genetic code (Table 3-1)

    – The genetic code is the collection of codons that specify all the amino acids found in proteins.

Table 3-1. The Genetic Code

First Base (5′)	Second Base				Third Base (3′)
	U	**C**	**A**	**G**	
U	Phe	Ser	Tyr	Cys	U
	Phe	Ser	Tyr	Cys	C
	Leu	Ser	Term	Term	A
	Leu	Ser	Term	Trp	G
C	Leu	Pro	His	Arg	U
	Leu	Pro	His	Arg	C
	Leu	Pro	Gln	Arg	A
	Leu	Pro	Gln	Arg	G
A	Ile	Thr	Asn	Ser	U
	Ile	Thr	Asn	Ser	C
	Ile	Thr	Lys	Arg	A
	Met	Thr	Lys	Arg	G
G	Val	Ala	Asp	Gly	U
	Val	Ala	Asp	Gly	C
	Val	Ala	Glu	Gly	A
	Val	Ala	Glu	Gly	G

– A **codon is a sequence of three bases** (triplet) in mRNA (5′ to 3′) that specifies (corresponds to) a particular amino acid. During translation, the successive codons in an mRNA determine the sequence in which amino acids add to the growing polypeptide chain.

1. **The genetic code is degenerate** (redundant). Each of the 20 common amino acids has at least one codon; many amino acids have numerous codons.

2. The genetic code is **nonoverlapping** (i.e., each nucleotide is used only once), beginning with a start codon (**AUG**) near the 5′ end of the mRNA and ending with a termination (stop) codon (**UGA, UAG,** or **UAA**) near the 3′ end.

3. The code is **commaless** (i.e., there are no breaks or markers to distinguish one codon from the next).

4. The code is **nearly universal.** The same codon specifies the same amino acid in almost all species studied; however, some differences have been found in the codons used in mitochondria.

5. The **start codon** (AUG) determines the **reading frame.** Subsequent nucleotides are read in sets of three, sequentially following this codon.

B. Effect of mutations on proteins

– Mutations in DNA are transcribed into mRNA and thus can cause changes in the encoded protein.

– The various types of mutations that occur in DNA have different effects on the encoded protein.

1. **Point mutations** occur when one base in DNA is replaced by another, altering the codon in mRNA.

   a. **Silent** mutations do not affect the amino acid sequence of a protein (e.g., CGA to CGG causes no change, since both codons specify arginine).

   b. **Missense** mutations result in one amino acid being replaced by another (e.g., CGA to CCA causes arginine to be replaced by proline).

   c. **Nonsense** mutations result in premature termination of the growing polypeptide chain (e.g., CGA to UGA causes arginine to be replaced by a stop codon).

2. **Insertions** occur when a base or a number of bases are added to DNA. They can result in a protein with more amino acids than normal.

3. **Deletions** occur when a base or a number of bases are removed from DNA. They can result in a protein with fewer amino acids than normal.

4. **Frameshift mutations** occur when the number of bases added or deleted is not a multiple of three. The reading frame is shifted so that completely different sets of codons are read beyond the point where the mutation starts.

C. Formation of aminoacyl-tRNAs (Figure 3-23)

– **Amino acids are activated and attached to** their corresponding **tRNAs** by highly specific enzymes known as aminoacyl-tRNA synthetases.

1. Each **aminoacyl-tRNA synthetase** recognizes a particular amino acid and the tRNAs specific for that amino acid.

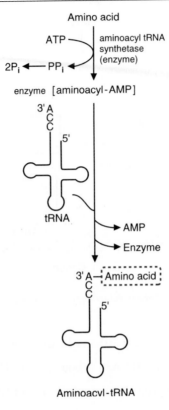

Figure 3-23. Formation of aminoacyl-tRNA.

2. An **amino acid** first reacts with ATP, forming an enzyme [aminoacyl-AMP] complex and pyrophosphate, which is cleaved to 2 P_i.

3. The **aminoacyl-AMP** then **forms an ester** with the 2′ or 3′ hydroxyl of a tRNA specific for that amino acid, producing an aminoacyl-tRNA and AMP.

4. Once an amino acid is attached to a tRNA, insertion of the amino acid into a growing polypeptide chain depends on the codon-anticodon interaction (Figure 3-24).

D. **Initiation of translation** (Figure 3-25)

1. **In eukaryotes, methionyl-tRNA$_i$^Met$ binds to the small ribosomal subunit.** The **5′ cap** of the mRNA binds to the small subunit and the first AUG codon base-pairs with the anticodon on the methionyl-tRNA$_i$^Met$. The methionine that initiates protein synthesis is subsequently removed from the N-terminus of the polypeptide.

a. **In bacteria,** the methionine that initiates protein synthesis is **formylated** and is carried by tRNA$_f$^Met$.

b. **Prokaryotes do not contain a 5′ cap** on their mRNA. An mRNA sequence upstream from the translation start site (the Shine-Dalgarno sequence) binds to the 3′ end of 16S rRNA.

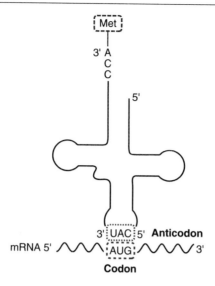

Figure 3-24. Antiparallel binding of aminoacyl-tRNA to mRNA.

2. The **large ribosomal subunit binds,** completing the initiation complex.

    a. The methionyl-tRNA$_i^{Met}$ is bound at the **P** (peptidyl) **site** of the complex.

    b. The **A** (acceptor or aminoacyl) **site** of the complex is unoccupied.

3. Initiation factors, ATP, and **GTP** are required for formation of the initiation complex.

    a. The **initiation factors** are designated IF-1, IF-2, and IF-3 in prokaryotes. In eukaryotes, they are designated eIF-1, eIF-2, and so on. Seven or more may be present.

    b. Release of the initiation factors involves hydrolysis of GTP to GDP and P$_i$.

E. Elongation of polypeptide chains (see Figure 3-25B)

    – The addition of each amino acid to the growing polypeptide chain involves binding of an aminoacyl-tRNA at the A site, formation of a peptide bond, and translocation of the peptidyl-tRNA to the P site.

1. Binding of aminoacyl-tRNA to the A site

    a. The **mRNA codon** at the A site determines which aminoacyl-tRNA will bind.

        (1) The **codon and the anticodon** bind by **base-pairing** that is **antiparallel** (see Figure 3-24).

        (2) Internal methionine residues in the polypeptide chain are added in response to AUG codons. They are carried by tRNA$_m^{Met}$, a second tRNA specific for methionine.

    b. An **elongation factor** (EF-Tu in prokaryotes and EF-1 in eukaryotes) and hydrolysis of GTP are required for binding.

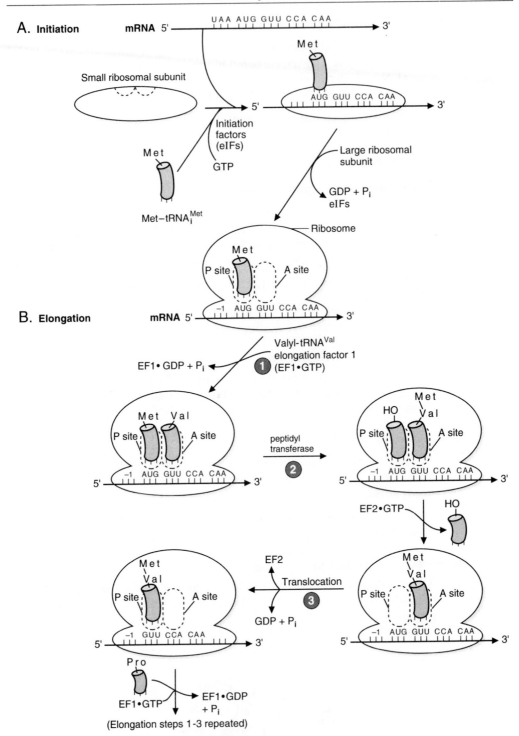

Figure 3-25. The initiation *(A)* and elongation *(B)* reactions of protein synthesis. eIFs are initiation factors in eukaryotes (IFs in prokaryotes). EF-1 and EF-2 are eukaryotic elongation factors corresponding with EF-Tu and EF-G in prokaryotes.

2. Formation of a peptide bond

a. A peptide bond forms between the amino group of the aminoacyl-tRNA at the **A site** and the carbonyl of the aminoacyl group attached to the tRNA at the **P site.** Formation of the peptide bond is catalyzed by **peptidyl transferase,** which is rRNA.

b. The tRNA at the P site now does not contain an amino acid. It is "uncharged."

c. The growing polypeptide chain is attached to the tRNA in the A site.

3. Translocation of peptidyl-tRNA

a. The peptidyl-tRNA (along with the attached mRNA) moves from the A site to the P site, and the uncharged tRNA is released from the ribosome. An **elongation factor** (EF-2 in eukaryotes or EF-G in prokaryotes) and the hydrolysis of **GTP** are required for translocation.

b. The next codon in the mRNA is now in the A site.

c. The elongation and translocation steps are repeated until a termination codon moves into the A site.

F. Termination of translation

– When a termination codon (UGA, UAG, or UAA) occupies the A site, release factors cause the newly synthesized polypeptide to be released from the ribosome, and the ribosomal subunits dissociate from the mRNA.

G. Polysomes (Figure 3-26)

1. More than one ribosome can be attached to a single mRNA at any given time. The complex of mRNA with multiple ribosomes is known as a **polysome.**

2. Each ribosome carries a nascent polypeptide chain that grows longer as the ribosome approaches the 3′ end of the mRNA.

H. Posttranslational processing

– After synthesis is completed, **proteins can be modified** by phosphorylation, glycosylation, ADP-ribosylation, hydroxylation, and addition of other groups.

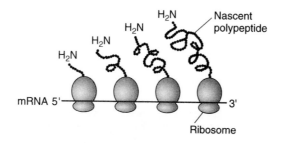

Figure 3-26. A polysome.

I. Synthesis and release of secretory proteins

1. **Secretory proteins,** destined for release from the cell, are synthesized on ribosomes attached to the rough endoplasmic reticulum (**RER**) in eukaryotic cells.

2. A **hydrophobic signal sequence** at the N-terminus of a secretory protein causes the nascent protein to pass into the lumen of the RER. The signal sequence is cleaved from the N-terminus, and the protein may be glycosylated within the RER.

3. The protein travels in vesicles to the **Golgi,** where it may be glycosylated further and is packaged in secretory vesicles.

4. **Secretory vesicles** containing the protein travel from the Golgi to the cell membrane. The protein is released from the cell by **exocytosis.**

V. Regulation of Protein Synthesis

- Regulation of protein synthesis in prokaryotes occurs mainly at the transcriptional level and involves genetic units known as operons.
  - Operons contain promoter regions where proteins bind and facilitate or inhibit the binding of RNA polymerase.
  - When RNA polymerase transcribes the structural genes of an operon, a polycistronic mRNA (i.e., an mRNA that codes for more than one polypeptide) is produced.
- In eukaryotes, regulation of protein synthesis can occur by modification of DNA or at the level of transcription, processing of mRNA, or translation.
  - Genes can be deleted from cells or they can be amplified, rearranged, or modified (e.g., methylated).
  - Histones nonspecifically repress transcription of genes.
  - Regulatory elements in DNA sequences control the expression of genes that produce proteins. They include the basal promoter (TATA box and other sequences near the start site), enhancers, and silencers.
  - Inducers cause proteins to bind to DNA sequences (response elements) and stimulate transcription of specific genes.
  - Regulation occurs during processing of hnRNA to form mRNA and involves the use of alternative start sites for transcription, alternative splice sites for removal of introns, alternative polyadenylation sites for addition of the poly(A) tail, and RNA editing.
  - Synthesis of proteins can be regulated at the level of translation.

A. Regulation of protein synthesis in prokaryotes

1. **Relationship of protein synthesis to nutrient supply**

   a. **Prokaryotes** respond to changes in their supply of **nutrients** in a way that allows them to obtain or conserve energy most efficiently.
      - Prokaryotes, such as *E. coli,* require a source of **carbon,** which is usually a sugar that is oxidized for energy.
      - A source of **nitrogen** is also required for the synthesis of amino acids from which structural proteins and enzymes are produced.

   b. *E. coli* uses **glucose** preferentially whenever it is available. The enzymes in the pathways for glucose utilization are made **constitutively** (i.e., they are constantly being produced).

c. **If glucose is not present** in the medium but another sugar is available, *E. coli* produces the enzymes and other proteins that allow the cell to derive energy from that sugar. The process by which synthesis of the enzymes is regulated is called **induction.**

d. **If an amino acid is present** in the medium, *E. coli* does not need to synthesize that amino acid and conserves energy by ceasing to produce the enzymes required for its synthesis. The process by which synthesis of these enzymes is regulated is called **repression.**

2. **Operons**

a. An operon is a **set of genes** that are **adjacent** to one another in the genome and are **coordinately controlled**; that is, the genes are either all turned on or all turned off (Figure 3-27).

b. The **structural genes** of an operon **code** for a series of different **proteins.**

A. **In the absence of inducer**

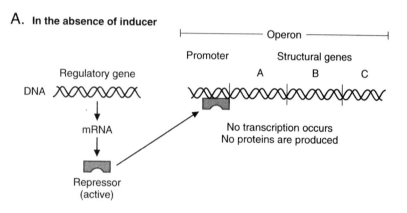

B. **In the presence of inducer**

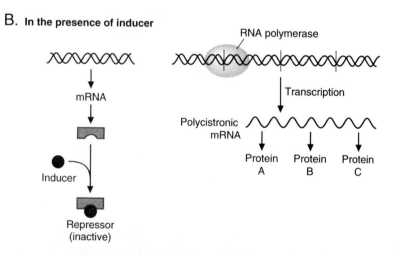

Figure 3-27. An inducible operon (e.g., the *lac* operon). If the inducer is absent, the repressor is active and binds to the operator, preventing RNA polymerase from binding. Thus, transcription does not occur. If the inducer is present, it binds to and inactivates the repressor, which then does not bind to the operator. Therefore, RNA polymerase can bind and transcribe the structural genes.

- A single **polycistronic mRNA** is transcribed from an operon. This single mRNA codes for all the proteins of the operon.
- A series of **start** and **stop codons** on the polycistronic mRNA allows a number of different proteins to be produced at the translational level from the single mRNA.

c. Transcription begins near a **promoter region,** located upstream from the group of structural genes.

d. Associated with the promoter is a short sequence, the **operator,** which determines whether or not the genes are expressed.

e. **Binding of a repressor protein** to the operator region prevents binding of RNA polymerase to the promoter and **inhibits transcription** of the structural genes of the operon.

- Repressor proteins are encoded by regulatory genes, which may be located anywhere in the genome.

3. **Induction** (see Figure 3-27*B*)

a. Induction is the process whereby an **inducer** (a small molecule) **stimulates transcription** of an operon.

b. The inducer is frequently a sugar (or a metabolite of the sugar), and the proteins produced from the inducible operon allow the sugar to be metabolized.

   (1) The inducer binds to the **repressor,** inactivating it.

   (2) The **inactive repressor does not bind** to the operator.

   (3) **RNA polymerase,** therefore, can **bind** to the promoter and **transcribe** the operon.

   (4) The structural **proteins** encoded by the operon are **produced.**

c. The lactose (***lac***) operon is **inducible.**

   (1) A metabolite of lactose, **allolactose,** is the inducer.

   (2) Proteins produced by the genes of the *lac* operon allow the cell to oxidize lactose as a source of energy. Gene Z produces a **β-galactosidase;** gene Y, a lactose permease; and gene A, a transacetylase.

   (3) The *lac* operon is induced only in the **absence of glucose.** It exhibits **catabolite repression** (see V A 6)

4. **Repression**

a. Repression is the process whereby a **corepressor** (a small molecule) **inhibits transcription** of an operon.

b. The **corepressor** is usually an amino acid, and the proteins produced from the repressible operon are involved in the synthesis of the amino acid.

   (1) The **corepressor binds to the repressor,** activating it.

   (2) The **active repressor binds to the operator.**

   (3) **RNA polymerase,** therefore, cannot bind to the promoter, and the operon is not transcribed.

(4) The cell stops producing the structural proteins encoded by the operon.

c. The tryptophan (***trp***) operon is **repressible**.

   (1) Tryptophan is the corepressor.

   (2) The proteins encoded by the *trp* operon are involved in the synthesis of tryptophan.

   (3) The *trp* operon is repressed in the presence of tryptophan, since cells do not need to make the amino acid if it is present in the growth medium.

5. Positive control

   a. Some operons are turned on by mechanisms that **activate transcription.**

   b. When the repressor of the arabinose (*ara*) operon binds arabinose, it changes conformation and becomes an activator that stimulates binding of RNA polymerase to the promoter. The operon is then transcribed, and the proteins required for oxidation of arabinose are produced.

6. Catabolite repression (Figure 3-28)

   a. Cells preferentially use **glucose** when it is available.

   b. Some operons (e.g., *lac* and *ara*) are not expressed when glucose is present in the medium. These operons require **cAMP** for their expression.

   (1) Glucose causes cAMP levels in the cells to decrease.

   (2) When **glucose decreases, cAMP levels rise**.

   (3) cAMP binds to the catabolite-activator protein (**CAP**).

   (4) The **cAMP-protein complex** binds to a site near the **promoter** of the operon and facilitates binding of RNA polymerase to the promoter

   c. The ***lac* operon** exhibits catabolite repression.

   (1) In the **presence of lactose** and the **absence of glucose**, the *lac* repressor is inactivated and the high levels of cAMP facilitate binding of RNA polymerase to the promoter.

   (2) The **operon is transcribed**, and the proteins that allow the cells to utilize lactose are produced.

7. Attenuation

   a. In bacterial cells, **transcription and translation** occur **simultaneously**.

   b. Attenuation occurs by a mechanism by which **rapid translation** of the nascent transcript causes **termination of transcription**.

   c. As the transcript is being produced, if ribosomes attach and **rapidly translate** the transcript, a secondary structure is generated in the mRNA that is a **termination signal** for RNA polymerase.

   d. If **translation is slow**, this termination structure does not form, and **transcription continues**.

A. **In the presence of inducer and glucose**

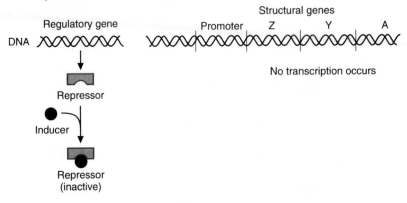

B. **In the presence of inducer and absence of glucose**

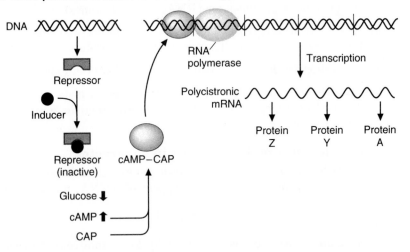

Figure 3-28. Catabolite repression. The operon is transcribed only when glucose is low. Cyclic adenosine monophosphate (cAMP) is elevated, and the inducer binds to the repressor, inactivating it. Under these conditions, the cAMP-CAP complex forms and binds to the DNA, facilitating the initiation of transcription by RNA polymerase. The *lac* operon exhibits catabolite repression.

   (1) Multiple codons for the amino acid are located near the translation start site of the mRNA.

   (2) When cells contain low levels of the amino acid (which is produced by the enzymes encoded by the operon), less aminoacyl-tRNA is available to bind to these codons, and translation slows.

   e. The *trp* operon is regulated by attenuation.

8. **Factors, such as sigma, affect RNA polymerase activity.** These factors bind to the core RNA polymerase and increase its ability to bind to specific promoters.

B. Differences between eukaryotes and prokaryotes

1. **Eukaryotic cells undergo differentiation,** and the organisms go through various developmental stages.

2. **Eukaryotes contain nuclei.** Therefore, transcription is separated from translation. In prokaryotes, transcription and translation occur simultaneously.

3. **DNA is complexed with histones in eukaryotes**, but not in prokaryotes.

4. The **mammalian genome** contains about **1000 times more DNA** than *E. coli* (10^9 versus 10^6 base pairs).

5. Most **mammalian** cells are **diploid.**

6. The **major part of the genome** of mammalian cells **does not code for proteins.**

7. **Some eukaryotic genes**, like most bacterial genes, **are unique** (i.e., they exist in one or a small number of copies per genome).

8. **Other eukaryotic genes,** unlike bacterial genes, have **many copies** in the genome (e.g,. genes for tRNA, rRNA, histones).

9. Relatively **short, repetitive DNA sequences** are dispersed throughout the eukaryotic genome. They do not code for proteins (e.g., Alu sequences).

10. **Eukaryotic genes contain introns.** Bacterial genes do not.

11. **Bacterial genes** are organized in **operons** (sets that are under the control of a single promoter). **Each eukaryotic gene has its own promoter.**

C. Regulation of protein synthesis in eukaryotes

– Regulation can result from changes in genes or from mechanisms that affect transcription, processing and transport of mRNA, mRNA translation, or mRNA stability.

1. Changes in genes

a. **Genes can be lost** (or partially lost) from cells, so that functional proteins can no longer be produced (e.g., during differentiation of red blood cells).

b. **Genes can be amplified.** For example, the drug methotrexate causes hundreds of copies of the gene for the enzyme dihydrofolate reductase to be produced, which results in resistance to the drug.

c. **Segments of DNA can move** from one location to another on the genome, associating with each other in various ways so that different proteins are produced.

   (1) A number of different potential sequences (or arrangements) occur for various portions of an antibody-producing gene (Figure 3-29).

   (2) During differentiation of lymphocytes, specific sequences are selected and rearranged so that they are adjacent to each other in the genome and can act as a single transcriptional unit for a specific antibody.

d. **Modification** of the **bases in DNA** affects the **transcriptional activity** of a gene.

   (1) Cytosine can be methylated at its 5 position.

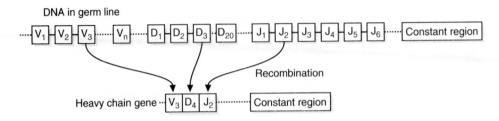

Figure 3-29. Rearrangement of DNA. Specific V, D, and J segments from among a large number of potential sequences in the DNA of precursor cells combine to form the heavy chain gene from which lymphocytes produce immunoglobulins (antibodies).

(2) The greater the extent of methylation, the less readily a gene is transcribed.

– Globin genes are more extensively methylated in nonerythroid cells than in erythroid cells, in which they are expressed.

2. Regulation of the level of transcription

a. Histones, which are small, basic proteins associated with the DNA of eukaryotes, act as nonspecific repressors.

b. The **expression** of specific genes is stimulated by **positive** mechanisms.

c. Inducers (e.g., steroid hormones) enter cells, bind to protein receptors, interact with chromatin in the nucleus, and **activate specific genes** (see Chapter 8).

d. Some genes have **more than one promoter.** Thus, the promoter that is used can differ under different physiologic conditions or in different cell types.

3. Regulation during processing and transport of mRNA

– Regulatory mechanisms that occur during capping, polyadenylation, and splicing can alter the amino acid sequence or the quantity of the protein produced from the mRNA. Editing of mRNA also occurs, and the rate of degradation of mRNA is also regulated.

a. Alternative splice sites can be used to produce different mRNAs.

– The use of different splice sites results in the production of different proteins from the calcitonin gene in the thyroid gland and the brain (Figure 3-30).

b. Alternative polyadenylation sites can be used to generate different mRNAs.

(1) Lymphocytes produce a membrane-bound IgM antibody at one stage of development and a soluble form that is secreted at a later stage. The gene for this antibody contains two polyadenylation sites, one after the last two exons (which code for a hydrophobic amino acid sequence) and one before these exons.

(2) When cleavage and poly(A) addition occur after the last two exons, the antibody contains a hydrophobic region that anchors it in the cell membrane. When polyadenylation occurs at the first site, the antibody lacks the hydrophobic tail and is secreted from the cell.

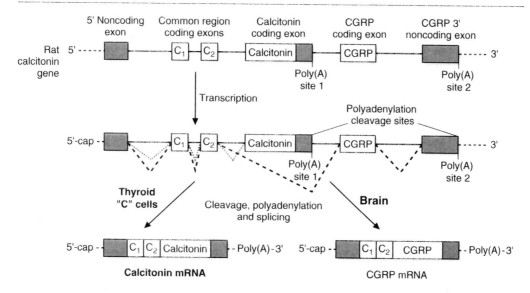

Figure 3-30. Alternative splicing of the calcitonin gene. In thyroid cells, hnRNA transcribed from the calcitonin gene is processed to form the mRNA that produces calcitonin. In the brain, the same transcript of this gene is spliced differently. The first polyadenylation site is cleaved out, and a second polyadenylation site is used. The protein product is the calcitonin gene-related protein (CGRP).

   c. mRNAs can be degraded by nucleases after their synthesis in the nucleus and before their translation in the cytoplasm.
   (1) mRNAs have different half-lives. Some are degraded more rapidly than others.
   (2) Interferon stimulates synthesis of 2′,5′-oligo(A), which activates a nuclease that degrades mRNA.

   d. RNA editing involves the alteration ("editing") of bases in mRNA after transcription (Figure 3-31).

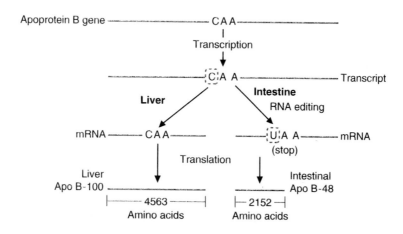

Figure 3-31. RNA editing. In liver, the apoprotein B (Apo B) gene produces a protein (Apo B-100) that contains more than 4000 amino acids. It is the major apoprotein of very low density lipoprotein (VLDL). In intestinal cells, the same gene produces a protein that contains only 48% of this number of amino acids. This protein (Apo B-48) is the major apoprotein of chylomicrons. "Editing" of mRNA (conversion of a C to a U) generates a stop codon in the intestinal mRNA.

4. **Protein synthesis** can be **regulated at the translational level**, during the initiation or elongation reactions.

   a. **Heme** stimulates the synthesis of globin by preventing the phosphorylation and consequent inactivation of eIF-2, a factor involved in initiation of protein synthesis.

   b. **Interferon** stimulates the phosphorylation of eIF-2, causing inhibition of initiation.

VI. Biotechnology Involving Recombinant DNA

- Newly developed techniques in molecular biology are being used for research, medical diagnosis, and production of therapeutic proteins. They provide hope as future therapy for diseases that currently are considered incurable.
- Restriction enzymes, which cleave within short, specific sequences of DNA, can be used to obtain DNA fragments for study or for insertion into DNA from other sources. The fusion product is known as chimeric DNA.
- Because DNA strands can base-pair with complementary strands of DNA or RNA, a technique known as hybridization has been developed. Labeled DNA can be used as a probe to identify homologous (complementary sequences of) DNA or RNA.
- Gel electrophoresis separates DNA fragments.
- The nucleotide sequence of DNA can be determined and used to deduce the amino acid sequence of the protein produced from the DNA.
- Large quantities of DNA can be produced by polymerase chain reaction (PCR).
- Fragments of DNA obtained, for example, from genomic DNA or DNA copied from mRNA (cDNA), can be amplified by PCR and cloned (i.e., inserted into another organism, where the foreign DNA can be replicated and expressed). The effects of the protein product can then be studied or, in some cases, large quantities of the protein product can be obtained.
- In medicine, recombinant DNA techniques permit the production of specific proteins that are used for therapy or as vaccines. The techniques are also used to diagnose disease, to predict the risk of genetic defects, and to determine parentage or other types of relationships. Ultimately, they will be used to treat disease (gene therapy).

A. Strategies for obtaining copies of genes or fragments of DNA

1. Short sequences of DNA (**oligonucleotides**) can be synthesized in vitro and used as **primers** for DNA synthesis or as **probes** for detection of DNA or RNA sequences.

2. **Restriction endonucleases** cleave DNA into fragments.

   a. Restriction endonucleases recognize short sequences in DNA and cleave both strands within this region (Figure 3-32).

   b. Most of the DNA sequences recognized by these enzymes are **palindromes** (i.e., both strands of DNA have the same base sequence in the 5′ to 3′ direction).

      (1) The enzyme *Eco*RI cleaves a region between an A and a G on each strand, generating two products.

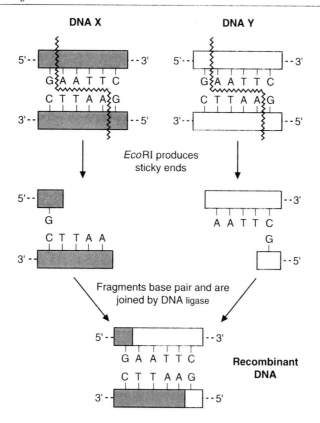

Figure 3-32. Action of restriction enzymes. *Eco*RI cleaves a palindrome (5′-GAATTC-3′). Two fragments are produced that contain complementary single-stranded regions (sticky ends). If two different DNAs (e.g., X and Y) are cleaved by *Eco* RI, the sticky ends can pair to form a recombinant DNA.

(2) The single-stranded regions of the products allow them to reanneal or to recombine with other DNA that has been cleaved by the same restriction endonuclease.

  c. A **DNA fragment,** which contains a **specific gene,** can be isolated from the cellular genome with restriction enzymes. Genes isolated from eukaryotic cells usually contain **introns,** whereas those from bacteria do not.

3. The **mRNA** for a gene can be isolated, and a DNA copy (**cDNA**) can be produced by **reverse transcriptase.** cDNA does not contain introns.

B. Techniques for identifying DNA sequences

1. Use of probes to detect specific DNA or RNA sequences

  a. A **probe** is a single strand of DNA that can **hybridize (base pair)** with a **complementary sequence** on another single-stranded polynucleotide composed of DNA or RNA.

  b. The probe must contain a **label,** so that it can detect complementary DNA or RNA. The label may be radioactive (so it can be detected by autoradiography) or a chemical that can be identified, for example, by fluorescence.

2. Gel electrophoresis of DNA

– Gel electrophoresis **separates** DNA **chains** of varying length. Poly-acrylamide gels can be used to separate short DNA chains that differ in length by only one nucleotide. Agarose gels separate chains of larger size.

a. Because DNA contains negatively charged phosphate groups, it will **migrate** in an electric field **toward the positive electrode**.

b. Shorter chains migrate more rapidly through the pores of the gel, so **separation depends on length**.

c. DNA **bands** in the gel can be **visualized** by various techniques including staining with dyes (e.g., ethidium bromide) and autoradiography (if the gel contains a radioactive compound, which reacts with a photographic film). **Labeled probes** (see VI B1) detect **specific DNA sequences**.

d. Blots of gels can be made using nitrocellulose paper (Figure 3-33).

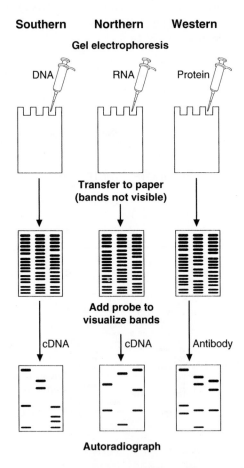

Figure 3-33. Southern, Northern, and Western blots. In Southern blots, DNA is electrophoresed, denatured with alkali, transferred to nitrocellulose paper ("blotted"), and hybridized with a DNA probe. In Northern blots, RNA is electrophoresed and hybridized with a DNA probe. (In this case, alkali is not used because RNA is already single-stranded, and alkali would hydrolyze the RNA.) Western blots involve electrophoresis of proteins that are visualized by binding to antibodies. The nucleic acids and proteins can only be seen on the gel after the gel is treated with a labeled probe (i.e., labeled DNA or antibodies).

(1) **Southern blots** are produced when a radioactive **DNA** probe hybridizes with **DNA** on a nitrocellulose blot of a gel.

(2) **Northern blots** are produced when a radioactive **DNA** probe hybridizes with **RNA** on a nitrocellulose blot of a gel.

(3) A **Western blot** is a related technique in which **proteins** are separated by gel electrophoresis and probed with **antibodies** that bind a specific protein.

3. **DNA sequencing** by the Sanger dideoxynucleotide method (Figure 3-34)

a. **Dideoxynucleotides** are added to solutions in which DNA polymerase is catalyzing polymerization of a DNA chain.

b. Because a dideoxynucleotide does not contain a 3′-hydroxyl group, **polymerization of the chain is terminated** wherever a dideoxynucleotide is incorporated into the growing chain.

c. Because the dideoxynucleotide competes with the normal nucleotide for incorporation into the growing chain, **DNA chains of varying lengths are produced**. The shortest chains are nearest the 5′ end of the DNA chain (which grows 5′ to 3′).

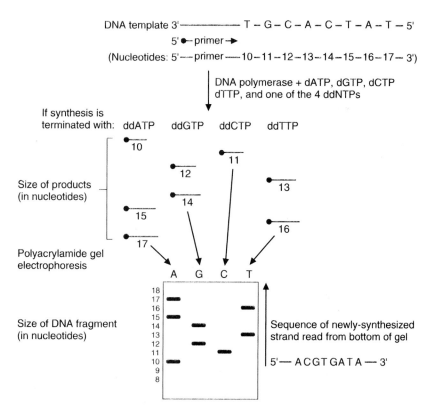

Figure 3-34. DNA sequencing by the dideoxynucleotide method. A DNA template is hybridized with a primer. DNA polymerase is added plus dATP, dGTP, dCTP, and dTTP. Either the primer or the nucleotides must have a radioactive label, so bands can be visualized on the gel by autoradiography. Samples are placed in each of four tubes, and one of the four dideoxyribonucleotides (ddNTPs) is added to each tube to cause random termination of DNA synthesis. Strands of different sizes are produced in each tube, electrophoresed, and visualized. The sequence of the newly synthesized strand is read from the bottom to the top of the gel.

    d. The sequence of the growing chain can be read (5′ to 3′) from the bottom to the top of the gel on which the DNA chains are separated.

C. Techniques for amplifying DNA sequences

1. Polymerase chain reaction (PCR)

– PCR is an **in vitro technique** used for rapidly producing large amounts of DNA (Figure 3-35). It is suitable for clinical or forensic testing because only a very small sample of DNA is required as the starting material.

2. Cloning of DNA (Figure 3-36)

– DNA from one organism (**"foreign" DNA**, obtained as described earlier) can be **inserted into a DNA vector** and used to **transform** cells from another organism, usually a bacterium, that grows rapidly, replicating the foreign DNA, as well as its own.

– Large quantities of the foreign DNA can be isolated or, under the appropriate conditions, the DNA can be expressed, and its protein product can be obtained in large quantities.

D. Use of recombinant DNA techniques to detect polymorphisms

– Humans differ in their genetic composition. **Polymorphisms** (variations in DNA sequences) occur frequently in the genome both in coding and in noncoding regions. Point mutations cause the simplest type of polymorphisms, but insertions and deletions of varying lengths also occur.

1. Restriction fragment length polymorphism (RFLP)

    a. Occasionally, a **mutation** occurs **in a restriction enzyme cleavage site** that is within or tightly linked to a gene. The enzyme can cleave the normal DNA at this site, but not the mutant. Thus, two smaller restriction fragments will be obtained from this region of the normal DNA, compared with only one larger fragment from the mutant.

    b. Sometimes, **a mutation creates a restriction site** that is not present in or near the normal gene. In this case, two smaller restriction fragments will be obtained from the mutant, and only one larger fragment from the normal (Figure 3-37).

    c. Normal human DNA has many regions that contain a highly variable number of tandem repeats (**VNTR**). The number of repeats differs from one individual to another (and from one allele to another). Restriction enzymes that cleave on the left and right flanks of a VNTR produce **DNA fragments of variable length**. The length depends on the number of repeats that the DNA contains (Figure 3-38). Fragments produced by various restriction enzymes from a number of different loci can be used to identify individuals with the accuracy of a fingerprint. Therefore, a technique called **"DNA fingerprinting"** is used to determine parentage or other genetic relationships, or to implicate suspects in criminal cases.

2. Detection of mutations by allele-specific oligonucleotide probes

    a. An **oligonucleotide probe** is synthesized that is **complementary** to a region of DNA that contains a **mutation**. A different probe is made for the normal DNA (Figure 3-39).

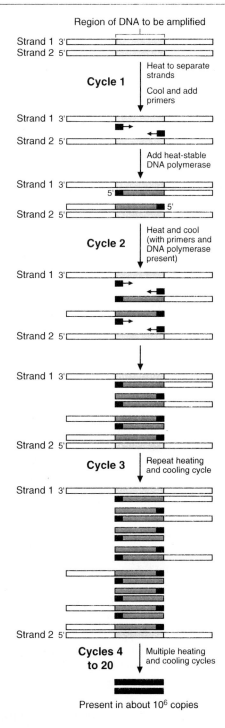

Figure 3-35. Polymerase chain reaction (PCR). The original DNA sample (strands 1 and 2) is denatured by heat. Large quantities of primers (the short, dark rectangles) are added that bind to each DNA strand when the solution is cooled. A heat-stable DNA polymerase (Taq) is added, and polymerization is allowed to proceed. The gray areas represent the regions that are replicated by extension of the primers. Heating and cooling cycles are repeated until the DNA is amplified many times.

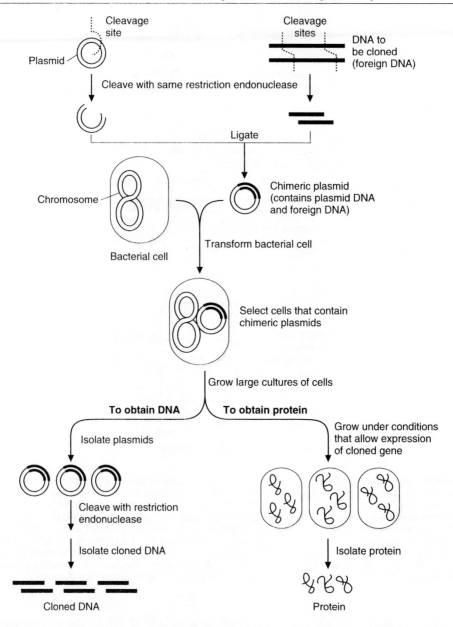

Figure 3-36. A simplification of the method for cloning foreign DNA in bacteria. A vector for transferring the foreign DNA into the bacterium, such as a plasmid, is cleaved with the same restriction endonuclease as the foreign DNA. The plasmid and foreign DNA, both cleaved by the same restriction enzyme, are mixed together and treated with DNA ligase. Some of the interactions produce chimeric plasmids, containing the foreign DNA integrated into the plasmid DNA. The plasmids are introduced into bacterial host cells (transformation). Clones that contain the chimeric plasmid are selected and cultured. To obtain large quantities of the foreign DNA, the plasmids are isolated from cells and treated with the restriction enzyme to release the foreign DNA, which is then isolated. To obtain large quantities of the protein product of the foreign DNA, the cells are grown under conditions that promote synthesis of the protein, and the protein is isolated from the cells. The DNA used to produce foreign proteins in bacterial cells must not contain introns because bacteria cannot remove them. Bacterial promoters must be inserted into the DNA so that the gene can be expressed.

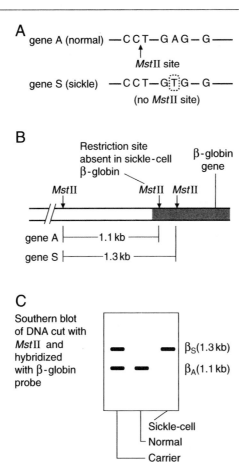

Figure 3-37. Restriction fragment length polymorphism (RFLP) caused by loss of a restriction site. If a mutation occurs in a cleavage site for a restriction enzyme, the pattern of restriction fragments differs from normal. *(A)* The mutation that causes sickle cell anemia results in the loss of an *Mst*II site in the β-globin gene. *(B)* Samples of DNA from individuals are treated with restriction endonucleases and then subjected to electrophoresis on gels. With the Southern blot technique, the restriction fragments on the gel are hybridized with a radioactive cDNA probe for the β-globin gene. The sickle cell allele produces a fragment of 1.3 kilobases (kb) when treated with *Mst*II. A normal allele produces a fragment of 1.1 kb (plus a fragment of 0.2 kb that is not seen on the gel). For a person with sickle cell disease, both alleles produce 1.3-kb restriction fragments. In a normal person, both alleles produce 1.1-kb fragments. For a carrier, both the 1.3- and 1.1-kb fragments are observed.

   b. If the mutant probe binds to a sample of DNA, the sample contains DNA from a mutant allele. If the normal probe binds, the sample contains DNA from a normal allele. If both probes bind, the sample contains DNA from both a mutant and a normal allele (i.e, the person providing the DNA sample is a carrier of the mutation).

3. Testing for mutations by PCR

   – An oligonucleotide complementary to a mutant region is used as a **primer for PCR**. If the primer binds to a DNA sample (i.e., if the sample contains the mutation), amplification of the DNA occurs (i.e., the primer is extended). If the primer does not bind, extension does not occur (i.e., the DNA is normal).

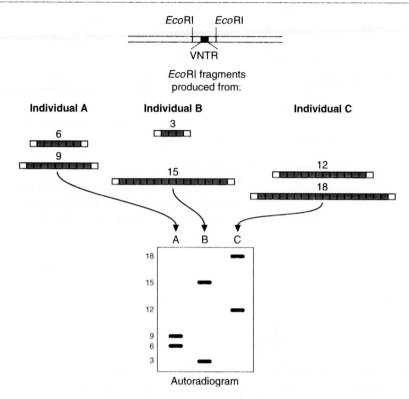

Figure 3-38. Restriction fragments produced from a gene with a variable number of tandem repeats (VNTR). DNA from three individuals, each with two alleles for this gene and a different number of repeats in each allele, was cleaved, electrophoresed, and treated with a probe for this gene. The length of the fragments depends on the number of repeats that they contain.

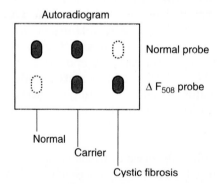

Figure 3-39. The use of oligonucleotide probes to test for cystic fibrosis (CF). Oligonucleotide probes complementary to the region where a 3-base deletion is located in the CF gene were synthesized. One probe binds only to the mutant (ΔF_{508}), and the other probe binds only to the normal region. DNA was isolated from individuals and amplified by polymerase chain reaction. Two spots were placed on nitrocellulose paper for each person. One spot was treated with the probe for the mutant region of the gene, and the other spot was treated with the probe for the normal region. Dark spots indicate binding of a probe. Only the normal probe binds to the DNA from a normal person, and only the mutant probe binds to the DNA from a person with CF. Both probes bind to DNA from a carrier. In carriers, one allele is normal and the other has the CF mutation.

E. Alterations in the genetic composition of animals

- If a **gene** from another organism is **inserted into a fertilized egg**, a **transgenic animal** can be produced. Such animals can be used for research or for other purposes, ranging from the production of human proteins in the milk of transgenic sheep to generation of larger and stronger species.
- The removal or disruption of genes (**gene knockout**) can be used to develop strains of animals that lack the protein product of the gene. The effects of loss of the protein can then be studied.

F. Mapping of the human genome

- A massive effort has been mounted to **sequence the entire human genome**. The results are expected to provide a better understanding of normal function and to elucidate the specific defects that result in inherited disease.

G. Gene therapy

- Ultimately, recombinant DNA technology will be used to treat genetic diseases. Already, some diseases (e.g., adenosine deaminase deficiency) have responded to efforts to introduce normal genes into individuals with defective genes.

VII. Clinical Correlations

A. Diseases related to abnormal hemoglobin

Sickle cell anemia results from a **point mutation** (GAG to GTG) that causes valine to replace glutamate at position 6 in the β-globin chain. Hydrophobic interactions between these valine residues on different hemoglobin molecules cause polymerization of sickle cell hemoglobin, which alters the shape of the red blood cells and results in hemolysis. In **hemoglobin Wayne**, deletion of a base causes a **frameshift** that produces the wrong sequence of amino acids in the chain beyond position 127.

In the **thalassemias** (a group of hemolytic anemias), mutations affect all steps of RNA metabolism. Substitutions in the **TATA box** decrease promoter function. Mutations in **splice junctions** create alternative splice sites. A change in the **polyadenylation site** (AATAAA to AATAGA) results in incorrect processing of the hnRNA, and the abnormal mRNA is degraded. A change from CAG to TAG produces a **stop codon** at position 39 that causes a shortened, nonfunctional protein to be synthesized. These mutations cause insufficient quantities of globin chains to be produced, and an anemia results.

B. Cancer

Cancer is a group of diseases in which cells are not responsive to the normal restraints on growth. The major causes of cancer are **radiation, chemicals,** and **viruses.** Radiation and chemicals cause **damage to DNA**, which, if not repaired rapidly, produces **mutations** that can result in cancer.

Burning organic material (e.g., cigarettes) produces chemicals such as **benzo(a)pyrene** that covalently bind to the bases in DNA, producing mutations that lead to **lung cancer. Ultraviolet light**, including that from the sun, produces **pyrimidine dimers** in DNA that lead to **skin cancer.** This condition is particularly pronounced in people with **xeroderma pigmentosum** because their DNA repair system does not function normally.

Oncogenes are genes that cause cancer. Their counterparts in normal cells, **proto-oncogenes**, are involved in **normal growth** and **development**. If oncogenes enter cells as a consequence of viral infection or if the normal proto-oncogenes are altered or expressed abnormally, **cancer** can result. Many oncogenes encode proteins that are related to **growth factors**, to receptors for growth factors, or to proteins produced by growth factors. Some oncogene products enter the nucleus and **activate genes**. According to the oncogene theory, **viruses cause cancer** by inserting **additional or abnormal copies** of proto-oncogenes into cells or by inserting strong **promoters** into regions that regulate the expression of these genes. Proto-oncogenes can be **amplified**. The gene for the proto-oncogene or its control region may undergo **mutations** due to radiation or chemicals. Alteration of the product or of the level of expression of a proto-oncogene produces changes in the growth characteristics of cells that can result in cancer.

Cancer can also result from alterations in genes that produce proteins which act as **suppressors of cell growth**. Decreased expression of these **suppressor genes** (e.g., p53, the retinoblastoma gene) results in increased cell growth.

The **treatment** of **cancer** frequently involves **drugs that interfere with DNA synthesis**. For example, 5-fluorouracil (**5-FU**) prevents the conversion of dUMP to dTMP, reducing the level of thymine nucleotides required for DNA synthesis. **Methotrexate** prevents formation of tetrahydrofolate from its more oxidized precursors. As a result, the formation of both thymine for DNA synthesis and the purines for DNA and RNA synthesis is inhibited.

Adriamycin contains a series of rings that intercalate (slip) between DNA base pairs. When adriamycin is present, DNA cannot act as a template for replication or transcription.

C. Treatment of viral infections

When viruses infect cells, they convert the cells' DNA-, RNA-, and protein-producing machinery to the generation of viral genes and proteins (i.e., to the production of new viruses). Few drugs are currently effective against viral infections.

Azidothymidine (**AZT**), an analogue of thymidine, is phosphorylated in the cell and **inhibits retroviral reverse transcriptase** (which is used to make DNA copies of viral RNA) by serving as a **DNA chain terminator**. It has been used to treat **HIV** infections associated with **AIDS**. Other nucleotide analogues, such as dideoxyinosine (**ddI**), also serve as chain terminators. More recently, **inhibitors of the HIV protease** have been produced. These inhibitors prevent the protease from cleaving a polyprotein produced from the viral genome into structural proteins and enzymes required for assembly of viral particles. A combination of protease inhibitors and DNA chain terminators currently provides the most successful therapy for HIV infections.

D. Compounds that inhibit RNA synthesis

Antibiotics that selectively affect bacterial function and have minimal side effects in humans are usually selected to treat bacterial infections. **Rifampicin**, which **inhibits the initiation of prokaryotic RNA synthesis**, is used to treat tuberculosis.

α-Amanitin, derived from the poisonous mushroom *Amanita phalloides,* inhibits **eukaryotic** RNA polymerases. Ingestion of small amounts of α-amanitin initially causes gastrointestinal problems but can rapidly result in death.

E. Compounds that inhibit protein synthesis

Streptomycin, tetracycline, chloramphenicol, and erythromycin inhibit protein synthesis **on prokaryotic (70S) ribosomes** and are used to treat a variety of infections. Because **mitochondria contain 70S-type ribosomes** that function similarly to those in prokaryotic cells, these compounds also **inhibit mitochondrial protein synthesis.** Chloramphenicol is particularly damaging to mitochondrial ribosomes and must be used with caution.

Streptomycin binds to the 30S ribosomal subunit of prokaryotes and causes misreading of mRNA, thus preventing formation of the initiation complex.

Tetracycline binds to the 30S ribosomal subunit of prokaryotes and inhibits binding of aminoacyl-tRNA to the A site. **Chloramphenicol** inhibits the peptidyl transferase activity of the 50S ribosomal subunit of prokaryotes. **Erythromycin** binds to the 50S ribosomal subunit of prokaryotes and prevents translocation. Some inhibitors of protein synthesis are not used clinically but are useful tools for research. **Puromycin** binds at the A site, forms a peptide bond with the growing peptide chain, and prematurely terminates synthesis. It acts in both prokaryotes and eukaryotes. **Cycloheximide** inhibits peptidyl transferase in eukaryotes.

F. Protein synthesis inhibitors that cause disease

Diphtheria toxin is produced from phage genes incorporated into the bacterium *Corynebacterium diphtheriae.* The toxin causes diphtheria, a lethal disease of the respiratory tract. The A fragment of the toxin catalyzes the **ADP-ribosylation** of **EF-2,** thus inhibiting translocation in eukaryotes.

G. Clinical uses of biotechnology

Biotechnology is currently being used in the **diagnosis of disease** (e.g., sickle cell anemia, cystic fibrosis, phenylketonuria). Recombinant DNA techniques are used to produce the probes (e.g., cDNA) for **screening human samples,** and they are used to generate large quantities of **proteins for use in therapy** (e.g., human insulin, growth hormone, tissue plasminogen activator, erythropoietin, factor VIII for hemophilia) or as **vaccines** (e.g., hepatitis B). Ultimately, these techniques will be used to introduce normal genes into individuals with defective genes (i.e., in **gene therapy** for inherited disease).

Review Test

Directions: Each of the numbered items or incomplete statements in this section is followed by answers or by completions of the statement. Select the **one** lettered answer or completion that is **best** in each case.

1. In DNA, on a molar basis

(A) adenine equals thymine
(B) adenine equals uracil
(C) guanine equals adenine
(D) cytosine equals thymine
(E) cytosine equals uracil

2. Which of the following sequences is complementary to the DNA sequence 5'-AAGTC-CGA-3'?

(A) 5'-AAGUCCGA-3'
(B) 3'-TTCAGGCT-5'
(C) 5'-TTCAGGCT-3'
(D) 3'-TCGGACTT-5'

3. DNA contains which one of the following components?

(A) Nitrogenous bases joined by phosphodiester bonds
(B) Negatively charged phosphate groups in the interior of the molecule
(C) Base pairs stacked along the central axis of the molecule
(D) Two strands that run in the same direction
(E) The sugar ribose

4. Which RNA contains 7-methylguanine at the 5' end?

(A) 5S RNA
(B) rRNA
(C) hnRNA
(D) tRNA

5. Thymine is present in which type of RNA?

(A) mRNA
(B) rRNA
(C) hnRNA
(D) tRNA

6. The action of DNA polymerases requires

(A) a 5'-hydroxyl group
(B) dUTP
(C) NAD⁺ as a cofactor
(D) a 3'-hydroxyl group
(E) CTP

7. Which of the following statements concerning replication of DNA is TRUE?

(A) It progresses in both directions away from each point of origin on the chromosome
(B) It requires a DNA template that is copied in its 5' to 3' direction
(C) It occurs during the M phase of the cell cycle
(D) It produces one newly synthesized double helix and one composed of the two parental strands

8. When base-pairing occurs in loops of RNA, adenine is hydrogen-bonded to

(A) guanine
(B) thymine
(C) cytosine
(D) uracil

Questions 9–13

Use the figure below to answer questions 9–13.

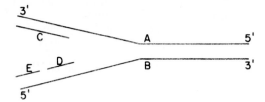

9. When synthesis of segment C begins, which other segment is also being synthesized?

(A) A
(B) B
(C) C
(D) D
(E) E

10. Segment C is synthesized

(A) from the middle toward both ends simultaneously
(B) toward the replication fork
(C) away from the replication fork
(D) in a 3' to 5' direction

91

11. Segment E is synthesized

(A) from the middle toward both ends simultaneously
(B) toward the replication fork
(C) away from the replication fork
(D) after segment D

12. The enzyme that joins segments D and E is

(A) the replicative DNA polymerase
(B) RNA polymerase
(C) an endonuclease
(D) DNA ligase
(E) a repair DNA polymerase

13. If adenine is the first base on the template strand corresponding to the initiation point for segment E, which precursor molecule would serve as the substrate that formed the first nucleotide in segment E?

(A) dUTP
(B) UTP
(C) dTTP
(D) TTP
(E) dTMP

14. Which of the following statements concerning Okazaki fragments is TRUE?

(A) They are produced by restriction enzymes
(B) They are synthesized on the leading strand during replication
(C) They are regions of DNA that do not code for the amino acids in a protein
(D) They are relatively short polydeoxyribonucleotides with a few ribonucleotide residues at the 5′ end
(E) They are products of the action of RNase on hnRNA

15. A bacterial mutant grows normally at 32°C but at 42°C accumulates short segments of newly synthesized DNA. Which of the following enzymes is most likely to be defective in this mutant?

(A) An endonuclease
(B) DNA polymerase
(C) An exonuclease
(D) An unwinding enzyme (helicase)
(E) DNA ligase

16. Which of the following phrases describes nucleosomes?

(A) Single ribosomes attached to mRNA
(B) Complexes of DNA and newly-transcribed RNA
(C) Subunits of chromatin
(D) Structures that contain DNA in the core with histones wrapped around the surface
(E) Complexes of protein and the 45S rRNA precursors found in the nucleolus

17. The base pair shown is normally found in

(A) DNA
(B) RNA
(C) both DNA and RNA
(D) neither DNA nor RNA

18. In an embryo that lacked nucleoli, the synthesis of which type of RNA would be most directly affected?

(A) tRNA
(B) rRNA
(C) mRNA
(D) 5S RNA
(E) hnRNA

19. Eukaryotic genes that produce mRNA

(A) contain a TATA box downstream from the start site of transcription
(B) can contain a CAAT box in the 5′ flanking region
(C) are transcribed by RNA polymerase III
(D) contain long stretches of thymine nucleotides that produce the poly(A) tail of mRNA
(E) do not contain introns

20. If a fragment of DNA containing the sequence 5'-AGCCAATT-3' serves as the template for transcription, the RNA that is produced will have the sequence

(A) 5'-AGCCAAUU-3'
(B) 5'-UCGGUUAA-3'
(C) 5'-UUAACCGA-3'
(D) 5'-AAUUGGCU-3'

21. A person ate mushrooms picked in a wooded area. Shortly thereafter, he was rushed to the hospital, where he died. He had no previous medical problems. The cause of his death was most likely the RNA polymerase inhibitor

(A) rifampicin
(B) α-amanitin
(C) streptolydigin
(D) actinomycin D

22. When benzo(a)pyrene (a carcinogen in cigarette smoke) binds to DNA, it forms a bulky covalent adduct on guanine residues. The consequence is that

(A) cells are rapidly transformed into cancer cells
(B) glycosylases remove the benzpyrene residues
(C) a repair process usually removes and replaces the damaged region of DNA
(D) UV light cleaves the benzpyrene from the guanine residue

23. Patients with xeroderma pigmentosum suffer DNA damage when they are exposed to ultraviolet (UV) light because UV light causes the formation of

(A) purine dimers in DNA
(B) pyrimidine dimers in DNA
(C) deoxyribose dimers in DNA
(D) anhydride bonds between phosphate groups in DNA

24. Patients with xeroderma pigmentosum develop skin cancer when they are exposed to sunlight because they have a deficiency in

(A) the primase enzyme of the replication complex
(B) a recombinase that permits chromosomes to exchange segments
(C) a glycosylate that removes damaged bases from DNA
(D) an enzyme that acts early in the nucleotide excision repair pathway
(E) an enzyme essential to repair mismatched bases

25. A common mutagenic event is the deamination of cytosine in DNA to form uracil. If the damaged strand is replicated, a CG base pair in DNA will be converted to a

(A) TA base pair
(B) GC base pair
(C) GG base pair
(D) UG base pair

26. If cytosine in DNA is deaminated, the uracil residue that results may be removed by

(A) an endonuclease
(B) an exonuclease
(C) a glycosylase
(D) DNA ligase
(E) a repair DNA polymerase

27. An aminoacyl-tRNA exhibits which one of the following characteristics?

(A) It is produced by a synthetase that is specific for the amino acid, but not the tRNA
(B) It is composed of an amino acid esterified to the 5' end of the tRNA
(C) It requires GTP for its synthesis from an amino acid and a tRNA
(D) It contains an anticodon that is complementary to the codon for the amino acid

28. Which one of the following changes in mRNA (caused by a point mutation) would result in translation of a protein identical to the normal protein?

(A) UCA → UAA
(B) UCA → CCA
(C) UCA → UCU
(D) UCA → ACA
(E) UCA → GCA

29. The structure shown is

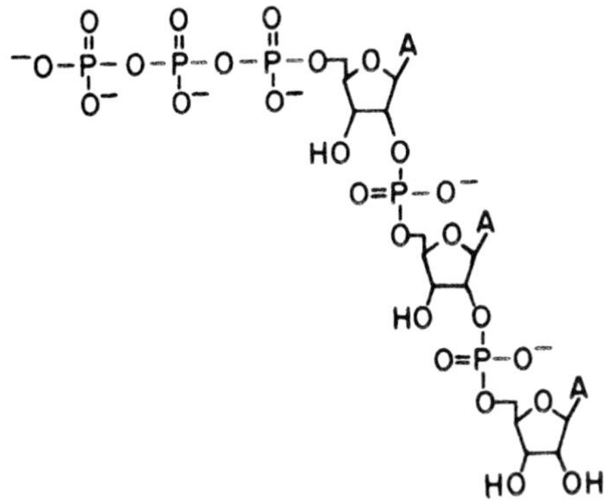

(A) a segment of the poly(A) tail of mRNA
(B) a region of DNA that, when transcribed to mRNA, codes for phenylalanine
(C) a sequence found at the 3′ end of all tRNAs
(D) not found in DNA or RNA

30. Which of the following statements about methionine is TRUE?

(A) It is the amino acid used for initiation of the synthesis of all proteins
(B) It is generally found at the N-terminus of proteins isolated from cells
(C) It requires a codon other than AUG to be added to growing polypeptide chains
(D) It is formylated when it is bound to tRNA in eukaryotic cells

31. Which of the following statements about bacteria is correct?

(A) They contain 80S ribosomes
(B) They initiate protein synthesis with methionyl-tRNA
(C) They are insensitive to chloramphenicol
(D) They synthesize proteins on mRNA that is in the process of being transcribed

32. Which of the following is required for initiation of protein synthesis in the cytosol of eukaryotic cells?

(A) A 40S ribosomal subunit
(B) IF-2
(C) Methionyl-tRNA$_f^{Met}$
(D) UTP
(E) EF-2

33. Which of the following is required for the elongation reactions of protein synthesis in eukaryotes?

(A) Peptidyl transferase
(B) CTP
(C) Formylmethionyl-tRNA
(D) Elongation factor G (EF-G)
(E) hnRNA

34. The mechanism for termination of protein synthesis in eukaryotes requires

(A) a peptidyl-tRNA that cannot bind at the P site
(B) the codon UGA, UAG, or AUG in the A site
(C) nuclease cleavage of mRNA
(D) release factors

35. Proteins that are secreted from cells

(A) contain methionine as the N-terminal amino acid
(B) are produced from translation products that have a signal sequence at the C-terminal end
(C) are synthesized on ribosomes that bind to proteins on the endoplasmic reticulum
(D) contain a hydrophobic sequence that is embedded in the membrane of secretory vesicles
(E) contain carbohydrate residues that bind to receptors on the interior of lysosomal membranes

36. Tetracycline, streptomycin, and erythromycin are effective antibiotics because they inhibit

(A) RNA synthesis in prokaryotes
(B) RNA synthesis in eukaryotes
(C) protein synthesis in prokaryotes
(D) protein synthesis on cytosolic ribosomes of eukaryotes
(E) protein synthesis on mitochondrial ribosomes of eukaryotes

Questions 37 and 38

In the year 2020, a new antibiotic will be available. Studies performed using an in vitro protein-synthesizing system produced the expected polypeptide in response to a synthetic mRNA with the following sequence:

AUGUUCUUCUUCUUCUUCUUCUAA

37. The polypeptide produced in the in vitro system was
(A) Met-Phe-Phe-Phe-Phe-Phe-Phe
(B) Met-Ser-Ser-Ser-Ser-Ser-Ser
(C) Met-Leu-Leu-Leu-Leu-Leu-Leu
(D) Met-Phe-Ser-Leu-Phe-Ser-Leu

38. When this in vitro protein-synthesizing system was treated with the new antibiotic, the only product was methionyl-phenylalanyl-tRNA. What process in protein synthesis is inhibited by the antibiotic?

(A) Binding of an aminoacyl-tRNA to the A site of the ribosome
(B) Initiation
(C) Translocation
(D) Peptidyl transferase catalyzed formation of a peptide bond

39. In bacterial operons that are inducible

(A) the inducer binds to the repressor and activates it
(B) the inducer stimulates binding of RNA polymerase to the promoter
(C) a regulatory gene produces an inactive repressor
(D) structural genes that are adjacent on the DNA are coordinately expressed in response to the inducer
(E) each of the structural genes produces a separate mRNA

40. When cyclic adenosine monophosphate (cAMP) levels are relatively high in *Escherichia coli*

(A) lactose is not required for transcription of the *lac* operon
(B) glucose levels in the medium are low
(C) the repressor is bound to the *lac* operon if lactose is present
(D) the enzymes for the metabolism of lactose are not induced

41. Which of the following statements about regulation of protein synthesis in eukaryotes is correct?

(A) A gene that is methylated is transcribed more readily than one that is not methylated
(B) Genes cannot undergo rearrangements that allow cells to produce new proteins
(C) Red blood cells do not produce hemoglobin mRNA because they lack the appropriate gene
(D) Recognition of alternative polyadenylation sites allows cells to produce proteins that have different N-terminal regions
(E) Steroid hormones activate genes that are specifically repressed by histones

42. Gene transcription rates and mRNA levels were determined for an enzyme that is induced by glucocorticoids. Compared with untreated levels, glucocorticoid treatment caused a 10-fold increase in the gene transcription rate and a 20-fold increase in both mRNA levels and enzyme activity. These data indicate that a primary effect of glucocorticoid treatment is to decrease

(A) the activity of RNA polymerase II
(B) the rate of mRNA translation
(C) the ability of nucleases to act on mRNA
(D) the rate of binding of ribosomes to mRNA

43. Use the following figure to answer question 43.

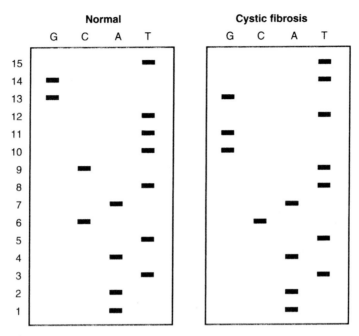

The gene for cystic fibrosis (CF) has been isolated and sequenced. The gel pattern for the DNA sequence of the region that differs from the normal gene is shown above. The positions of the bases, starting at the 5′ end of this sequence, are indicated on the left. In this region

(A) there is no homology between the normal and CF genes
(B) the first nine bases of the CF gene are the same as the normal gene
(C) the four bases at positions 12–15 of the normal gene are the same as those at positions 9–12 of the CF gene
(D) the CF gene has a 3-base insertion
(E) the CF gene has a 4-base deletion

44. Use the following figure to answer question 44.

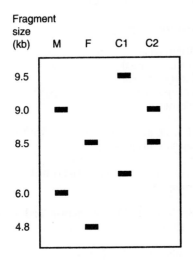

Fragment size (kb)   M   F   C1   C2

Two male infants were born on the same day in the same hospital. Because of concern that the infants had been switched in the hospital nursery, genetic tests based on a DNA restriction fragment that exhibits polymorphism (RFLP, restriction fragment length polymorphism) were performed. Blood was drawn from the parents and the infants, the DNA extracted, and polymerase chain reaction (PCR) performed. The DNA was then treated with the restriction enzyme *BanI*, and the fragments were separated by gel electrophoresis. The results of a Southern blot test are shown on the left. A radioactive probe was used that bound to a sequence within the *BanI* fragments that exhibited polymorphism. Which of the two infants, C1 or C2, is the genetic offspring of this mother (M) and father (F)?

(A) C1 could be the offspring of these parents
(B) C2 could be the offspring of these parents
(C) Both infants could be the offspring of these parents (i.e., this test cannot discriminate)
(D) Either of these infants could be related to the mother, but neither could be related to the father
(E) Neither infant could be related to this mother or this father

45. Which region (A to D) of the DNA strands shown could serve as the template for transcription of the region of an mRNA that contains the initial codon for translation of a protein 300 amino acids in length?

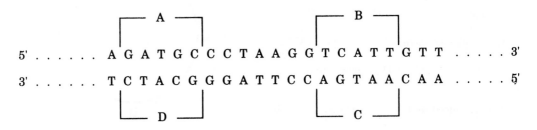

(A) A
(B) B
(C) C
(D) D

Directions: Each group of items in this section consists of lettered options followed by a set of numbered items. For each item, select the **one** lettered option that is most closely associated with it. Each lettered option may be selected once, more than once, or not at all.

Questions 46–49

(A) DNA polymerase
(B) RNA polymerase
(C) DNA ligase
(D) Reverse transcriptase

Match each characteristic below with the most appropriate enzyme.

46. Used by retroviruses to copy their RNA genome

47. Uses a nucleotide containing uracil as a precursor

48. Initiates the synthesis of polynucleotide strands

49. Does not produce inorganic pyrophosphate

Questions 50–53

(A) mRNA
(B) hnRNA
(C) rRNA
(D) tRNA

For each characteristic below, select the most appropriate RNA of eukaryotes.

50. Contains introns and a cap at the 5′ end

51. Contains no introns but has a poly (A) tail

52. Does not travel from the nucleus to the cytoplasm

53. Is produced by RNA polymerase I

Questions 54–56

(A) Introns
(B) Exons
(C) TGA
(D) TAA

Match each description below with the most appropriate term.

54. Generally absent from bacterial genes

55. Removed from transcripts by a splicing process

56. Codes for amino acids in proteins

Questions 57–61

(A) Rifampicin
(B) 5-Fluorouracil
(C) Erythromycin
(D) Streptomycin
(E) Tetracycline

Match each of the effects below with the most appropriate drug.

57. Prevents formation of the translation initiation complex

58. Binds to RNA polymerase and prevents transcription

59. Inhibits translocation

60. Prevents synthesis of DNA

61. Prevents binding of aminoacyl-tRNAs to the A site of ribosomes.

Questions 62–65

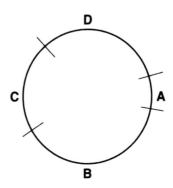

In the diagram above, the letters indicate the phases of the cell cycle. For each statement, select the letter corresponding to the most appropriate phase.

62. Colchicine prevents formation of the mitotic spindle

63. Anticancer drugs inhibit replication

64. Screening tests for chromosomal abnormalities can be performed

65. Liver cells enter this phase when they have been stimulated to divide

Questions 66–68

DNA was isolated from each member of a family (the father, mother and three children), amplified by PCR, and two spots were placed on nitrocellulose paper for each individual. One spot was treated with a probe that hybridizes with the mutant region of the cystic fibrosis (CF) gene, and the other with a probe that hybridizes to the corresponding region of the normal gene. The dark spots on the figure indicate binding of the probe.

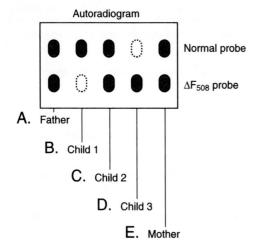

From the figure, choose the child who best fits each description.

66. has cystic fibrosis

67. is normal

68. is a carrier for cystic fibrosis

Answers and Explanations

1–A. On a molar basis, DNA contains equal amounts of adenine and thymine and of guanine and cytosine. Uracil is not found in DNA.

2–B. Complementary sequences base-pair with each other. The strands run in opposite directions. 5′-AAGTCCGA-3′ base-pairs with 3′-TTCAGGCT-5′ (or with the RNA sequence 3′-UUCAGGCU-5′).

3–C. DNA chains are composed of nucleotides joined by 3′, 5′- phosphodiester bonds. Each nucleotide consists of a nitrogenous base linked to deoxyribose that contains a phosphate group. Two DNA chains, oriented in opposite directions, base-pair with each other and are twisted to form a double helix. The base pairs are stacked on top of each other, forming a "spiral staircase" in the center of the molecule, and the sugar-phosphate backbone, in which the phosphates are negatively charged, is wrapped around the outside.

4–C. hnRNA is capped at its 5′ end during transcription. The cap, which contains 7-methylguanine, is retained when hnRNA is converted to mRNA.

5–D. Each tRNA contains one thymine residue in the ribothymidine that is found in the TψC loop.

6–D. DNA polymerase requires dATP, dTTP, dGTP, and dCTP as precursors that add to the 3′-hydroxyl group at the 3′ end of the growing chain.

7–A. Replication occurs during the S phase of the cell cycle. "Bubbles" on the parental DNA serve as points of origin from which replication proceeds in both directions simultaneously. (Replication is bidirectional.) DNA template strands are always copied in a 3′ to 5′ direction. New strands are synthesized 5′ to 3′. The daughter molecules each contain one parental strand and one newly synthesized strand. (Replication is semiconservative.)

8–D. RNA contains uracil instead of thymine. Uracil base-pairs with adenine.

9–E. Segment C is synthesized in a 5′ to 3′ direction. When synthesis of C begins, E is also being synthesized.

10–B. Segment C is synthesized in a 5′ to 3′ direction, toward the replication fork.

11–C. Segment E is synthesized in a 5′ to 3′ direction (following the template 3′ to 5′) away from the replication fork. Segment E is synthesized before segment D. Therefore, the overall direction of synthesis of the lagging strand is toward the replication fork; this occurs as short fragments are synthesized in the opposite direction and then are joined together.

12–D. DNA ligase joins DNA chains together. Polymerases can only add one nucleotide at a time to the 3′ end of a growing chain. An endonuclease cleaves DNA strands.

13–B. The first nucleotide to be added must base-pair with adenine. However, DNA polymerase cannot initiate synthesis of strands. RNA polymerase (the primase) produces a short primer that DNA polymerase can extend. Therefore, the first nucleotide must be a ribonucleotide that base-pairs with adenine, that is, UTP. Nucleoside triphosphates serve as precursors for the polymerases.

14–D. Okazaki fragments are synthesized on the lagging strand. They consist of a few ribonucleotides (added by RNA polymerase) to which deoxyribonucleotides were added by DNA polymerase.

15–E. The short segments of newly synthesized DNA that accumulate at 42°C are Okazaki fragments. They are usually joined together by DNA ligase, which is probably temperature-sensitive in this mutant. If the ligase is not functioning, Okazaki fragments would not be joined during replication, so the cells would contain short fragments of DNA. Endonucleases and exonucleases cleave DNA strands in the middle and at the ends, respectively. They do not join fragments together, nor does DNA polymerase. Unwinding enzymes "unzip" the parental strands.

16–C. Nucleosomes are subunits of chromatin (the complex of DNA and proteins in the nucleus). They consist of a core composed of two molecules of each of the four histones–H2A, H2B, H3, and H4–with 140 base pairs of DNA wrapped around the surface. Histone H1 binds to the linker DNA that joins one nucleosome core to the next.

17–B. The figure shows adenine on the right base-paired to uracil on the left. Uracil is present in RNA but not in DNA.

18–B. In nucleoli, rRNA genes are transcribed to produce the 45S rRNA precursor, which is trimmed, modified, and complexed with proteins to form ribosomal subunits. Therefore, the synthesis of rRNA would be most directly affected. The embryo probably would not survive.

19–B. Eukaryotic genes contain a TATA box and often contain a CAAT box in the 5′ flanking region, upstream from the start site for transcription. RNA polymerase II transcribes these genes, producing hnRNA, which is modified and processed to form mRNA. A cap is added at the 5′ end and poly (A) is added to the 3′ end posttranscriptionally; they are not encoded in the DNA. These genes contain introns, which are removed during processing of hnRNA.

20–D. The RNA will run in the opposite direction and will be complementary: A pairing with T, U with A, G with C, and C with G. Thus, the RNA will be 3′-UCGGUUAA-5′ (which is 5′-AAUUGGCU-3′).

21–B. The poison in poisonous mushrooms is α-amanitin, an inhibitor of eukaryotic RNA polymerases.

22–C. If the damage is repaired rapidly enough, transformation does not occur. Bulky lesions in DNA are repaired by the process of nucleotide excision. A short segment of nucleotides is removed and replaced, with the undamaged strand serving as the template.

23–B. UV light causes the formation of pyrimidine dimers in DNA.

24–D. The damage to DNA caused by ultraviolet light (pyrimidine dimers) can be repaired by the nucleotide excision repair pathway. In some cases, the missing enzyme is a repair endonuclease.

25–A. When the DNA is replicated, U in the template strand will pair with A in the daughter strand. Subsequent rounds of replication will cause the original CG base pair to become a TA base pair.

26–C. Although other enzymes are involved in the repair of DNA, only glycosylases remove bases by cleaving *N*-glycosidic bonds.

27–D. Aminoacyl-tRNA synthetases react with ATP and an amino acid to form an enzyme [aminoacyl-AMP] complex. The amino acid is then transferred to the 3′ end of tRNA. These enzymes are very specific for both the amino acid and the tRNA. The codon on mRNA for the amino acid is complementary to the anticodon on the tRNA.

28–C. UCA is a codon for serine. It is converted to a termination codon by A, to a proline codon by B, to a threonine codon by D, and to an alanine codon by E. Only C would produce no change in the protein, since UCU is also a codon for serine.

29–D. The structure contains 2′,5′-phosphodiester bonds, so it is not part of DNA or RNA, both of which have 3′,5′-phosphodiester bonds. This compound, 2′,5′-oligo (A), is produced in response to interferon and activates a nuclease that degrades mRNA.

30–A. Methionine, the amino acid that initiates the synthesis of proteins, is subsequently cleaved from the protein. The only codon for methionine is AUG, which serves as the codon for methionine residues within a protein as well as the initiating residue. The methionyl-tRNA for initiation is formylated in bacterial cells and in mitochondria.

31–D. Bacteria contain 70S ribosomes that are sensitive to chloramphenicol. They initiate protein synthesis with methionine that is formylated. Because bacteria do not have nuclei, ribosomes bind to mRNA as it is being synthesized, so that translation begins before transcription is completed.

32–A. Methionyl-tRNA (not formylated Met-tRNA), initiation factor eIF-2, and GTP bind to the 40S ribosomal subunit. The cap of mRNA binds, and the ribosomal subunit moves along the mRNA until the first AUG codon pairs with the anticodon on the tRNA. The 60S subunit is added, and protein synthesis is initiated. EF-2 is used during the elongation process in eukaryotes, and IF-2 is a prokaryotic initiation factor.

33–A. mRNA supplies the codons, aminoacyl-tRNA and GTP provide energy, peptidyl transferase catalyzes the formation of peptide bonds, and elongation factor 2 (EF-G) translocates the peptidyl-tRNA. Formylmethionyl-tRNA is involved in initiation of protein synthesis in prokaryotes. EF-G is a prokaryotic elongation factor. hnRNA is the precursor of mRNA.

34–D. Protein synthesis is normally terminated by release factors, not by nuclease cleavage of mRNA or peptidyl-tRNA that cannot bind at the P site. UGA and UAG are stop codons, but AUG is the initiation codon.

35–C. Proteins destined for secretion contain a signal sequence at the N-terminal end that causes the ribosomes on which they are being synthesized to bind to the rough endoplasmic reticulum (RER). As they are being produced, they enter the cisternae of the RER, where the signal sequence, including the initial methionine, is removed. Carbohydrate groups can be attached in the RER or the Golgi. Secretory vesicles bud from the Golgi, and the proteins are secreted from the cell by the process of exocytosis. If the proteins have a hydrophobic sequence that embeds in the membrane, they remain attached and are not secreted. If carbohydrate residues bind to lysosomal receptors, the proteins remain in lysosomes.

36–C. These antibiotics inhibit protein synthesis in prokaryotes; thus, they can be used to treat bacterial infections. One of their undesirable side effects, however, is that they also inhibit protein synthesis on mitochondrial ribosomes (which are of the 70S prokaryotic class).

37–A. AUG is the initiation codon for methionine. The subsequent bases, read sequentially in sets of three, would all produce phenylalanine, except the termination codon UAA.

38–C. Initiation and formation of the first peptide bond occurred; therefore, A, B, and D were not affected. The antibiotic most likely affects the translocation step.

39–D. In induction, a regulatory gene produces an active repressor, which is inactivated by binding to the inducer. The inducer prevents binding of the repressor to the operator rather than stimulating binding of RNA polymerase. The structural genes are coordinately expressed. Transcription yields a single, polycistronic mRNA, which is translated to produce a number of different proteins.

40–B. cAMP is involved in catabolite repression. Bacterial cells preferentially use glucose. When glucose is low, cAMP rises. cAMP forms a complex with the CAP protein, and the complex binds near the *lac* promoter region, facilitating the binding of RNA polymerase. Lactose must be present to inactivate the repressor, so that the operon can be expressed.

41–C. A gene that is methylated is less readily transcribed than one that is not methylated. In cells that become antibody-producing lymphocytes, segments of genes are rearranged to form the V, D, and J regions of the gene that will produce an antibody in the mature cell. Red blood cells have lost their nuclei, so they do not produce mRNA. Polyadenylation sites are at the C-terminus of a protein. Histones are nonspecific repressors of gene expression.

42–C. If the rate of degradation of the mRNA is not altered by glucocorticoids, the increase in mRNA levels should reflect the increase in transcription rate. Because the increase in mRNA level is greater than the increase in transcription rate, the glucocorticoids must also be increasing mRNA stability (i.e., decreasing the rate of degradation by nucleases). The activity of RNA polymerase II is increased (transcription is increased), and the rate of translation (the binding of ribosomes to mRNA) is increased (the enzyme activity is increased).

43–C. Sequences are read from the bottom to the top of the gel. In this region, the sequences of the CF and normal genes are identical for the first eight bases. Positions 12–15 of the normal gene and 9–12 of the CF gene are identical. Therefore, there is a 3-base deletion in the CF gene corresponding to bases 9–11 of the normal gene.

44–B. Every chromosome has a homologue. Therefore, there will be two copies of every DNA sequence in the genome. Child C2 could have obtained the 9-kb restriction fragment from this mother, and the 8.5-kb fragment from this father. According to this test, child C1 is not genetically related to either this mother or this father.

45–B. Although D contains the sequence 3′-TAC-5′, which produces a start codon (5′-AUG-3′) in the mRNA, there is a sequence (3′-ATT-5′ in the DNA) that would produce a stop codon (5′-UAA-3′) in the mRNA in frame with this start codon. Sequence B, read 3′ to 5′ (from right to left), would produce a start codon in the mRNA transcribed from it. There are no stop codons in this sequence, so it *could* produce a protein 300 amino acids in length. Sequences A and C do not contain triplets corresponding to the start codon in mRNA.

46–D. Reverse transcriptase produces a DNA copy of an RNA template.

47–B. UTP is a substrate for RNA polymerase.

48–B. Only RNA polymerase can initiate the synthesis of strands.

49–C. When nucleoside triphosphates add to growing DNA or RNA strands in reactions catalyzed by polymerases or reverse transcriptase, pyrophosphate is released. Ligase joins two polynucleotide strands together.

50–B. Both hnRNA and mRNA are capped, but only hnRNA contains introns.

51–A. Both hnRNA and mRNA contain poly(A) tails, but hnRNA contains introns that are removed as it is processed to form mRNA.

52–B. Only hnRNA does not travel from the nucleus to the cytoplasm.

53–C. RNA polymerase I produces the large rRNA precursor. Polymerase II produces hnRNA (and consequently mRNA). Polymerase III produces tRNA and 5S rRNA.

54–A. Bacterial genes generally do not contain introns.

55–A. Introns are removed from RNA transcripts by splicing mechanisms.

56–B. Exons code for amino acids in proteins. Introns do not. TGA and TAA produce stop codons in mRNA.

57–D. Streptomycin causes misreading of mRNA codons and, thus, prevents formation of the initiation complex in prokaryotes.

58–A. Rifampicin binds to RNA polymerase and prevents initiation of transcription in prokaryotes.

59–C. Erythromycin prevents translocation during protein synthesis in prokaryotes.

60–B. 5-Fluorouracil prevents conversion of dUMP to dTMP. DNA synthesis is inhibited because of a lack of thymine nucleotides, so this compound is used to treat cancer.

61–E. Tetracycline prevents the binding of aminoacyl-tRNAs to the A site on ribosomes.

62–A. The mitotic spindle functions during mitosis (M phase), which is the shortest phase of the cycle.

63–C. Replication occurs during the S phase.

64–A. Condensed chromosomes can be observed under the microscope during the M phase (mitosis).

65–B. Liver cells in a nondividing state (G_0) can be stimulated to reenter the cell cycle at the G_1 phase.

66–D. Child 3 has CF. Only the mutant probe binds to the child's DNA.

67–B. Child 1 is normal. Only the normal probe binds to the child's DNA.

68–C. Child 2 is a carrier. One allele of the gene is normal (and binds the normal probe). The other allele has the CF mutation (and binds the CF probe).

4

Generation of ATP from Metabolic Fuels

Overview

- Adenosine triphosphate (ATP) transfers energy from the processes that produce it to those that use it.
- Most carbons of glucose, fatty acids, glycerol, and amino acids are ultimately converted to acetyl CoA. ATP is produced by these reactions (Figure 4-1).
- Acetyl CoA is oxidized in the tricarboxylic acid (TCA) cycle. CO_2 is released, and electrons are passed to NAD^+ and FAD, producing NADH and $FADH_2$.
- NADH and $FADH_2$ transfer the electrons to O_2 via the electron transport chain. Energy from this transfer of electrons is used to produce ATP by the process of oxidative phosphorylation.

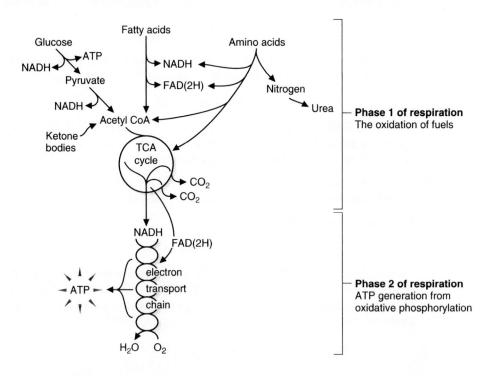

Figure 4-1. The generation of adenosine triphosphate (ATP) from fuels in the blood.

- Cofactors, many of which are minerals or compounds produced from vitamins, aid the enzymes that catalyze the reactions of these metabolic pathways.

I. Bioenergetics

- For a biochemical reaction,

$$aA + bB \rightleftharpoons cC + dD$$

the change in free energy (ΔG) is related to the concentrations of the substrates and products and to the change in the standard free energy of the reaction at pH 7 ($\Delta G^{o\prime}$). The change in standard free energy is determined by the chemical bonds that are being broken and formed.

- Reactions with a negative ΔG proceed spontaneously; those with a positive ΔG do not.
  If $\Delta G = 0$, the reaction is at equilibrium, and

$$K_{eq} = \frac{[C]^c [D]^d}{[A]^a [B]^b}$$

where the substrates and products are at their equilibrium (eq) concentrations. Therefore,

$$\Delta G^{o\prime} = -RT \ln K_{eq}$$

- The change in free energy indicates the direction in which a reaction will proceed, but not the speed of the reaction. Enzymes determine the speed.

A. The change in free energy in biologic systems

1. The **change in free energy** (the energy available to do **useful work** at constant pressure and temperature) is defined by the equation

$$\Delta G = \Delta H - T\Delta S$$

where ΔG is the change in free energy; ΔH is the change in enthalpy (heat content); ΔS is the change in entropy (randomness or disorder); and T is the absolute temperature in degrees Kelvin (K).

2. For a biochemical reaction, the change in free energy can be used to predict the **direction** in which the reaction will proceed.

3. For the reaction in which

$$aA + bB \rightleftharpoons cC + dD$$

(where the upper-case letters symbolize the molecule; the lower-case letters indicate the number of molecules) the free energy change depends on the concentrations of substrates and products and on the value of the constant $\Delta G^{o\prime}$.

$$\Delta G = \Delta G^{o\prime} + RT \ln \frac{[C]^c [D]^d}{[A]^a [B]^b}$$

where **$\Delta G^{o\prime}$ is the standard free energy change at pH 7**; R is the gas constant; T is the absolute temperature, and [ ] means concentration.

4. If ΔG is negative, the reaction will proceed spontaneously with the release of energy. If ΔG is positive, the reaction will not proceed spontaneously. If ΔG = 0, the reaction is at equilibrium, and, although substrates react to form products and products react to form substrates, there is no net change in the concentrations.

B. The equilibrium constant and the change in free energy

1. At **equilibrium, ΔG = 0** and

$$\Delta G^{o\prime} = -RT \ln \frac{[C]^c \, [D]^d}{[A]^a \, [B]^b}$$

2. The **equilibrium constant** (K_{eq})is related to the **concentrations** of substrates and products **at equilibrium,**

$$K_{eq} = \frac{[C]^c \, [D]^d}{[A]^a \, [B]^b}$$

Therefore, $\Delta G^{o\prime} = -RT \ln K_{eq}$.
– If $K_{eq} = 1$, $\Delta G^{o\prime} = 0$.
– If $K_{eq} > 1$, $\Delta G^{o\prime}$ is negative.
– If $K_{eq} < 1$, $\Delta G^{o\prime}$ is positive.

3. The larger and more negative the $\Delta G^{o\prime}$, the less substrate relative to product is required to produce a negative ΔG (i.e., the more likely the reaction is to proceed spontaneously).

4. For a sequence of reactions that have common intermediates, the **standard free energy changes are additive** (Table 4-1).

C. The relevance of free energy changes to biologic systems

1. The rate of a reaction is not related to its free energy change.

a. A reaction with a large negative free energy change does not necessarily proceed rapidly.

b. The **speed** of a reaction depends on the properties of the **enzyme** that catalyzes the reaction.

– An enzyme increases the rate at which a reaction reaches equilibrium. It does not affect K_{eq} (the relative concentrations of substrates and products at equilibrium).

2. Most biochemical reactions exist in pathways; therefore, other reactions are constantly adding substrate and removing product.

– The relative activities of the enzymes that catalyze the individual reactions of a pathway differ.

Table 4-1. Additive Nature of Free Energy Changes

glucose + P_i → glucose-6-P + H_2O	$\Delta G^{o\prime}$ = +3.3 kcal/mole
ATP + H_2O → ADP + P_i	$\Delta G^{o\prime}$ = –7.3 kcal/mole
Sum: glucose + ATP → glucose-6-P + ADP	$\Delta G^{o\prime}$ = –4.0 kcal/mole

– Some reactions are near equilibrium ($\Delta G = 0$). Their direction can be readily altered by small changes in the concentrations of their substrates or products.

– Other reactions are far from equilibrium. Allosteric factors that alter the activity of these enzymes can change the overall flux through the pathway.

II. Properties of Adenosine Triphosphate

- ATP contains the base adenine, the sugar ribose, and three phosphate groups joined to each other by two anhydride bonds.
- ATP is produced from adenosine diphosphate (ADP) and inorganic phosphate (P$_i$) mainly by the process of oxidative phosphorylation.
- The free energy released when ATP is hydrolyzed is used to drive reactions that require energy.
- ATP can transfer phosphate groups to other compounds such as glucose, forming ADP.
- ADP can accept phosphate groups from compounds such as phosphocreatine, forming ATP.

A. The structure of ATP

– ATP consists of the base **adenine**, the sugar **ribose**, and **three phosphate groups** (Figure 4-2).

1. **Adenosine** (a nucleoside) contains the base adenine linked to ribose.

2. Adenosine monophosphate (**AMP**) is a nucleotide that contains adenosine with a phosphate group esterified to the 5′-hydroxyl of the sugar.

3. **ADP** contains a second phosphate group attached by an anhydride bond.

4. **ATP** contains a third phosphate group.

B. The functions of ATP

– ATP plays a central role in **energy exchanges** in the body.

1. ATP is constantly being **consumed and regenerated**.

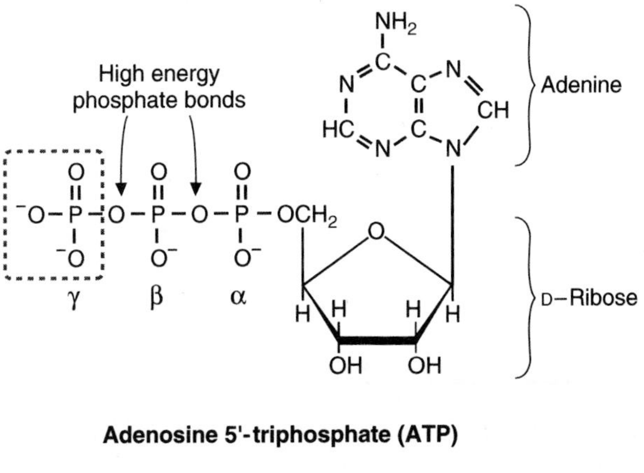

Adenosine 5′-triphosphate (ATP)

Figure 4-2. The structure of adenosine triphosphate (ATP).

    a. It is consumed by processes such as muscular contraction, active transport, and biosynthetic reactions.

    b. It is regenerated by the oxidation of foodstuffs.

2. The **free energy** released when ATP is hydrolyzed is used to drive reactions that require energy.

    a. ATP can be hydrolyzed to **ADP** and inorganic phosphate (P_i) or to **AMP** and pyrophosphate (PP_i). ATP, ADP, and AMP are interconverted by the adenylate kinase reaction.

$$ATP + AMP \rightleftharpoons 2ADP$$

    b. Other nucleoside triphosphates (GTP, UTP, and CTP) are sometimes used to drive biochemical reactions. They can be derived from ATP.

3. For the **hydrolysis of ATP to ADP and P_i, $\Delta G^{o'}$ = –7.3 kcal/mole**.

    a. The anhydride bonds of ATP are often called "high-energy bonds."

    b. **$\Delta G^{o'}$ is large,** however, not because a single bond is broken, but because the products of hydrolysis are more stable than ATP.

4. **ATP** can transfer phosphate groups to compounds such as glucose, forming ADP.

5. **ADP** can accept phosphate groups from compounds such as phosphoenolpyruvate, phosphocreatine, or 1,3-bisphosphoglycerate, forming ATP.

III. Electron Carriers and Vitamins

- Certain cofactors of enzymes are involved in the transfer of electrons from foodstuffs to O_2, a process that generates energy for the production of ATP.
- NAD^+ (derived from the vitamin niacin) and FAD (derived from the vitamin riboflavin) pass electrons to the electron transport chain. In this chain, flavin mononucleotide (FMN) and coenzyme Q (ubiquinone) pass the electrons to heme-containing cytochromes, which transfer the electrons to O_2. As a consequence of these processes, ATP is produced.
- Other cofactors involved in deriving energy from food include coenzyme A (synthesized from the vitamin pantothenate), thiamine pyrophosphate (synthesized from the vitamin thiamine), and lipoic acid.
- Additional cofactors derived from water-soluble vitamins are involved in a variety of metabolic reactions. These cofactors include NADPH (derived from the vitamin niacin), biotin, pyridoxal phosphate (derived from vitamin B_6), tetrahydrofolate (derived from the vitamin folate), vitamin B_{12}, and vitamin C.
- The fat-soluble vitamins (A, D, E, and K) are also involved in metabolism.

A. Major cofactors in the generation of ATP from foodstuffs

    – As food is oxidized to CO_2 and H_2O, electrons are transferred mainly to nicotinamide adenine dinucleotide (**NAD^+**) and flavin adenine dinucleotide (**FAD**).

1. **NAD$^+$** accepts a hydride ion, which reacts with its nicotinamide ring (Figure 4-3). NAD$^+$ is reduced; the substrate (RH$_2$) is oxidized; and a proton is released.

$$NAD^+ + RH_2 \rightleftharpoons NADH + H^+ + R$$

   a. NAD$^+$ is frequently involved in oxidizing a hydroxyl group to a ketone.

$$\underset{\overset{|}{\underset{}{R - CH - R_1}}}{\overset{OH}{}} + NAD^+ \rightleftharpoons \underset{\overset{||}{\underset{}{R - C - R_1}}}{\overset{O}{}} + NADH + H^+$$

   b. The **nicotinamide ring** of NAD$^+$ is derived from the vitamin **niacin** (nicotinic acid) and, to a limited extent, from the amino acid **tryptophan**.

2. **FAD** accepts two hydrogen atoms (with their electrons) (Figure 4-4). FAD is reduced, and the substrate is oxidized.

$$FAD + RH_2 \rightleftharpoons FADH_2 + R$$

   a. FAD is frequently involved in reactions that produce a double bond.

$$R\text{-}CH_2\text{-}CH_2\text{-}R_1 + FAD \rightleftharpoons R\text{-}CH{=}CH\text{-}R_1 + FADH_2$$

   b. FAD is derived from the vitamin **riboflavin**.

B. Components of the electron transport chain

   – The reduced cofactors, NADH and FADH$_2$, transfer electrons to the electron transport chain.

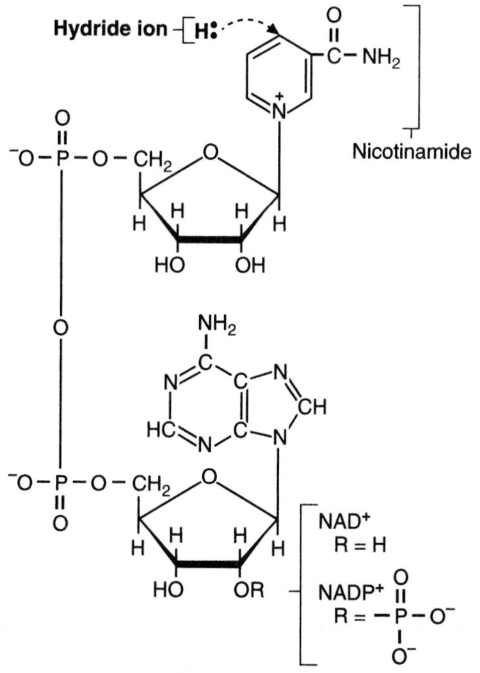

Figure 4-3. The structure of NAD$^+$ and NADP$^+$. R differs for NAD$^+$ and NADP$^+$ as indicated. The arrow shows the position where a hydride ion (H$^-$; H:) covalently binds when NAD$^+$ or NADP$^+$ is reduced.

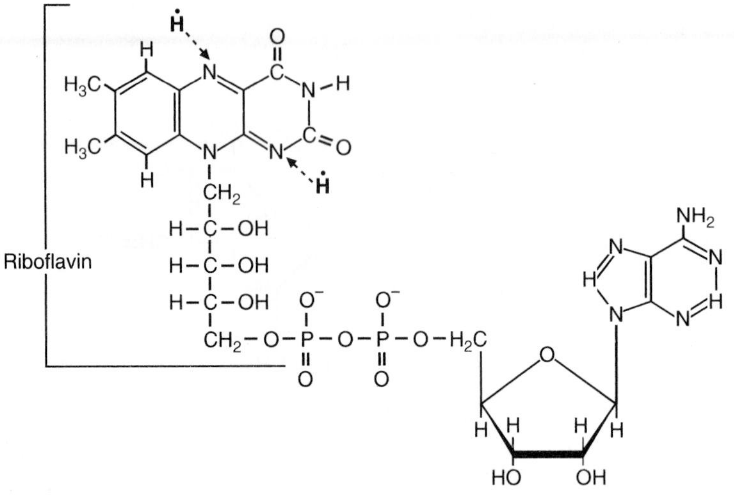

Figure 4-4. The structure of flavin adenine dinucleotide (FAD). *Arrows* indicate positions where hydrogens ($\dot{H}$) covalently bind when FAD is reduced to $FADH_2$. FMN consists only of the riboflavin moiety plus one phosphate.

1. **FMN** receives electrons from NADH and transfers them through Fe-S centers to coenzyme Q (Figure 4- 5).
   – FMN is derived from **riboflavin**.

2. **Coenzyme Q** (CoQ) receives electrons from FMN and also through Fe-S centers from $FADH_2$
   – $FADH_2$ is not free in solution like NAD^+ and NADH; it is tightly bound to enzymes.
   – Coenzyme Q can be synthesized in the body. It is not derived from a vitamin.

3. **Cytochromes** receive electrons from the reduced form of coenzyme Q.
   – Each cytochrome consists of a **heme** group (Figure 4-6) associated with a protein.

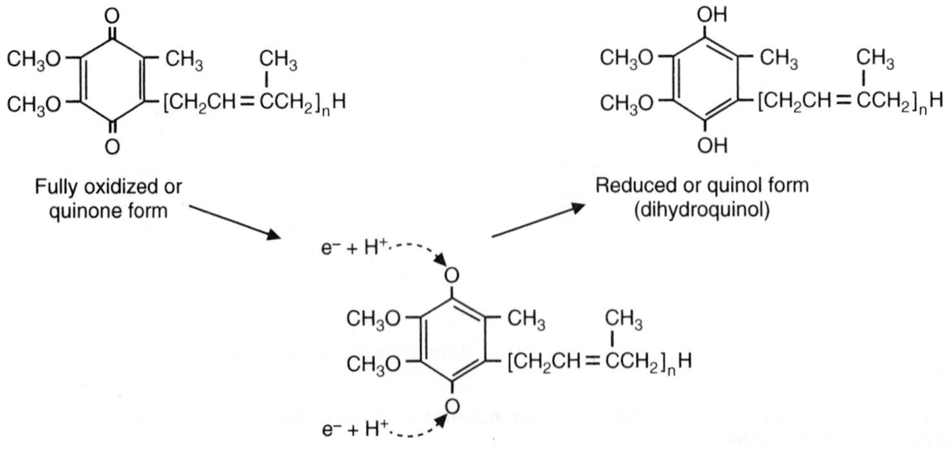

Figure 4-5. The structure of coenzyme Q (CoQ), or ubiquinone. Hydrogen atoms can bind, one at a time, as indicated by the arrows.

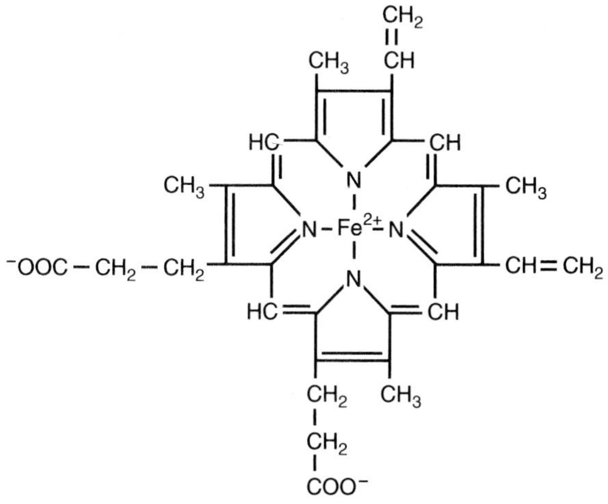

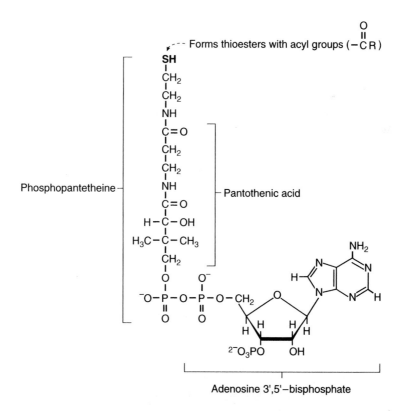

Figure 4-6. The general structure of the heme group, which is present in hemoglobin, myoglobin, and the cytochromes b, c, and c_1.

Figure 4-7. The structure of coenzyme A. The arrow indicates where acyl (e.g., acetyl, succinyl, and fatty acyl) groups bind to form thioesters.

- The **iron** of the heme group is reduced when the cytochrome accepts an electron.

$$Fe^{3+} \rightleftharpoons Fe^{2+}$$

- Heme is synthesized from glycine and succinyl CoA in humans. It is not derived from a vitamin.

4. **Oxygen** (O_2) ultimately receives the electrons at the end of the electron transport chain and is reduced to H_2O.

C. Coenzyme A

- **Coenzyme A (CoASH)** contains a sulfhydryl group that reacts with carboxylic acids to form **thioesters,** such as acetyl CoA, succinyl CoA, and palmitoyl CoA (Figure 4-7).

1. The $\Delta G^{o\prime}$ for hydrolysis of the thioester bond is –7.5 kcal/mole (a high-energy bond).

2. Coenzyme A contains the vitamin **pantothenic acid.**
   - Pantothenic acid is also present in the fatty acid synthase complex.

D. Thiamine and lipoic acid, cofactors for α-ketoacid dehydrogenases

- **α-Keto acid dehydrogenases** catalyze **oxidative decarboxylations** in a sequence of reactions involving thiamine pyrophosphate, lipoic acid, coenzyme A, FAD, and NAD^+.
- The major α-ketoacid dehydrogenases are:
  - **pyruvate dehydrogenase**, the enzyme complex that oxidatively decarboxylates pyruvate, forming acetyl CoA
  - **α-ketoglutarate dehydrogenase**, which catalyzes the conversion of α-ketoglutarate to succinyl CoA
  - the **α-keto acid dehydrogenase** complex involved in the oxidation of the branched chain amino acids.

1. **Thiamine pyrophosphate** (Figure 4-8*A*) is involved in the **decarboxylation of α-keto acids.**

   a. The α-carbon of the α-keto acid becomes covalently attached to thiamine pyrophosphate, and the carboxyl group is released as CO_2.

   b. Thiamine pyrophosphate is also the cofactor for the **transketolase** of the pentose phosphate pathway.

   c. Thiamine pyrophosphate is formed from ATP and the vitamin **thiamine.**

2. **Lipoic acid** oxidizes the keto group of the decarboxylated α-keto acid (Figure 4-9).

   a. After an α-keto acid is decarboxylated, the remainder of the compound is oxidized as it is transferred from thiamine pyrophosphate to lipoic acid, which is reduced in the reaction.

   b. The oxidized compound, which forms a thioester with lipoate, is then transferred to the sulfur of coenzyme A.

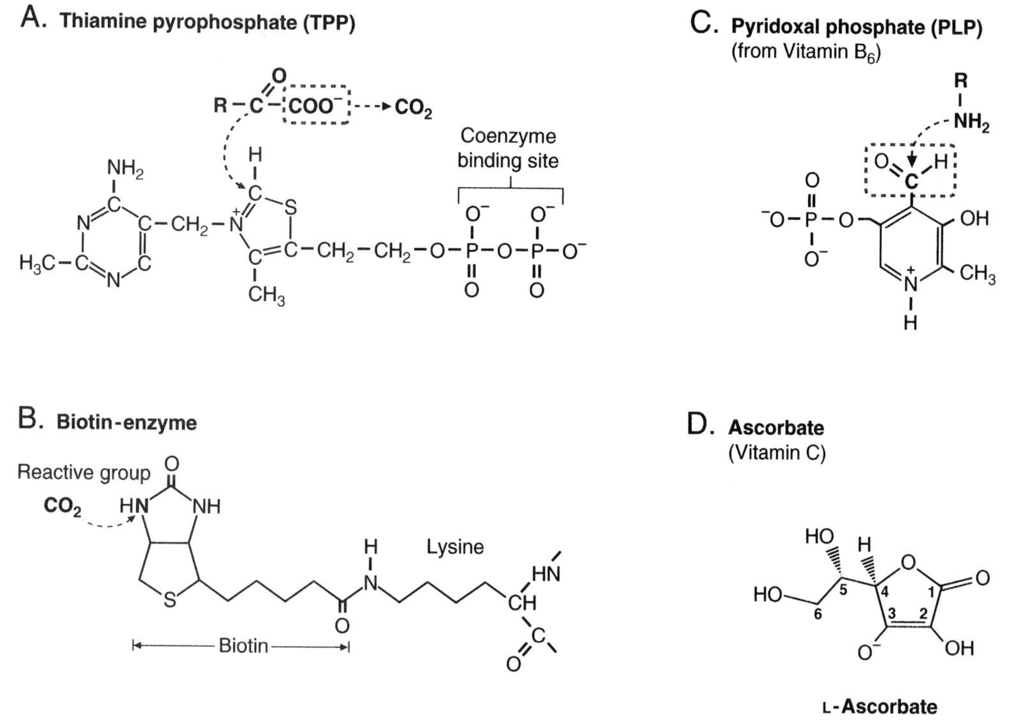

A. **Thiamine pyrophosphate (TPP)**

C. **Pyridoxal phosphate (PLP)**
(from Vitamin B_6)

B. **Biotin-enzyme**

D. **Ascorbate**
(Vitamin C)

L-Ascorbate

Figure 4-8. The structures of thiamine pyrophosphate *(A)*, biotin *(B)*, pyridoxal phosphate *(C)*, and ascorbate *(D)*. *Arrows* indicate the reactive sites. When an α-keto acid binds to thiamine pyrophosphate, the keto group attaches and the carboxyl group is released as CO_2.

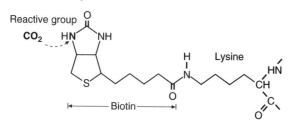

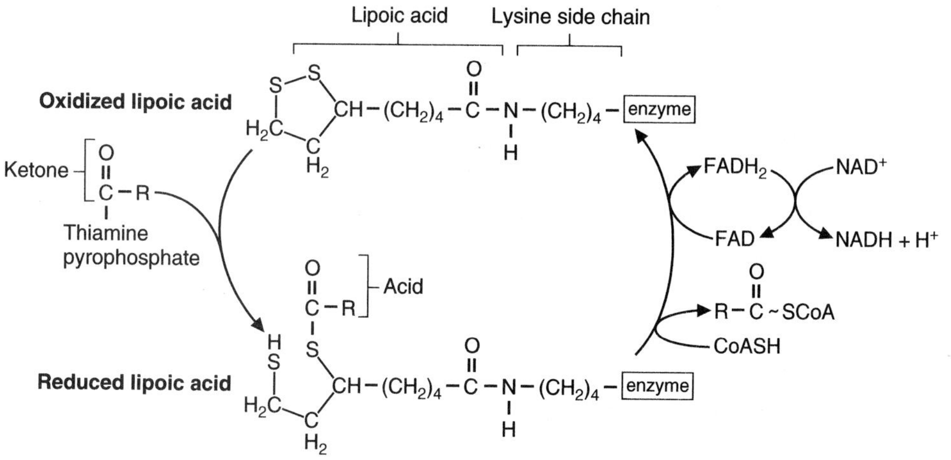

Figure 4-9. Role of lipoic acid in oxidative decarboxylation of α-keto acids.

   c. Because there is a limited amount of lipoate in the cell, reduced lipoate must be reoxidized so that it can be reutilized in these types of reactions. It is reoxidized by FAD, which becomes reduced to $FADH_2$ and is subsequently reoxidized by NAD^+.

   d. Lipoic acid is not derived from a vitamin.

E. Other cofactors derived from water-soluble vitamins

1. **NADPH** (the reduced form of NADP$^+$) provides reducing equivalents for the synthesis of **fatty acids** and other compounds and for the reduction of **glutathione**.
   - NADP$^+$ is identical to NAD$^+$ except that it contains an additional phosphate group (see Figure 4-3).

2. **Biotin** is involved in the **carboxylation** of **pyruvate** (which forms oxaloacetate), **acetyl CoA** (which forms malonyl CoA), and **propionyl CoA** (which forms methylmalonyl CoA).
   - The vitamin biotin is covalently linked to a lysyl residue of the enzyme (see Figure 4-8*B*).

3. **Pyridoxal phosphate**, an aldehyde, interacts with an amino acid to form a Schiff base. Various products can be generated, depending on the enzyme (see Figure 4-8*C*).
   a. Amino acids are **transaminated, decarboxylated**, or **deaminated** in pyridoxal phosphate-requiring reactions.
   b. Pyridoxal phosphate is derived from **vitamin B$_6$** (pyridoxine).

4. **Tetrahydrofolate** (see Figure 7-14) **transfers one-carbon units** (that are more reduced than CO$_2$) from compounds such as serine to compounds such as dUMP (to form dTMP).
   - Tetrahydrofolate is synthesized from the **vitamin folate.**

5. **Vitamin B$_{12}$** (see Figure 7-17), which contains cobalt, is involved in two reactions in the body.
   a. It **transfers methyl groups** from tetrahydrofolate to homocysteine (to form methionine).
   b. It is involved in the **conversion of methylmalonyl CoA to succinyl CoA**.

6. **Vitamin C** (ascorbic acid) has at least three functions in the body (see Figure 4-8*D*).
   a. It is involved in **hydroxylation reactions**, such as the hydroxylation of prolyl residues in the precursor of collagen.
   b. It functions in the **absorption of iron**.
   c. It is an **antioxidant**.

F. Fat-soluble vitamins (Figure 4-10)

1. **Vitamin K** is involved in the activation of precursors of prothrombin and other **clotting factors** by carboxylation of glutamate residues.

2. **Vitamin A** is necessary for the light reactions of **vision,** for normal **growth** and **reproduction**, and for differentiation and maintenance of **epithelial tissues**.
   a. Δ^{11}-*cis*-Retinal binds to the protein opsin, forming rhodopsin.
      - Light causes Δ^{11}-*cis*-retinal in rhodopsin to be converted to all-trans-retinal, which dissociates from opsin, causing changes that allow light to be perceived by the brain.

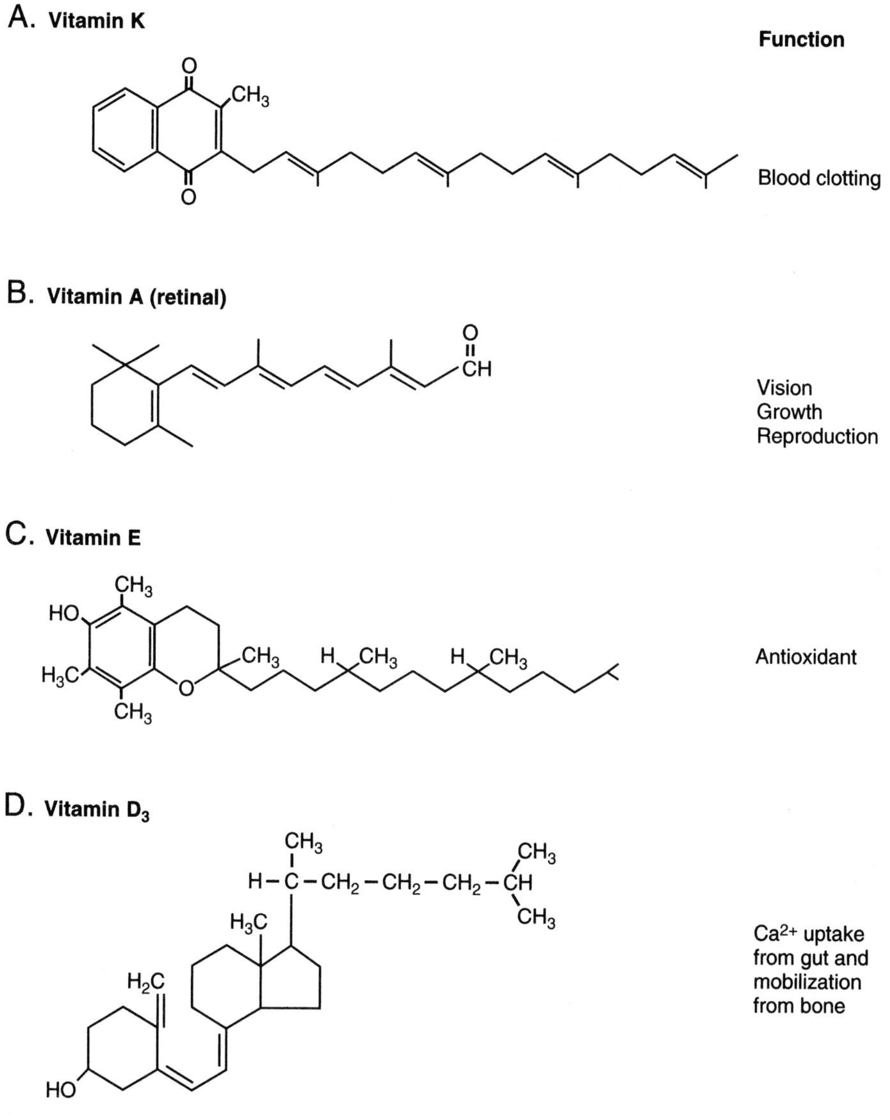

A. Vitamin K

Function

Blood clotting

B. Vitamin A (retinal)

Vision
Growth
Reproduction

C. Vitamin E

Antioxidant

D. Vitamin D₃

Ca²⁺ uptake
from gut and
mobilization
from bone

Figure 4-10. The fat-soluble vitamins and their major functions.

> **b.** Retinoic acid, the most oxidized form of vitamin A, acts like a steroid hormone (see Chapter 8).

3. Vitamin E serves as an **antioxidant**.

> **a.** It prevents free radicals from oxidizing compounds such as polyunsaturated fatty acids.

> **b.** A major consequence is that the integrity of membranes, which contain fatty acid residues in phospholipids, is maintained.

4. Vitamin D (as 1,25-dihydroxycholecalciferol) is involved in **calcium metabolism** (see Chapter 8).

IV. TCA Cycle

- The tricarboxylic acid (TCA) cycle, also known as the citric acid cycle or the Krebs cycle, is the major energy-producing pathway in the body. The cycle occurs in mitochondria.
- Foodstuffs feed into the cycle as acetyl CoA and are oxidized for energy.
- The cycle also serves in the synthesis of fatty acids, amino acids, and glucose.
- The cycle starts with the 4-carbon compound oxaloacetate, adds 2 carbons from acetyl CoA, loses 2 carbons as CO_2, and regenerates the 4-carbon compound oxaloacetate.
- Electrons are transferred by the cycle to NAD^+ and FAD.
- As the electrons subsequently are passed to O_2 by the electron transport chain, ATP is generated by the process of oxidative phosphorylation.
- ATP is also generated from GTP, produced in one reaction of the cycle by substrate level phosphorylation.

A. The reactions of the TCA cycle (Figure 4-11)

– All the enzymes of the TCA cycle are in the **mitochondrial matrix** except succinate dehydrogenase, which is in the inner mitochondrial membrane.

1. **Acetyl CoA** and **oxaloacetate** condense, forming citrate.

   a. Enzyme: **citrate synthase**.

   b. Cleavage of the high energy thioester bond in acetyl CoA provides the energy for this condensation.

   c. Citrate (the product) is an inhibitor of this reaction.

2. **Citrate** is isomerized to isocitrate by a rearrangement of the molecule.

   a. Enzyme: **aconitase**.

   b. Aconitate serves as an enzyme-bound intermediate.

3. **Isocitrate** is oxidized to α-ketoglutarate in the first oxidative decarboxylation reaction. CO_2 is produced, and the electrons are passed to NAD^+ to form NADH + H^+.

   a. Enzyme: **isocitrate dehydrogenase**.

   b. This key regulatory enzyme of the TCA cycle is allosterically activated by ADP and inhibited by NADH.

4. **α-Ketoglutarate** is converted to succinyl CoA in a second oxidative decarboxylation reaction. CO_2 is released, and succinyl CoA, NADH, and H^+ are produced.

   a. Enzyme: **α-ketoglutarate dehydrogenase**.

   b. This enzyme requires five cofactors: thiamine pyrophosphate, lipoic acid, CoASH, FAD, and NAD^+ (see III D).

5. **Succinyl CoA** is cleaved to succinate. Cleavage of the high-energy thioester bond of succinyl CoA provides energy for the substrate level phosphorylation of GDP to GTP. Since this does not involve the electron transport chain, it is not an oxidative phosphorylation.

   a. Enzyme: **succinate thiokinase**.

   b. The enzyme is also called **succinyl CoA synthetase**.

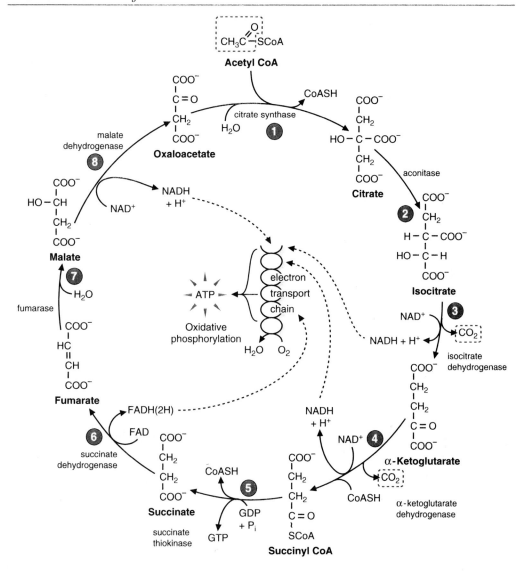

Figure 4-11. The tricarboxylic acid (TCA) cycle.

6. **Succinate** is oxidized to fumarate. Succinate transfers two hydrogens together with their electrons to FAD, which forms $FADH_2$.

   a. Enzyme: **succinate dehydrogenase**.

   b. This enzyme is present in the inner mitochondrial membrane. The other enzymes of the cycle are in the matrix.

7. **Fumarate** is converted to malate by the addition of water across the double bond.

   – Enzyme: **fumarase**.

8. **Malate** is oxidized, regenerating **oxaloacetate** and thus completing the cycle. Two hydrogens along with their electrons are passed to NAD^+, producing $NADH + H^+$.

   – Enzyme: **malate dehydrogenase**

B. Energy production by the TCA cycle

1. The NADH and $FADH_2$ (produced by the cycle) donate electrons to the electron transport chain. For each **NADH**, approximately **3ATP** are generated, and for each **$FADH_2$** approximately **2ATP** are generated by the passage of these electrons to O_2 (oxidative phosphorylation). In addition, GTP is produced when succinyl CoA is cleaved. **GTP** produces ATP

$$(GTP + ADP \rightleftharpoons ATP + GDP).$$

2. The **total energy** generated by one round of the cycle, starting with 1 acetyl CoA, is approximately **12 ATP.**

C. Regulation of the TCA cycle

– The TCA cycle is regulated by the **cell's need for energy** in the form of ATP. The TCA cycle acts in concert with the electron transport chain and the ATP synthase in the inner mitochondrial membrane to produce ATP.

1. The cell has limited amounts of adenine nucleotides (ATP, ADP, and AMP).

2. When ATP is utilized, ADP and inorganic phosphate (P_i) are produced.

3. **When ADP levels are high** relative to ATP—that is, when the cell needs energy—the reactions of the electron transport chain are accelerated. NADH is rapidly oxidized; consequently, the **TCA cycle speeds up.**

   – One aspect of this process is that ADP allosterically activates isocitrate dehydrogenase.

4. **When the concentration of ATP is high**—that is, when the cell has an adequate energy supply—the electron transport chain slows down, NADH builds up, and consequently **the TCA cycle is inhibited**.

   a. NADH allosterically inhibits isocitrate dehydrogenase. Isocitrate accumulates, and because the aconitase equilibrium favors citrate, the concentration of citrate rises. Citrate inhibits citrate synthase, the first enzyme of the cycle.

   b. High NADH (and low NAD^+) levels also affect the reactions of the cycle that generate NADH, resulting in a slowing of the cycle by mass action.

      – Oxaloacetate is converted to malate when NADH is high and, therefore, less substrate (OAA) is available for the citrate synthase reaction.

D. Vitamins required for reactions of the TCA cycle

1. **Niacin** is used for the synthesis of the nicotinamide portion of **NAD**, which is used in the isocitrate dehydrogenase, α-ketoglutarate dehydrogenase, and malate dehydrogenase reactions.

2. **Riboflavin** is used for the synthesis of **FAD**, which is the cofactor for succinate dehydrogenase. FAD is also required by α-ketoglutarate dehydrogenase.

3. **α-Ketoglutarate dehydrogenase**, a multienzyme complex (see III D), contains lipoic acid and four other cofactors that are synthesized from vitamins.

   a. **Thiamine** is used for the synthesis of **thiamine pyrophosphate.**

   b. **Pantothenate** for **CoASH.**

    c. Riboflavin for **FAD.**

    d. Niacin for **NAD⁺.**

E. Pyruvate dehydrogenase complex

– In order for carbons from glucose to enter the TCA cycle, glucose is first converted to pyruvate by glycolysis, then pyruvate forms acetyl CoA.

    1. Reaction sequence

        a. Pyruvate dehydrogenase, a multienzyme complex located exclusively in the mitochondrial matrix, catalyzes the oxidative decarboxylation of pyruvate, forming acetyl CoA.

        b. The reactions catalyzed by the pyruvate dehydrogenase complex are analogous to those catalyzed by the α-ketoglutarate dehydrogenase complex. These enzyme complexes require the same five coenzymes, four of which contain vitamins (see IV D 3).

    2. Regulation of pyruvate dehydrogenase

        a. In contrast to α-ketoglutarate dehydrogenase, pyruvate dehydrogenase exists in a phosphorylated (inactive) form and a dephosphorylated (active) form.

        b. A **kinase** associated with the multienzyme complex phosphorylates the pyruvate decarboxylase subunit, inactivating the pyruvate dehydrogenase complex.

            – The products of the pyruvate dehydrogenase reaction, **acetyl CoA** and **NADH**, activate the kinase, and the substrates, **CoASH** and **NAD⁺**, inactivate the kinase. The kinase is also inactivated by ADP.

        c. A **phosphatase** dephosphorylates and activates the pyruvate dehydrogenase complex.

        d. When the concentration of substrates is high, the dehydrogenase is active, and pyruvate is converted to acetyl CoA. When the concentration of products is high, the dehydrogenase is relatively inactive.

F. Synthetic functions of the TCA cycle (Figure 4-12)

– **Intermediates** of the TCA cycle are utilized in the fasting state in the liver for the production of **glucose** and in the fed state for the synthesis of **fatty acids**. Intermediates of the TCA cycle are also used to synthesize **amino acids** or to convert one amino acid to another.

    1. Anaplerotic reactions replenish intermediates of the TCA cycle as they are removed for the synthesis of glucose, fatty acids, amino acids, or other compounds.

        a. A key anaplerotic reaction is catalyzed by **pyruvate carboxylase**, which carboxylates pyruvate, forming oxaloacetate.

            (1) Pyruvate carboxylase requires **biotin**, a cofactor that is commonly involved in CO_2 fixation reactions.

            (2) Pyruvate carboxylase, found in liver, brain, and adipose tissue (but not in muscle), is **activated by acetyl CoA.**

        b. Amino acids produce intermediates of the TCA cycle through anaplerotic reactions.

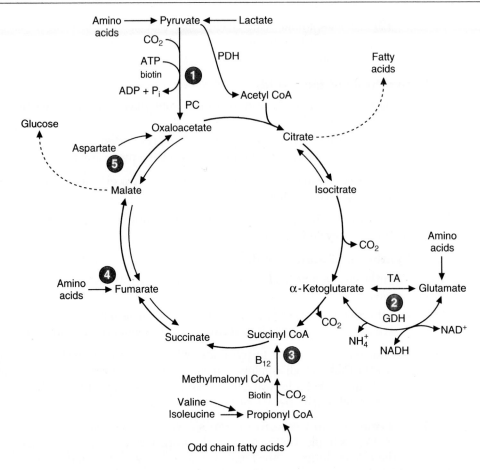

Figure 4-12. Anaplerotic and biosynthetic reactions involving the tricarboxylic acid (TCA) cycle intermediates. Synthetic reactions that form fatty acids and glucose are indicated by *dashed lines*. GDH = glutamate dehydrogenase; PDH = pyruvate dehydrogenase; TA = transamination; ❶ to ❺ = anaplerotic reactions; PC = pyruvate carboxylase.

(1) **Glutamate** is converted to α-ketoglutarate.

  – Amino acids that form glutamate include glutamine, proline, arginine, and histidine.

(2) **Aspartate** is transaminated to form oxaloacetate. Asparagine can produce aspartate.

(3) **Valine, isoleucine, methionine,** and **threonine** produce propionyl CoA, which is converted to methylmalonyl CoA and subsequently, to succinyl CoA, an intermediate of the TCA cycle.

(4) **Phenylalanine, tyrosine, and aspartate** form fumarate.

2. Synthesis of glucose

  a. The synthesis of glucose occurs by the pathway of **gluconeogenesis**, which involves intermediates of the TCA cycle.

  b. As glucose is synthesized, **malate or oxaloacetate** is removed from the TCA cycle and replenished by anaplerotic reactions.

  (1) Pyruvate, produced from lactate or alanine, is converted by pyruvate carboxylase to oxaloacetate, which forms malate.

   (2) Various amino acids that supply carbon for gluconeogenesis are
   converted to intermediates of the TCA cycle, which form malate
   and, thus, glucose.

3. Synthesis of fatty acids

   – The pathway for fatty acid synthesis from glucose includes reactions of
   the TCA cycle.

   a. From glucose, pyruvate is produced and converted to oxaloacetate (by
   pyruvate carboxylase) and to acetyl CoA (by pyruvate dehydrogenase).

   b. Oxaloacetate and acetyl CoA condense to form **citrate**, which is used
   for fatty acid synthesis.

   c. Pyruvate carboxylase catalyzes the anaplerotic reaction that replenishes
   the TCA cycle intermediates.

4. Synthesis of amino acids

   – Synthesis of amino acids from glucose involves intermediates of the TCA
   cycle.

   a. Glucose is converted to pyruvate, which forms oxaloacetate, which by
   transamination forms **aspartate** and, subsequently, **asparagine**.

   b. Glucose is converted to pyruvate, which forms both oxaloacetate and
   acetyl CoA, which condense, forming citrate. Citrate forms isocitrate
   and then α-ketoglutarate, from which **glutamate, glutamine, proline,** and **arginine** are produced.

5. Interconversion of amino acids involves intermediates of the TCA
   cycle. For example, the carbons of **glutamate** can feed into the TCA cycle
   at the α-ketoglutarate level and traverse the cycle, forming oxaloacetate,
   which may be transaminated to **aspartate**.

V. Electron Transport Chain and Oxidative Phosphorylation

- ATP is generated as a result of the energy produced when electrons from
  NADH and $FADH_2$ are passed to molecular oxygen by a series of electron
  carriers, collectively known as the electron transport chain. The components
  of the chain include FMN, Fe-S centers, coenzyme Q, and a series of cytochromes (b, c_1, c, and aa_3).
- The energy derived from the transfer of electrons through the electron
  transport chain is used to pump protons across the inner mitochondrial
  membrane from the matrix to the cytosolic side. An electrochemical gradient
  is generated, consisting of a proton gradient and a membrane potential.
- Protons move back into the matrix through the ATP synthase complex,
  causing ATP to be produced from ADP and inorganic phosphate.
- ATP is transported from the mitochondrial matrix to the cytosol in exchange
  for ADP (the ATP-ADP antiport system).
- The oxidation of one NADH generates approximately 3 ATP, while the
  oxidation of one $FADH_2$ generates approximately 2 ATP.
- Because energy generated by the transfer of electrons through the electron
  transport chain to O_2 is used in the production of ATP, the overall process
  is known as oxidative phosphorylation.

- Electron transport and ATP production occur simultaneously and are tightly coupled.
- NADH and $FADH_2$ are oxidized only if ADP is available for conversion to ATP (i.e., if ATP is being utilized and converted to ADP).

A. Overview of the electron transport chain

– **NADH and $FADH_2$** are produced by glycolysis, β-oxidation of fatty acids, the TCA cycle, and other oxidative reactions. NADH and $FADH_2$ pass electrons to the components of the electron transport chain, which are located in the inner mitochondrial membrane.

– **NADH** freely diffuses from the matrix to the membrane, while **$FADH_2$** is tightly bound to enzymes that produce it within the inner mitochondrial membrane.

– **Mitochondria** are separated from the cytoplasm by two membranes. The soluble interior of a mitochondrion is called the **matrix.** The matrix is surrounded by the inner membrane, which contains infoldings known as **cristae**.

1. The **transfer of electrons** from NADH to O_2 occurs in three stages, each of which involves a large protein complex in the inner mitochondrial membrane.

2. Each complex uses the energy from electron transfer to **pump protons** to the cytosolic side of the membrane.

3. An **electrochemical potential** or proton-motive force is generated.

   a. The electrochemical potential consists of both a membrane potential and a pH gradient.

   b. The cytosolic side of the membrane is more acidic (i.e., has a higher $[H^+]$) than the matrix.

4. The inner mitochondrial membrane is impermeable to protons. The **protons can re-enter** the matrix only **through the ATP synthase** complex (the F_0- F_1/ATPase), **causing ATP to be generated.**

   – The ATP synthase complex contains proteins (F_o) that form a channel in the inner mitochondrial membrane, through which protons can flow, and a stalk that is attached to an ATP-synthesizing head (F_1) that projects into the matrix.

5. During the transfer of electrons through the electron transport chain, **some** of the **energy is lost as heat**.

6. The electron transport chain has a large negative $\Delta G^{o\prime}$, thus electrons flow from NADH (or $FADH_2$) toward O_2.

B. The three major stages of electron transport (Figure 4-13)

1. **Transfer of electrons from NADH to coenzyme Q**

   a. **NADH** passes electrons via the **NADH dehydrogenase complex** to flavin mononucleotide (FMN).

   (1) NADH is produced by the α-ketoglutarate dehydrogenase, isocitrate dehydrogenase, and malate dehydrogenase reactions of the TCA cycle, by the pyruvate dehydrogenase reaction that converts pyruvate to acetyl CoA, by β-oxidation of fatty acids, and by other oxidation reactions.

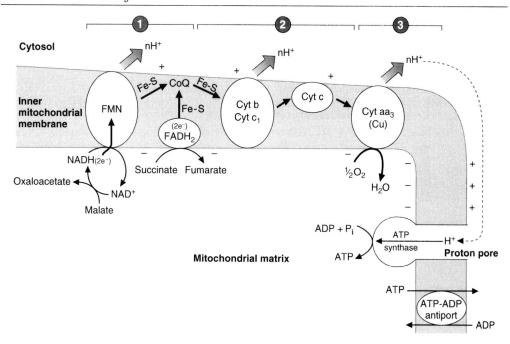

Figure 4-13. The electron transport chain and oxidative phosphorylation. *Heavy arrows* indicate the flow of electrons. CoQ = coenzyme Q (ubiquinone); Cyt = cytochrome; Fe-S = iron-sulfur centers; FMN = flavin mononucleotide. nH$^+$ indicates that an undetermined number of protons are pumped from the matrix to the cytosolic side. The *numbers* at the top of the figure correspond with the three major stages of electron transfer described in the text in V B.

(2) NADH produced in the mitochondrial matrix diffuses to the inner mitochondrial membrane where it passes electrons to FMN, which is tightly bound to a protein.

b. FMN passes the electrons through a series of iron-sulfur (Fe-S) complexes to **coenzyme Q** (CoQ), which accepts electrons one at a time, forming first the semiquinone and then ubiquinol.

c. The energy produced by these electron transfers is used to pump protons to the cytosolic side of the inner mitochondrial membrane.

d. As the protons flow back into the matrix through pores in the ATP synthase complex, approximately one ATP is generated for each NADH that transfers electrons to CoQ.

2. Transfer of electrons from coenzyme Q to cytochrome c

a. Coenzyme Q passes electrons through Fe-S centers to **cytochromes b and c$_1$**, which transfer the electrons to **cytochrome c**. The protein complex involved in these transfers is called **cytochrome reductase**.

(1) These cytochromes each contain heme as a prosthetic group but have different apoproteins.

(2) In the **ferric (Fe^{3+})** state, the heme iron can accept one electron and be reduced to the **ferrous (Fe^{2+})** state.

(3) Because the cytochromes can only carry one electron at a time, two molecules in each cytochrome complex must be reduced for every molecule of NADH that is oxidized.

    b. The energy produced by the transfer of electrons from coenzyme Q to cytochrome c is used to pump protons across the inner mitochondrial membrane.

    c. As the protons flow back into the matrix through pores in the ATP synthase complex, approximately one ATP is generated for every $CoQH_2$ that transfers two electrons to cytochrome c.

    d. Electrons from $FADH_2$, produced by reactions such as the oxidation of succinate to fumarate, **enter** the electron transport chain **at the CoQ level** (see Figure 4-13).

  3. Transfer of electrons from cytochrome c to oxygen

    a. Cytochrome c transfers electrons to the **cytochrome aa$_3$** complex, which transfers the electrons to molecular **oxygen**, reducing it to water. **Cytochrome oxidase** catalyzes this transfer of electrons.

      (1) Cytochromes a and a$_3$ each contain heme a and two different proteins that each contain **copper**.

      (2) Two electrons are required to reduce one atom of oxygen; therefore, for each NADH that is oxidized, one-half O_2 is converted to H_2O.

    b. The energy produced by the transfer of electrons from cytochrome c to oxygen is used to pump protons across the inner mitochondrial membrane.

    c. As the protons flow back into the matrix, approximately one ATP is generated for every two electrons that are transferred from cytochrome c to oxygen—that is, for every one-half O_2 that is reduced to H_2O.

C. ATP production

  – The production of ATP is coupled to the transfer of electrons through the electron transport chain to O_2. The overall process is known as **oxidative phosphorylation**.

  – The exact amount of ATP that is generated by this process has not been unequivocally established.

  1. For every NADH that is oxidized, one-half O_2 is reduced to H_2O and approximately 3 ATP are produced.

  2. For every $FADH_2$ that is oxidized, approximately 2 ATP are generated because the electrons from $FADH_2$ enter the chain via coenzyme Q, bypassing the NADH dehydrogenase step.

D. The ATP-ADP antiport

  – ATP produced within mitochondria is transferred to the cytosol in exchange for ADP by a transport protein in the inner mitochondrial membrane known as the ATP-ADP antiport (see Figure 4-13).

E. Inhibitors of electron transport and oxidative phosphorylation

  1. Agents that act on components of the electron transport chain

    – If there is a block at any point in the electron transport chain, all carriers before the block will accumulate in their reduced states, whereas those after the block will accumulate in their oxidized states. As a result, O_2 will not be consumed; ATP will not be generated; and the TCA cycle will slow down.

a. Rotenone, a fish poison, complexes with NADH dehydrogenase, causing NADH to accumulate. It does not block the transfer of electrons to the chain from $FADH_2$.

b. Antimycins (antibiotics) block the passage of electrons through the cytochrome b-c_1 complex.

c. Cyanide and carbon monoxide, poisons commonly used for suicide, combine with cytochrome oxidase and block the transfer of electrons to O_2.

2. Inhibitors of ATP synthesis

– Because the synthesis of ATP and electron transport are coupled, if the ATP synthase complex is inhibited or if an adequate supply of ADP is not available, ATP synthesis will be inhibited, O_2 will not be consumed, the components of the electron transport chain will accumulate in their reduced states, and the TCA cycle will slow down.

3. Uncoupling agents

a. Agents such as **dinitrophenol** are ionophores that allow protons from the cytosol to re-enter the matrix without going through the pore in the ATP synthase complex. Thus, they uncouple electron transport and ATP production.

b. Uncouplers **increase** the rate of O_2 consumption, **electron transport, the TCA** cycle, and CO_2 production.

c. ATP production decreases because the proton gradient across the inner mitochondrial membrane is dissipated.

d. The **energy** generated by the increased rate of respiration (electron transport and O_2 consumption) is **lost as heat**.

VI. Clinical Correlations

A. Vitamin deficiencies and excesses

Vitamin deficiencies (Table 4-2) usually occur because of an insufficient dietary intake or a decreased conversion of the vitamin to its coenzyme derivatives caused by drugs, diseases, or other factors. Decreased absorption from the gut, plasma transport, tissue storage, binding to proteins, or increased excretion may also play a role. Often multiple deficiencies occur, usually of the water-soluble vitamins, which are stored in limited amounts that may be depleted within weeks. Stores of the fat-soluble vitamins are larger and, therefore, are depleted more slowly. Toxicity due to excessive intake of the fat-soluble vitamins can develop.

B. Cyanide poisoning

Cyanide binds to Fe^{3+} in cytochrome aa_3. As a result, O_2 cannot receive electrons; respiration is inhibited; energy production is halted; and death occurs rapidly.

C. Malignant hyperthermia

The major inhalation anesthetics (halothane, ether, and methoxyflurane) trigger a reaction in susceptible people, which results in the uncoupling of oxidative phosphorylation from electron transport. ATP production decreases;

Table 4-2. Vitamin Deficiencies and Their Manifestations

Fat-Soluble Vitamins	Manifestations of Deficiency
Vitamin A	Night blindness, xerophthalmia
Vitamin D	Inadequate bone mineralization, rickets in children
Vitamin E	Reproductive failure, muscular dystrophy, neurologic abnormalities
Vitamin K	Defective blood coagulation

Water-Soluble Vitamins	Manifestations of Deficiency
Vitamin C	Scurvy
Thiamine	Beriberi
Riboflavin	Oral-buccal cavity lesions
Niacin	Pellagra (diarrhea, dermatitis, dementia, death)
Vitamin B_6 (pyridoxine)	Convulsions, dermatitis, anemia
Folate	Megaloblastic anemia (due to impaired cell division and growth)
Vitamin B_{12}	Megaloblastic anemia, neurologic symptoms (resulting from demyelination)
Biotin	Anorexia, nausea, vomiting, glossitis, alopecia, dry, scaly dermatitis
Pantothenic acid	Listlessness, fatigue, "burning feet" syndrome

heat is generated; and the temperature rises markedly. The TCA cycle is stimulated, and excessive CO_2 production leads to respiratory acidosis.

D. Acute myocardial infarction

Coronary arteries frequently become narrow because of **atherosclerotic plaques**. If **coronary occlusions** occur, regions of heart muscle may be deprived of blood flow and, therefore, of oxygen for prolonged periods of time. **Lack of oxygen** causes inhibition of the processes of electron transport and oxidative phosphorylation, which results in a decreased production of ATP. **Heart muscle**, suffering from a lack of energy required for contraction and maintenance of membrane integrity, becomes **damaged**. **Enzymes** from the damaged cells (including the MB fraction of creatine kinase) **leak into the blood**. If the damage is relatively mild, the person may recover. If heart function is severely compromised, death may result.

Review Test

Directions: Each of the numbered items or incomplete statements in this section is followed by answers or by completions of the statement. Select the **one** lettered answer or completion that is **best** in each case.

Questions 1 and 2

Refer to the following equation when answering questions 1 and 2.

fumarate + $H_2O \rightleftharpoons$ malate

1. When measured in the absence of fumarase, the $\Delta G^{\circ\prime}$ for this reaction is 0 kcal/mole (neglecting any terms associated with H_2O). The equilibrium constant for this reaction is

(A) 0
(B) 0.5
(C) 1.0
(D) 10.0
(E) 50.0

2. Fumarase was added to a solution that initially contained 20 μM fumarate. After the establishment of equilibrium, the concentration of malate was

(A) 2 μM
(B) 5 μM
(C) 10 μM
(D) 20 μM
(E) 50 μM

Questions 3 and 4

Refer to the following reactions and associated values when answering questions 3 and 4.

Reaction	Approximate $\Delta G^{\circ\prime}$ (kcal/mole)
Acetate + 2 $O_2 \rightarrow$ 2 CO_2 + 2 H_2O	−243
NADH + H^+ + ½ $O_2 \rightarrow NAD^+$ + H_2O	−53
$FADH_2$ + ½ $O_2 \rightarrow$ FAD + H_2O	−41
GTP $\rightarrow$ GDP + P_i	−8
ATP $\rightarrow$ ADP + P_i	−8

3. Of the total energy available from the oxidation of acetate, what percentage is transferred via the TCA cycle to NADH, $FADH_2$, and GTP?

(A) 38%
(B) 42%
(C) 82%
(D) 86%
(E) 100%

4. What percentage of the energy available from the oxidation of acetate is converted to ATP?

(A) 3%
(B) 30%
(C) 40%
(D) 85%
(E) 100%

5. A genetic mutation caused the cellular concentration of an enzyme to increase 100-fold for a biochemical reaction. Therefore, the equilibrium constant for the reaction catalyzed by the enzyme

(A) decreased two-fold
(B) remained the same
(C) increased in proportion to the enzyme concentration
(D) changed inversely with the enzyme concentration

6. Which of the following conditions is caused by a vitamin deficiency characterized by diarrhea, dermatitis, and dementia?

(A) Pellagra
(B) Beriberi
(C) Scurvy
(D) Rickets

7. The principal function of the TCA cycle is to

(A) generate CO_2
(B) transfer electrons from the acetyl portion of acetyl CoA to NAD^+ and FAD
(C) oxidize the acetyl portion of acetyl CoA to oxaloacetate
(D) generate heat from the oxidation of the acetyl portion of acetyl CoA
(E) dispose of excess pyruvate and fatty acids

Question 8

Refer to the following compounds to answer question 8.

$$\overset{\displaystyle OH}{\underset{\displaystyle \underset{COO^-}{|}}{^-OOC - CH - CH - CH_2 - COO^-}}$$

Compound A

$$^-OOC - CH = CH - COO^-$$
Compound B

8. The segment of the TCA cycle in which Compound A is converted to Compound B

(A) yields 5 moles of high-energy phosphate bonds per mole of A
(B) requires a coenzyme synthesized in the human from niacin (nicotinamide)
(C) is catalyzed by enzymes located solely in the mitochondrial membrane
(D) produces 1 mole of CO_2 for every mole of Compound A oxidized
(E) requires GTP to drive one of the reactions

9. The reactions of the TCA cycle oxidizing succinate to oxaloacetate

(A) require coenzyme A
(B) include an isomerization reaction
(C) produce one high-energy phosphate bond
(D) require both NAD^+ and FAD
(E) produce one GTP from GDP + P_i

10. In the tricarboxylic acid cycle, thiamine pyrophosphate

(A) accepts electrons from the oxidation of pyruvate and α-ketoglutarate
(B) accepts electrons from the oxidation of isocitrate
(C) forms a covalent intermediate with the α-carbon of α-ketoglutarate
(D) forms a thioester with the sulfhydryl group of CoASH
(E) forms a thioester with the sulfhydryl group of lipoic acid

11. During exercise, stimulation of the tricarboxylic acid cycle results principally from

(A) allosteric activation of isocitrate dehydrogenase by increased NADH
(B) allosteric activation of fumarase by increased ADP
(C) a rapid decrease in the concentration of four-carbon intermediates
(D) product inhibition of citrate synthase
(E) stimulation of the flux through a number of enzymes by a decreased $NADH/NAD^+$ ratio

12. CO_2 production by the tricarboxylic acid cycle would be increased to the greatest extent by a genetic abnormality that resulted in

(A) a 50% increase in the concentration of ADP in the mitochondrial matrix
(B) a 50% increase in the oxygen content of the cell
(C) a 50% decrease in the V_m of α-ketoglutarate dehydrogenase
(D) a 50% increase in the K_m of isocitrate dehydrogenase

13. The enzyme pyruvate dehydrogenase

(A) contains only one polypeptide chain
(B) requires thiamine pyrophosphate as a cofactor
(C) produces oxaloacetate from pyruvate
(D) is converted to an active form by phosphorylation
(E) is activated when NADH levels increase

14. Alcoholics frequently develop thiamine deficiencies because ethanol decreases absorption of the vitamin. Which of the following enzymes would be most affected by a thiamine deficiency?

(A) α-Ketoglutarate dehydrogenase
(B) Succinate dehydrogenase
(C) Fumarase
(D) Malate dehydrogenase
(E) Pyruvate carboxylase

15. Which of the following vitamins is required for synthesis of a cofactor required for reactions in the oxidation of pyruvate to CO_2 and H_2O?

(A) Biotin
(B) Vitamin K
(C) Pantothenate
(D) Ascorbate
(E) Pyridoxine

16. Which of the following components of the electron transport chain only accepts electrons?

(A) Cytochrome b
(B) Oxygen
(C) Coenzyme Q
(D) FMN

17. A man presents to the emergency room after ingesting an insecticide. His respiration rate is very low. Information from the Poison Control Center indicates that this particular insecticide binds to and completely inhibits cytochrome c. Therefore, in this man's mitochondria

(A) coenzyme Q would be in the oxidized state
(B) cytochromes a and a_3 would be in the reduced state
(C) the rate of ATP synthesis would be approximately zero
(D) the rate of CO_2 production would be increased

18. Which one of the following statements best describes the consequence of ingesting a compound that stimulates ATP hydrolysis by plasma membrane Na^+-K^+ ATPase?

(A) The pH gradient across the mitochondrial membranes would increase
(B) The rate of conversion of NADH to NAD^+ in the mitochondria would decrease
(C) Heat production would decrease
(D) The transfer of electrons to O_2 would increase

19. A chemist wanting to lose weight obtained dinitrophenol (DNP). Before using the DNP, the chemist consulted her physician and was informed that DNP was an uncoupling agent and was dangerous to use for weight loss. Which of the following changes would have occurred in her mitochondria if she had ingested enough DNP?

(A) O_2 consumption would decrease
(B) CO_2 production would decrease
(C) The proton gradient would increase
(D) NADH would be oxidized more rapidly
(E) Temperature would decrease

20. A patient suffering a heart attack was brought to the emergency room. An atherosclerotic plaque had blocked a major coronary artery, preventing blood from reaching a region of her heart. As a result, in cells of the affected heart muscle, there was an increase in

(A) the rate of CO_2 production
(B) the rate of electron transport by the electron transport chain
(C) the concentration of ADP
(D) the proton gradient across the inner mitochondrial membrane
(E) the rate of O_2 consumption

Directions: Each group of items in this section consists of lettered options followed by a set of numbered items. For each item, select the **one** lettered option that is most closely associated with it. Each lettered heading may be selected once, more than once, or not at all.

Questions 21–25

(A) Riboflavin
(B) Pantothenic acid
(C) Niacin
(D) Vitamin B_6

Match each cofactor with the vitamin that is required for its synthesis.

21. NAD^+

22. FAD

23. Coenzyme A

24. FMN

25. Pyridoxal phosphate

Questions 26–29

(A) Blood clotting
(B) Calcium metabolism
(C) Collagen synthesis
(D) Vision

Each process above is affected by a vitamin deficiency. Match each process with the appropriate vitamin.

26. Vitamin A

27. Vitamin C

28. Vitamin D

29. Vitamin K

Questions 30–34

(A)
$$\text{OH}$$
$$|$$
$$^-OOC - CH_2 - CH - COO^-$$

(B)
$$\text{O}$$
$$||$$
$$^-OOC - CH_2 - CH_2 - C - COO^-$$

(C)
$$\text{OH}$$
$$|$$
$$^-OOC - CH_2 - C - CH_2 - COO^-$$
$$|$$
$$\text{COO}^-$$

(D)
$$^-OOC - CH_2 - CH_2 - COO^-$$

Match each description with the appropriate compound.

30. An intermediate in the conversion of isocitrate to succinyl CoA in the TCA cycle

31. Converted to isocitrate by the enzyme aconitase

32. Formed by the addition of water across the double bond of fumarate

33. Oxidized to oxaloacetate by malate dehydrogenase

34. Generated in a reaction that produces GTP

Questions 35–39

(A) Thiamine
(B) Niacin
(C) Thiamine and niacin
(D) Neither thiamine nor niacin

Match each enzyme below with the vitamin or vitamins required for its activity.

35. Pyruvate dehydrogenase

36. Malate dehydrogenase

37. Pyruvate carboxylase

38. α-Ketoglutarate dehydrogenase

39. Succinate dehydrogenase

Questions 40–43

(A) Isocitrate dehydrogenase
(B) Malate dehydrogenase
(C) Both isocitrate and malate dehydrogenase
(D) Neither dehydrogenase

Match each item below with the appropriate enzyme or enzymes.

40. Regulated allosterically by ADP

41. Liberates CO_2

42. Reduces a cofactor that transfers electrons to the electron transport chain

43. Utilizes FAD as a cofactor

Answers and Explanations

1–C. $\Delta G^{\circ\prime} = 0 = -1400 \log K_{eq}$. Therefore, $K_{eq} = 1$. Log $K_{eq} = \log 1 = 0$.

2–C. $K_{eq} = 1 = $ [Malate]/[Fumarate] $= X/(20\text{-}X)$. Therefore, $(20\text{-}X) = X$, $20 = 2X$, and $X = 10$.

3–D. In the TCA cycle, 3 NADHs are produced ($3 \times 53 = 159$ kcal), 1 $FADH_2$ (41 kcal), and 1 GTP (8 kcal). The percentage of the total energy available from oxidation of acetate that is transferred to these compounds is, therefore, 208/243 kcal or 86%.

4–C. About 12 ATP are produced by the TCA cycle (12×8 kcal $= 96$ kcal). The percentage of the total energy available from oxidation of acetate that is converted to ATP is 96/243, or 40%.

5–B. An enzyme increases the rate at which a reaction reaches equilibrium but does not change the concentration of reactants and products at equilibrium; that is, the K_{eq} is not affected by an enzyme.

6–A. Pellagra (due to a niacin deficiency) is characterized by the 4 Ds (i.e., the three listed above plus death). The other conditions and their associated vitamin deficiencies are: beriberi (thiamine), scurvy (vitamin C: ascorbate), and rickets (vitamin D).

7–B. Although the TCA cycle produces CO_2 and oxaloacetate and generates heat, these are not its major functions. It does not "dispose" of excess pyruvate and fatty acids; it oxidizes them in a controlled manner to generate energy. The principal function of the cycle is to pass electrons to NAD^+ and FAD, which transfer them to the electron transport chain. The net result is the production of ATP.

8–B. In the conversion of isocitrate (Compound A) to fumarate (Compound B), 2 CO_2, 2 NADH (which contains niacin), 1 GTP, and 1 $FADH_2$ are produced. A total of approximately 9 ATP are generated. The enzymes for these reactions are all located in the mitochondrial matrix except succinate dehydrogenase, which is in the inner mitochondrial membrane. GTP does not drive any of the reactions but is produced in the conversion of succinyl CoA to succinate.

9–D. FAD is required for conversion of succinate to fumarate, and NAD^+ is required for conversion of malate to oxaloacetate. Five ATP are generated. Coenzyme A is not required, and no isomerization reactions occur. GTP is produced in the previous step of the cycle, when succinyl CoA is converted to succinate.

10–C. Thiamine pyrophosphate forms a covalent intermediate with the α-carbon of α-ketoglutarate.

11–E. NADH decreases during exercise (if it increased, it would slow the cycle). Fumarase is not activated by ADP. Four-carbon intermediates of the cycle are recycled. Their concentration does not decrease. Product inhibition of citrate synthase would slow the cycle. During exercise, the tricarboxylic acid cycle is stimulated because the NADH/NAD^+ ratio decreases and stimulates flux through isocitrate dehydrogenase, α-ketoglutarate dehydrogenase, and malate dehydrogenase.

12–A. If the V_m of α-ketoglutarate dehydrogenase decreased, flux through the tricarboxylic acid cycle would decrease; therefore, CO_2 production would decrease. If the K_m of isocitrate dehydrogenase increased, higher concentrations of isocitrate would be required for the cycle to operate at its normal rate. O_2 is normally present in excess and is not rate-limiting. The only change that would increase the rate of CO_2 production by the cycle would be an increase of ADP, which would allosterically activate isocitrate dehydrogenase.

13–B. Pyruvate dehydrogenase converts pyruvate to acetyl CoA. It contains multiple subunits: a dehydrogenase component that oxidatively decarboxylates pyruvate, a dihydrolipoyl transacetylase that transfers the acetyl group to coenzyme A, and a dihydrolipoyl dehydrogenase that reoxidizes lipoic acid. Thiamine pyrophosphate, lipoic acid, coenzyme A, NAD^+, and FAD serve as cofactors for these reactions. In addition, a kinase is present that phosphorylates and inactivates the decarboxylase component. Acetyl CoA and NADH activate this kinase, thus inactivating pyruvate dehydrogenase. A phosphatase dephosphorylates the kinase, thereby reactivating pyruvate dehydrogenase.

14–A. α-Ketoglutarate dehydrogenase is the only one of these enzymes that requires thiamine (as thiamine pyrophosphate). It also requires lipoic acid, CoASH, FAD, and NAD^+.

15–C. Pantothenate is required for the synthesis of coenzyme A (CoASH). CoASH is a cofactor for pyruvate dehydrogenase, which converts pyruvate to acetyl CoA. Acetyl CoA enters the TCA cycle to be oxidized to CO_2 and H_2O. α-Ketoglutarate dehydrogenase, which converts α-ketoglutarate to succinyl CoA in the TCA cycle, also requires CoASH.

16–A. The cytochromes accept only electrons. The other components accept hydrogen and electrons.

17–C. If cytochrome c cannot function, all components of the electron transport chain between it and O_2 remain in the oxidized state, and the components of the chain before cytochrome c are reduced. The electron transport chain will not function; O_2 will not be consumed; a proton gradient will not be generated; and ATP will not be produced. NADH will not be oxidized, thus the TCA cycle will slow down and, therefore, CO_2 production will decrease.

18–D. If ATP were rapidly hydrolyzed, ADP levels would increase. Therefore, the rate of ATP synthesis would increase. The pH gradient across the mitochondrial membrane would decrease; the rate of electron transport would increase; O_2 consumption would increase; NADH would be oxidized more rapidly; and heat production would increase.

19–D. An "uncoupler" dissipates the proton gradient across the inner mitochondrial membrane. Therefore, ATP is not produced, and energy is liberated as heat. The low proton gradient causes the electron transport chain to speed up; O_2 consumption increases; NADH is rapidly oxidized; the TCA cycle speeds up; and CO_2 production increases.

20–C. A lack of blood flow decreased the flow of O_2, which slowed the electron transport chain. As NADH levels increased, the TCA cycle slowed down, and CO_2 production by the TCA cycle decreased. ATP was converted to ADP, but ATP could not be regenerated because the proton gradient decreased.

21–C. NAD^+ contains niacin.

22–A. FAD contains riboflavin.

23–B. Coenzyme A contains pantothenic acid.

24–A. FMN contains riboflavin.

25–D. Pyridoxal phosphate contains vitamin B_6.

26–D. Vitamin A is required for formation of the visual pigments.

27–C. Vitamin C is required for the hydroxylation of proline and lysine residues in the precursor of collagen. Defective collagen formation results in scurvy, which is characterized by bleeding gums.

28–B. Vitamin D stimulates calcium uptake from the intestine and resorption from bone and urine.

29–A. Vitamin K is required for blood clotting.

30–B. α-Ketoglutarate is an intermediate in the conversion of isocitrate to succinyl CoA.

31–C. Citrate is converted to isocitrate by aconitase.

32–A. Malate is formed by the addition of water across the double bond of fumarate.

33–A. Malate is oxidized to oxaloacetate by malate dehydrogenase.

34–D. Succinate is produced from succinyl CoA in a reaction that generates GTP.

35–C. Pyruvate dehydrogenase requires five coenzymes: thiamine pyrophosphate, lipoic acid, coenzyme A, FAD, and NAD^+ (which is synthesized from niacin).

36–B. Malate dehydrogenase requires NAD^+, which is synthesized from niacin.

37–D. Pyruvate carboxylase requires biotin.

38–C. α-Ketoglutarate dehydrogenase requires the same five coenzymes as pyruvate dehydrogenase.

39–D. Succinate dehydrogenase requires FAD.

40–A. Isocitrate dehydrogenase is allosterically activated by ADP.

41–A. Isocitrate dehydrogenase removes CO_2 from isocitrate to form α-ketoglutarate.

42–C. Isocitrate dehydrogenase and malate dehydrogenase produce NADH, which interacts with the electron transport chain.

43–D. Neither isocitrate dehydrogenase nor malate dehydrogenase utilizes FAD.

5
Carbohydrate Metabolism

Overview

- Dietary carbohydrates include starch, sucrose, lactose, and indigestible fiber.
- The major product of digestion of carbohydrates is glucose, but some galactose and fructose are also produced.
- Glucose is a major fuel source that is oxidized by cells for energy. After a meal, it is converted to glycogen or to triacylglycerols and stored.
- Glucose is also converted to compounds such as proteoglycans, glycoproteins, and glycolipids.
- When glucose enters cells, it is converted to glucose 6-phosphate, which is a pivotal compound in several metabolic pathways.
  - The major fate of glucose 6-phosphate is to enter the pathway of glycolysis, which produces pyruvate and generates NADH and ATP.
  - Glucose 6-phosphate can be converted to glucose 1-phosphate and then to UDP-glucose, which is used for the synthesis of glycogen or compounds such as the proteoglycans.
  - Glucose 6-phosphate can also enter the pentose phosphate pathway, which produces NADPH (for reactions such as the biosynthesis of fatty acids) and ribose for nucleotide production.
- Fructose and galactose are converted to intermediates in the pathways by which glucose is metabolized.
- Glycogen is the major storage form of carbohydrate in animals. The largest stores are in muscle and liver.
  - Muscle glycogen is used to generate ATP for muscle contraction.
  - Liver glycogen is used to maintain blood glucose during fasting or exercise.
- The maintenance of blood glucose is a major function of the liver.
  - The liver produces glucose by glycogenolysis and gluconeogenesis.

I. Carbohydrate Structure

- Carbohydrates are compounds that contain at least three carbon atoms, a number of hydroxyl groups, and usually an aldehyde or ketone group. They may contain phosphate, amino, or sulfate groups.
- In the body, monosaccharides, the simplest carbohydrates, are usually of the D-series.

- Monosaccharides form rings that usually contain five or six members and are called furanoses and pyranoses, respectively. The hydroxyl group on the anomeric carbon (the carbonyl carbon) may be in either the α or the β configuration.
- Monosaccharides are joined by *O*-glycosidic bonds to form disaccharides, oligosaccharides, and polysaccharides.
- Nucleotides contain *N*-glycosidic bonds.
- Monosaccharides can be oxidized to the corresponding acids or reduced to the corresponding polyols.

A. Monosaccharides

1. Nomenclature

a. The simplest monosaccharides have the formula $(CH_2O)_n$. Those with three carbons are called **trioses;** four, **tetroses;** five, **pentoses;** and six, **hexoses.**

b. They are called **aldoses** or **ketoses,** depending on whether their most oxidized functional group is an aldehyde or a ketone (Figure 5-1).

2. D and L sugars

a. The configuration of the asymmetric carbon atom farthest from the aldehyde or ketone group determines whether a monosaccharide belongs to the D or L series. In the D form, the hydroxyl group is on the right; in the L form, it is on the left (see Figure 5-1).

b. An **asymmetric carbon** atom has **four different chemical groups** attached to it.

c. **Sugars of the D** series, which are related to D-glyceraldehyde, are the most common in nature (Figure 5-2).

3. Stereoisomers, enantiomers, and epimers

a. **Stereoisomers** have the same chemical formula but differ in the position of the hydroxyl groups on one or more of their asymmetric carbons (see Figure 5-2).

b. **Enantiomers** are stereoisomers that are mirror images of each other (see Figure 5-1).

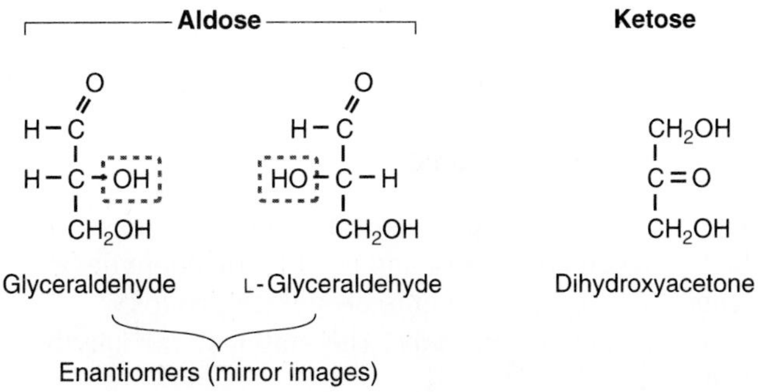

Figure 5-1. Examples of trioses, the smallest monosaccharides.

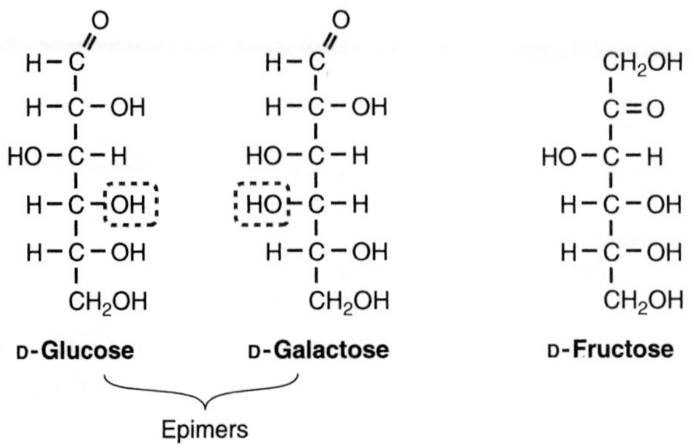

Figure 5-2. Common hexoses of the D configuration.

c. Epimers are stereoisomers that differ in the position of the hydroxyl group at only one asymmetric carbon. For example, D-glucose and D-galactose are epimers that differ at carbon 4 (see Figure 5-2).

4. Ring structures of carbohydrates

a. Although **monosaccharides** are often drawn as straight chains (Fischer projections), they exist mainly as ring structures in which the aldehyde or ketone group has reacted with a hydroxyl group in the same molecule (Figure 5-3).

b. Furanose and **pyranose** rings contain five and six members, respectively and are usually drawn as Haworth projections (see Figure 5-3).

c. The **hydroxyl group on the anomeric carbon** may be in the α or β configuration. In the **α configuration,** the hydroxyl group on the anomeric carbon is on the right in the Fischer projection and below the plane of the ring in the Haworth projection. In the **β configuration,** it is on the left in the Fischer projection and above the plane in the Haworth projection (Figure 5-4).

d. In solution, **mutarotation occurs.** The α and β forms equilibrate via the straight-chain aldehyde form (see Figure 5-4).

B. Glycosides

1. Formation of glycosides

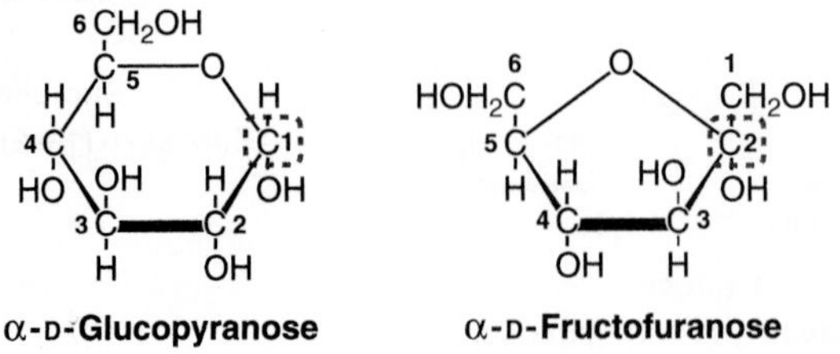

Figure 5-3. Furanose and pyranose rings. The anomeric carbons are surrounded by *dashed lines*.

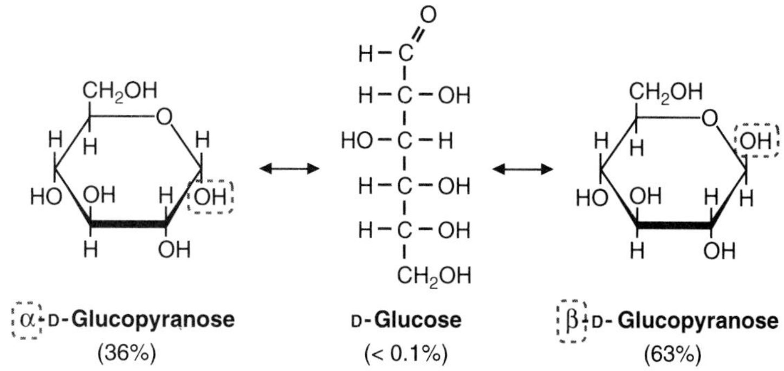

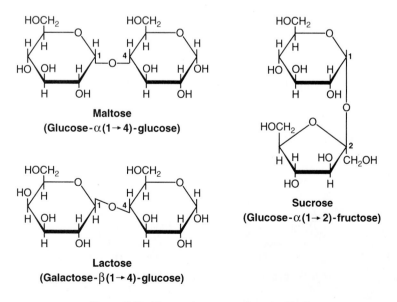

Figure 5-4. Mutarotation of glucose in solution. The percentage of each form is indicated.

   a. Glycosidic bonds form when the **hydroxyl** group on the anomeric carbon of a monosaccharide reacts with an -OH or -NH group of another compound.

   b. α-**Glycosides** or β-**glycosides** are produced depending on the position of the atom attached to the anomeric carbon of the sugar.

2. *O-Glycosides*

   a. Monosaccharides can be linked via *O*-glycosidic bonds to another monosaccharide, forming *O*-glycosides.

   b. Disaccharides contain two monosaccharides. Sucrose, lactose, and maltose are common disaccharides (Figure 5-5).

   c. Oligosaccharides contain up to approximately 12 monosaccharides (see II B and C).

   d. Polysaccharides contain more than 12 monosaccharides; for example, glycogen, starch, and glycosaminoglycans (see Figures 5-8 and 5-12).

Figure 5-5. The most common disaccharides.

3. *N*-Glycosides

– Monosaccharides can be linked via *N*-glycosidic bonds to compounds that are not carbohydrates. Nucleotides contain *N*-glycosidic bonds.

C. Derivatives of carbohydrates

1. Phosphate groups can be attached to carbohydrates.

a. Glucose and fructose can be phosphorylated on carbons 1 and 6.

b. Phosphate groups can link sugars to nucleotides, as in UDP-glucose (see Figure 5-13).

2. Amino groups, which are often acetylated, can be linked to sugars (e.g., glucosamine and galactosamine).

3. Sulfate groups are often found on sugars (e.g., chondroitin sulfate and other glycosaminoglycans) (see Figure 5-7).

D. Oxidation of carbohydrates

1. Oxidized forms

a. The anomeric carbon of an aldose (C1) can be oxidized to an acid.

– Glucose forms **gluconic acid** (gluconate). **6-Phosphogluconate** is an intermediate in the pentose phosphate pathway.

– Oxidation of glucose by glucose oxidase (a highly specific test for glucose) is used by clinical and other laboratories to measure the amount of glucose in solution.

b. Carbon 6 of a hexose can be oxidized to a uronic acid.

(1) Uronic acids are found in glycosaminoglycans of proteoglycans (see Figure 5-7).

(2) Glucose forms **glucuronic acid.** Conjugation with glucuronic acid makes lipid compounds more water soluble (e.g., bilirubin diglucuronide).

2. Test for reducing sugars

– Reducing sugars contain a free anomeric carbon that can be oxidized.

a. When the anomeric carbon is oxidized, another compound is reduced. If the reduced product of this reaction is colored, the intensity of the color can be used to determine the amount of the reducing sugar that has been oxidized.

b. This reaction is the basis of the reducing-sugar test, which is used by clinical laboratories. The test is not specific. Aldoses such as glucose give a positive test result. Ketoses such as fructose are also reducing sugars because they form aldoses under test conditions.

E. Reduction of carbohydrates

1. The aldehyde or ketone group of a sugar can be reduced to a hydroxyl group, forming a **polyol** (polyalcohol).

2. Glucose is reduced to **sorbitol** and galactose to **galactitol** (see Figure 5-28).

F. Glycosylation of proteins

– Aldehyde groups of sugars **nonenzymatically** form Schiff bases with amino groups of proteins. Subsequently, Amadori rearrangements form stable covalent interactions.

– A glycosylated fraction of hemoglobin, **HbA$_{1c}$**, is normally 6% of the total hemoglobin, but increases when red blood cells are exposed to high levels of blood glucose.

II. Proteoglycans, Glycoproteins, and Glycolipids

- Proteoglycans consist of long linear chains of glycosaminoglycans attached to a core protein. Each chain is composed of a repeating disaccharide that is usually negatively charged and contains a hexosamine and a uronic acid. Sulfate groups are often present.
  – The glycosaminoglycans are synthesized from UDP-sugars.
- Glycoproteins contain smaller polysaccharide chains that are usually branched.
  – In addition to glucose, galactose, and their amino derivatives, glycoproteins contain mannose, *L*-fucose, and *N*-acetylneuraminic acid (NANA).
  – For *O*-linked chains, the polysaccharide grows by the sequential addition of monosaccharide units from UDP-sugars to serine or threonine residues in a protein.
  – For *N*-linked chains, branched carbohydrates are synthesized on dolichol phosphate and transferred to the amide nitrogen of an asparagine residue in a protein.
- Glycolipids are members of the class of sphingolipids.
  – The carbohydrate portion is synthesized from UDP-sugars that add to the hydroxymethyl group of ceramide and then sequentially to the nonreducing end of the chain.
  – *N*-Acetylneuraminic acid (derived from CMP-NANA) often forms branches from the main chain.
- Proteoglycans, glycoproteins, and glycolipids are synthesized in the endoplasmic reticulum and Golgi complex; they are degraded by the action of lysosomes.

A. Proteoglycans are found in the extracellular matrix or ground substance of connective tissue, synovial fluid of joints, vitreous humor of the eye, secretions of mucus-producing cells, and in cartilage.

1. Structure of proteoglycans

a. Proteoglycans consist of a core protein with long unbranched polysaccharide chains (**glycosaminoglycans**) attached. The overall structure resembles a bottle brush (Figure 5-6).

b. These chains are composed of **repeating disaccharide units,** which usually contain a **uronic acid** and a **hexosamine** (Figure 5-7). The uronic acid is generally D-glucuronic or L-iduronic acid.

c. The amino group of the hexosamine is usually **acetylated**, and **sulfate** groups are often present on carbons 4 and 6.

d. A xylose and two galactose residues connect the chain of repeating disaccharides to the core protein.

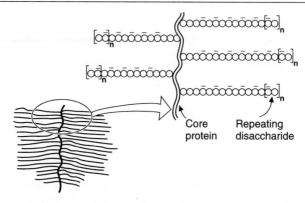

Figure 5-6. "Bottle brush" structure of a proteoglycan with a magnified segment.

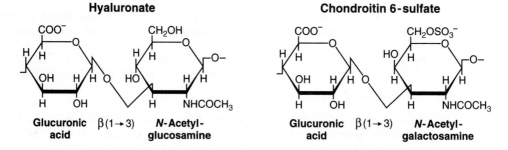

Figure 5-7. Examples of repeating disaccharides of glycosaminoglycans.

2. Synthesis of proteoglycans

a. The **protein** is synthesized on the endoplasmic reticulum (ER).

b. Glycosaminoglycans are produced by the addition of sugars to serine or threonine residues of the protein. UDP-sugars serve as the precursors.

c. In the ER and the Golgi, the glycosaminoglycan chains grow by sequential addition of sugars to the nonreducing end.

  (1) Sulfate groups, donated by 3'-phosphoadenosine 5'-phosphosulfate (PAPS), are added after the hexosamine is incorporated into the chain.

  (2) Because of the uronic acid and sulfate groups, the glycosaminoglycans are **negatively charged,** causing the chains to be heavily hydrated.

d. Proteoglycans are **secreted** from the cell.

e. Proteoglycans can associate noncovalently with **hyaluronic acid** (a glycosaminoglycan) forming large aggregates, which act as molecular sieves, that can be penetrated by small but not by large molecules.

3. Degradation of proteoglycans by lysosomal enzymes

a. Because proteoglycans are located outside the cell, they are taken up by **endocytosis.** The endocytic vesicles fuse with lysosomes.

    b. Lysosomal enzymes specific for each monosaccharide remove the sugars, one at a time, from the nonreducing end of the chain.

    c. Sulfatases remove the sulfate groups before the sugar residue is hydrolyzed.

B. Glycoproteins serve as enzymes, hormones, antibodies, and structural proteins. They are found in extracellular fluids and in lysosomes and are attached to the cell membrane. They are involved in cell-cell interactions.

  1. Structure of glycoproteins

    a. The **carbohydrate** portion of glycoproteins differs from that of proteoglycans in that it is **shorter** and often **branched** (Figure 5- 8).

      (1) Glycoproteins contain mannose, L-fucose, and N-acetylneuraminic acid (NANA) in addition to glucose, galactose, and their amino derivatives. NANA is a member of the class of sialic acids.

      (2) The antigenic determinants of the ABO and Lewis blood group substances are sugars at the ends of these carbohydrate branches.

    b. The carbohydrates are attached to the protein via the hydroxyl groups of **serine and threonine** residues or the amide N of **asparagine.**

  2. Synthesis of glycoproteins

    a. The protein is synthesized on the ER. In the ER and the Golgi, the **carbohydrate chain** is produced by the sequential addition of monosaccharide units to the nonreducing end. UDP-sugars, GDP-mannose, GDP-L-fucose, and CMP-NANA act as precursors.

    b. For *O*-linked glycoproteins, the initial sugar is added to a **serine or threonine** residue in the protein and the carbohydrate chain is then elongated.

    c. Dolichol phosphate is involved in the synthesis of *N*-linked glycoproteins in which the carbohydrate moiety is attached to the amide N of asparagine.

      (1) Dolichol phosphate, a long-chain alcohol containing about 20 five-carbon isoprene units, can be synthesized from acetyl CoA.

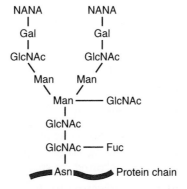

Figure 5-8. Example of the carbohydrate moiety of a glycoprotein. Note that, in this case, the carbohydrate is attached to an asparagine (*N*-linked). NANA = N-acetylneuraminic acid, Gal = galactose, GlcNAc = N-acetylglucosamine, Man = mannose, Fuc = fucose.

(2) Sugars are added sequentially to dolichol phosphate, which is associated with the membrane of the ER.

(3) The branched polysaccharide chain is transferred to an amide N of an asparagine residue in the protein.

(4) In the ER and the Golgi, sugars are removed from the chain and other sugars are added.

d. **Glycoproteins** are **segregated** into lysosomes within the cell, **attached** to the cell membrane, or **secreted** by the cell.

(1) **Lysosomal enzymes** are glycoproteins. A mannose phosphate residue targets these glycoproteins to lysosomes.

(2) When a glycoprotein is attached to the **cell membrane**, the carbohydrate portion extends into the extracellular space and a hydrophobic segment of the protein is anchored in the membrane.

3. **Degradation of glycoproteins**

– **Lysosomal enzymes** specific for each monosaccharide remove sugars sequentially from the nonreducing ends of the chains.

C. **Glycolipids**

1. Glycolipids (or **sphingolipids**) are derived from the lipid **ceramide** (see Figure 6-17). This class of compounds includes cerebrosides and gangliosides. Some bacterial toxins and viruses use glycolipids as receptors.

a. **Cerebrosides** are synthesized from ceramide and UDP-sugars.

b. **Gangliosides,** have *N*-acetylneuraminic acid residues (derived from CMP-NANA) branching from the linear oligosaccharide chain.

2. Glycolipids are found in the **cell membrane** with the carbohydrate portion extending into the extracellular space.

3. They are degraded by **lysosomal enzymes.**

III. Digestion of Carbohydrates

- The major dietary carbohydrates are starch, sucrose, and lactose.
- In the mouth, salivary α-amylase acts on starch, cleaving α-1,4 linkages between glucose residues.
- In the intestine, pancreatic α-amylase continues the digestion of starch.
- Enzymes associated with the brush border of intestinal epithelial cells digest sucrose, lactose, and the products generated from starch by α-amylase.
- The final products of carbohydrate digestion–glucose, fructose, and galactose–are absorbed by intestinal epithelial cells and enter the blood.

A. **Dietary carbohydrates** (mainly starch, sucrose, and lactose) constitute about 50% of the calories in the average diet in the United States.

1. **Starch,** the storage form of carbohydrate in plants, is similar in structure to glycogen (Figure 5-9).

– Starch contains amylose (long, unbranched chains with glucose units linked α-1,4) and amylopectin (α-1,4-linked chains with α-1,6-linked branches). Amylopectin has fewer branches than glycogen.

2. **Sucrose** (a component of table sugar and fruit) contains glucose and fructose residues linked via their anomeric carbons (see Figure 5-5).

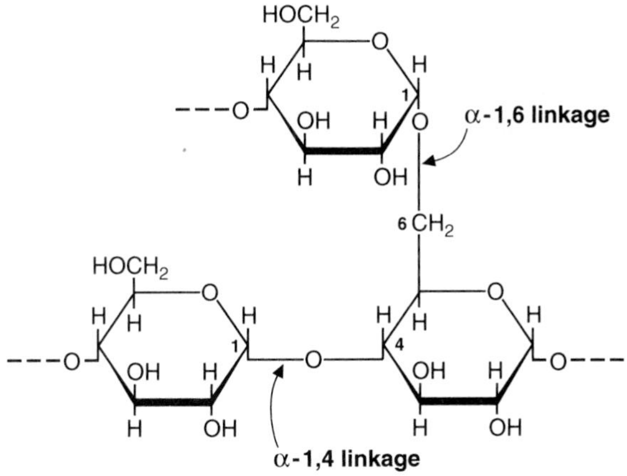

Figure 5-9. α-1,4 and α-1,6 linkages between glucose residues in starch and glycogen.

3. **Lactose** (milk sugar) contains galactose linked β-1,4 to glucose (see Figure 5-5).

B. **Digestion of dietary carbohydrates in the mouth** (Figure 5-10)
   – In the mouth, **salivary α-amylase** cleaves starch by breaking α-1,4 linkages between glucose residues within the chains (see Figure 5-9). Dextrins (linear and branched oligosaccharides) are the major products that enter the stomach.

C. **Digestion of carbohydrates in the intestine** (see Figure 5-10)
   – The stomach contents pass into the intestine where **bicarbonate** secreted by the pancreas neutralizes the stomach acid, raising the pH into the optimal range for the action of the intestinal enzymes.

   1. **Digestion by pancreatic enzymes** (see Figure 5-10)
      a. The pancreas secretes an **α-amylase** that acts in the lumen of the small intestine and, like salivary amylase, cleaves α-1,4 linkages between glucose residues.
      b. The products of pancreatic α-amylase are the disaccharides maltose and isomaltase, trisaccharides, and small oligosaccharides containing α-1,4 and α-1,6 linkages.

   2. **Digestion by enzymes of intestinal cells**
      – **Complexes of enzymes**, produced by intestinal epithelial cells and located in their **brush borders**, continue the digestion of carbohydrates (see Figure 5-10).
      a. **Glucoamylase (an α-glucosidase)** and other **maltases** cleave glucose residues from the nonreducing ends of oligosaccharides and also cleave the α-1,4 bond of maltose, releasing the two glucose residues.
      b. **Isomaltase** cleaves α-1,6 linkages, releasing glucose residues from branched oligosaccharides.
      c. **Sucrase** converts sucrose to glucose and fructose.
      d. **Lactase** (a β-galactosidase) converts lactose to glucose and galactose.

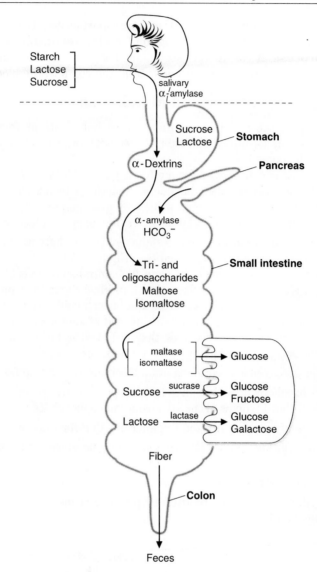

Figure 5-10. Digestion of carbohydrates. Starch is digested by salivary and pancreatic α-amylases and intestinal cell maltase and isomaltase. Sucrose and lactose are digested by intestinal enzymes.

D. Carbohydrates that cannot be digested

– Indigestible polysaccharides are part of the **dietary fiber** that passes through the intestine into the feces. For example, because enzymes produced by human cells cannot cleave the β-1,4 bonds of cellulose, this polysaccharide is indigestible.

E. Absorption of glucose, fructose, and galactose

– Glucose, fructose, and galactose, the final products generated by digestion of dietary carbohydrates, are absorbed by intestinal epithelial cells.

1. They are transported into the cells on **transport proteins,** moving down a concentration gradient.

2. Glucose also moves into cells on a transport protein that carries sodium ions in addition to the monosaccharide. This is **a secondary active transport process**. A Na$^+$-K$^+$ ATPase pumps Na$^+$ into the blood, and glucose moves down a concentration gradient from the cell into the blood.

IV. Glycogen Structure and Metabolism

- Glycogen, the major storage form of carbohydrate in animals, consists of chains of α-1,4-linked glucose residues with branches that are attached by α-1,6 linkages.
- Glycogen is synthesized from glucose (Figure 5-11).
  - UDP-glucose supplies the glucose moieties, which are added to the nonreducing ends of a glycogen primer by glycogen synthase.
  - Branches are produced by the branching enzyme, glucosyl 4:6 transferase.
- Glycogen degradation produces glucose 1-phosphate as the major product, but free glucose is also formed (see Figure 5-11).
  - Glucose units are removed from the nonreducing ends of glycogen chains by glycogen phosphorylase, which produces glucose 1-phosphate.
  - Three of the four glucose units at a branch point are moved by a glucosyl 4:4 transferase to the nonreducing end of another chain.
  - The remaining glucose unit that is linked α-1,6 at the branch point is released as free glucose by an α-1,6-glucosidase.
- Liver glycogen is used to maintain blood glucose during fasting or exercise.
  - Its breakdown is stimulated by glucagon and by epinephrine via a mechanism that involves cyclic adenosine monophosphate (cAMP).
- Muscle glycogen is utilized to generate ATP for muscle contraction.
  - Epinephrine, via cAMP, stimulates muscle glycogen breakdown.

A. Glycogen structure

- **Glycogen** is a large, **branched polymer** consisting of D-glucose residues (Figure 5-12).

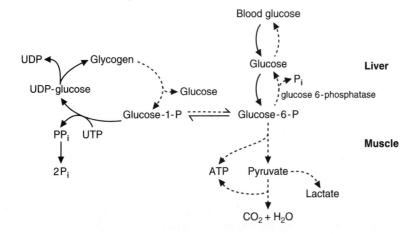

Figure 5-11. Overview of glycogen synthesis and degradation. *Solid arrows* = glycogen synthesis; *broken arrows* = glycogen degradation.

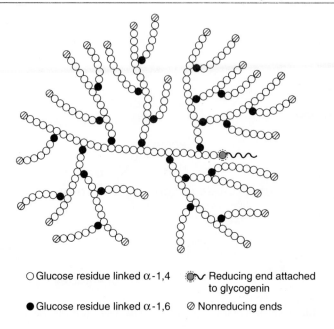

○ Glucose residue linked α-1,4   Reducing end attached
to glycogenin

● Glucose residue linked α-1,6   ⊘ Nonreducing ends

Figure 5-12. The structure of glycogen.

1. The **linkages** between glucose residues are **α-1,4** except at branch points where the linkage is **α-1,6.** Branching is more frequent in the interior of the molecule and less frequent at the periphery, the average being an α-1,6 branch every 8–10 residues.

2. One glucose unit, located at the reducing end of each glycogen molecule, is attached to the protein **glycogenin.**

3. The glycogen molecule branches like a tree and has **many nonreducing ends** at which addition and release of glucose residues occur during synthesis and degradation, respectively.

B. Glycogen synthesis

– **UDP-glucose** is the **precursor** for glycogen synthesis.

1. **Synthesis of UDP-glucose** (Figure 5-13)

a. Glucose enters cells and is phosphorylated to glucose 6-phosphate by **hexokinase** (or by **glucokinase** in the liver). ATP provides the phosphate group.

b. **Phosphoglucomutase** converts glucose 6-phosphate to glucose 1-phosphate.

c. Glucose 1-phosphate reacts with UTP, forming **UDP-glucose** in a reaction catalyzed by **UDP- glucose pyrophosphorylase.** Inorganic pyrophosphate (PP$_i$) is released in this reaction.

– **PP$_i$** is cleaved by a pyrophosphatase to 2 P$_i$. This removal of product helps to drive the process in the direction of glycogen synthesis.

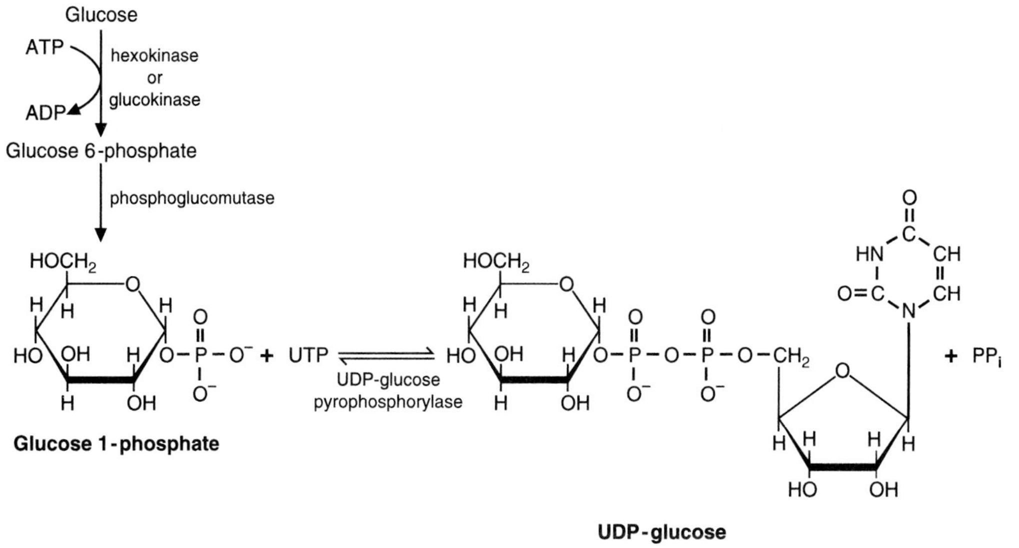

Figure 5-13. Formation of uridine diphosphate glucose (UDP-glucose) from glucose.

2. Action of glycogen synthase (Figure 5-14A)

a. Glycogen synthase is the key regulatory enzyme for glycogen synthesis. It transfers glucose residues from UDP-glucose to the nonreducing ends of a glycogen primer.
  – UDP is released and reconverted to UTP by reaction with ATP.

b. The primers, which are attached to glycogenin, are glycogen molecules that were partially degraded in liver during fasting or in muscle and liver during exercise.

3. Formation of branches (see Figure 5-14A)

a. When a chain contains 11 or more glucose residues, an **oligomer,** 6–8 residues in length, is removed from the nonreducing end of the chain. It is **reattached** via an **α-1,6 linkage** to a glucose residue within an α-1,4-linked chain.

b. These branches are formed by the branching enzyme, a **glucosyl 4:6 transferase** that breaks an α-1,4 bond and forms an α-1,6 bond.

c. The new branch points are at least 4 residues and an average of 7–11 residues from previously existing branch points.

4. Growth of glycogen chains

a. Glycogen synthase continues to add glucose residues to the nonreducing ends of newly formed branches as well as to the ends of the original chains.

b. As the chains continue to grow, additional branches are produced by the branching enzyme.

C. Glycogen degradation (see Figure 5-14B)

1. Action of glycogen phosphorylase

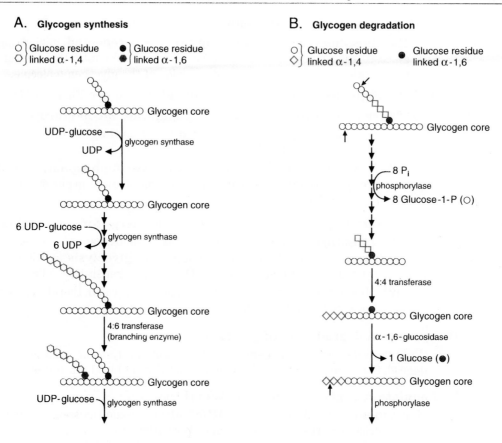

Figure 5-14. Glycogen synthesis and degradation.

a. Glycogen phosphorylase, the key regulatory enzyme for glycogen degradation, removes glucose residues, one at a time, from the nonreducing ends of glycogen molecules.

b. Phosphorylase uses inorganic phosphate (P_i) to cleave α-1,4 bonds, producing **glucose 1-phosphate.**

c. Phosphorylase can act only until it is four glucose units from a branch point.

2. Removal of branches

– The four units remaining at a branch are removed by the **debranching enzyme,** which has both glucosyl 4:4 transferase and α-1,6-glucosidase activity.

a. Three of the four glucose residues that remain at the branch point are removed as a trisaccharide and attached to the nonreducing end of another chain by a **4:4 transferase**, which cleaves an α-1,4 bond and forms a new α-1,4 bond.

b. The last glucose unit at the branch point, which is linked α-1,6, is hydrolyzed by **α-1,6-glucosidase**, forming free glucose.

3. **Degradation of glycogen chains**
   – The **phosphorylase/debranching process is repeated,** generating glucose 1-phosphate and free glucose in about a 10:1 ratio that reflects the length of the chains in the outer region of the glycogen molecule.

4. **Fate of glucosyl units released from glycogen** (see Figure 5-11)
   a. In the **liver,** glycogen is degraded to **maintain blood glucose.**
      (1) Glucose 1-phosphate is converted by **phosphoglucomutase** to glucose 6-phosphate.
      (2) Inorganic phosphate is released by **glucose 6-phosphatase,** and free glucose enters the blood. This enzyme also acts in gluconeogenesis (see VI A 3).

   b. In **muscle,** glycogen is degraded to provide **energy for contraction.**
      (1) Phosphoglucomutase converts glucose 1-phosphate to glucose 6-phosphate, which enters the pathway of **glycolysis** and is converted either to lactate or to CO_2 and H_2O, generating ATP.
      (2) Muscle does not contain glucose 6- phosphatase and, therefore, does not contribute to the maintenance of blood glucose.

D. **Lysosomal degradation of glycogen**
   – Glycogen is degraded by an **α-glucosidase** located in lysosomes. Lysosomal degradation is not necessary for maintaining normal blood glucose levels.

E. **Regulation of glycogen degradation** (Figure 5-15)
   – **Hormones** that use **3′,5′-cyclic AMP** (cAMP) as a second messenger stimulate a mechanism, resulting in the phosphorylation of enzymes.
   – Glycogen degradation is stimulated, and synthesis is inhibited when the enzymes of glycogen metabolism are phosphorylated.

1. **Glucagon** acts on liver cells and **epinephrine** (adrenaline) acts on both liver and muscle cells to stimulate glycogen degradation.
   – These hormones via G proteins activate **adenylate cyclase** in the cell membrane, which converts ATP to cAMP (Figure 5-16).
   – Adenylate cyclase is also called adenyl or adenylyl cyclase.

2. cAMP **activates protein kinase A** (see Figure 5-15), which consists of two regulatory and two catalytic subunits. cAMP binds to the regulatory (inhibitory) subunits, releasing the catalytic subunits in an active form.

3. **Protein kinase A** phosphorylates **glycogen synthase,** causing it to be less active, thus decreasing glycogen synthesis.

4. **Protein kinase A** phosphorylates **phosphorylase kinase.**

5. **Phosphorylase kinase** phosphorylates **phosphorylase b,** converting it to its active form, phosphorylase a.

6. **Phosphorylase a** cleaves glucose residues from the nonreducing ends of glycogen chains, producing glucose 1-phosphate, which is oxidized or, in the liver, converted to blood glucose.

7. **The cAMP cascade**
   – The cAMP-activated process is a cascade in which the initial **hormonal signal is amplified** many times.

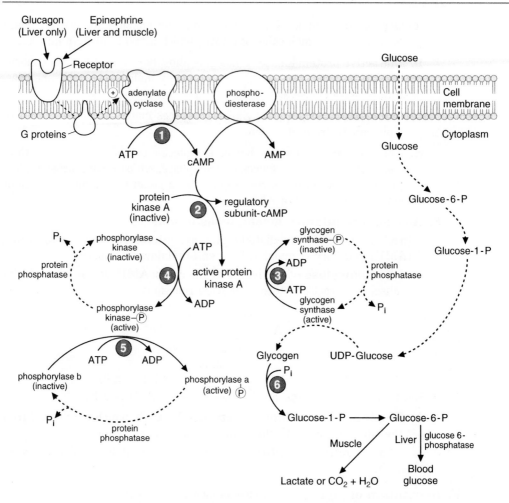

Figure 5-15. Hormonal regulation of glycogen synthesis and degradation. *Solid lines* indicate reactions that predominate when glucagon or epinephrine is elevated. Steps 1 through 6, indicated by *circled numbers,* correspond to IV E 1-6 in the text. *Dashed lines* indicate reactions that predominate when insulin is elevated. Note that protein kinase A phosphorylates both phosphorylase kinase and glycogen synthase.

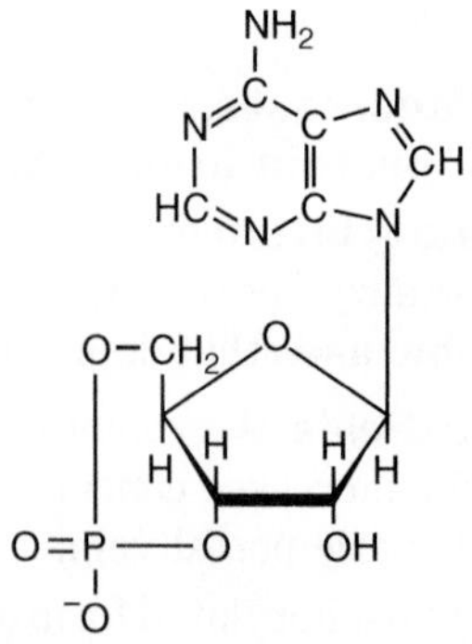

Figure 5-16. Cyclic adenosine monophosphate (cAMP).

a. One hormone molecule, by activating the enzyme adenylate cyclase, produces many molecules of cAMP, which activate protein kinase A.

b. One active protein kinase A molecule phosphorylates many phosphorylase kinase molecules, which convert many molecules of phosphorylase b to phosphorylase a.

c. One molecule of phosphorylase a produces many molecules of glucose 1-phosphate from glycogen.

d. The net result is that one hormone molecule can generate tens of thousands of molecules of glucose 1-phosphate, which form glucose 6-phosphate. Oxidation of glucose 6-phosphate generates hundreds of thousands of molecules of ATP.

8. Additional **regulatory mechanisms in muscle**

   – In addition to cAMP-mediated regulation, **adenosine monophosphate (AMP)** and **Ca^{2+}** stimulate glycogen breakdown in muscle.

   a. Phosphorylase b is activated by the rise in **AMP,** which occurs during muscle contraction by the following reactions:

$$2\ \text{ATP} \xrightarrow{\text{contraction}} 2\ \text{ADP} + 2\ P_i$$

$$2\ \text{ADP} \xrightarrow[\text{(myokinase)}]{\text{adenylate kinase}} \text{AMP} + \text{ATP}$$

$$\text{Sum: ATP} \longrightarrow \text{AMP} + 2\ P_i$$

   b. Phosphorylase kinase is activated by **Ca^{2+}**, which is released from the sarcoplasmic reticulum during muscle contraction.

   – Ca^{2+} binds to **calmodulin**, which serves as a subunit of phosphorylase kinase.

F. Regulation of glycogen synthesis (see Figure 5-15)

   – **Insulin,** which is elevated after a meal, stimulates the synthesis of glycogen in liver and muscle.

1. **Factors that promote glycogen synthesis in the liver**

   a. In the fed state, glycogen degradation decreases because **glucagon** is **low,** and the cAMP cascade is not activated.

   (1) cAMP is converted to AMP by a cell membrane **phosphodiesterase**.

   (2) As **cAMP decreases**, the regulatory subunits rejoin the catalytic subunits of **protein kinase A**, and the enzyme is **inactivated**.

   (3) Dephosphorylation of phosphorylase kinase and phosphorylase a causes these enzymes to be inactivated. **Insulin** causes activation of the **phosphatases** that dephosphorylate these enzymes.

   b. Glycogen synthesis is promoted by activation of **glycogen synthase** and by the increased concentration of glucose, which enters liver cells from the hepatic portal vein.

   – The inactive, phosphorylated form of glycogen synthase is dephosphorylated, causing the enzyme to become active. **Insulin** causes activation of the **phosphatase** that catalyzes this reaction.

2. Factors that promote glycogen synthesis in muscle

    a. After a meal, muscle will have low levels of cAMP, AMP, and Ca^{2+} if it is not contracting and epinephrine is low. Consequently, muscle glycogen degradation will not occur.

    b. Insulin stimulates glycogen synthesis by mechanisms similar to those in the liver.

    c. In addition, **insulin stimulates the transport of glucose** into muscle cells, providing increased substrate for glycogen synthesis.

V. Glycolysis

- Glycolysis is the pathway by which glucose is converted to pyruvate. It occurs in the cytosol of all cells of the body.
- In the initial reactions, a hexose is phosphorylated twice by ATP and then cleaved to yield two triose phosphates.
  - Glucose is phosphorylated to glucose 6-phosphate, which is isomerized to fructose 6-phosphate.
  - Fructose 6-phosphate is phosphorylated by the key regulatory enzyme, phosphofructokinase. The product is fructose 1,6-bisphosphate, which is cleaved, forming two triose phosphates.
- In the second sequence of reactions, the triose phosphates produce ATP.
- Overall, glycolysis produces ATP, NADH, and pyruvate.
  - ATP is produced directly by reactions catalyzed by phosphoglycerate kinase and pyruvate kinase.
  - Although NADH produced in the cytosol cannot directly enter mitochondria, reducing equivalents can be shuttled into this organelle, where they generate ATP.
  - Pyruvate can enter mitochondria and be converted to acetyl CoA, which is oxidized by the tricarboxylic acid (TCA) cycle, generating additional ATP.
  - Pyruvate can also be converted to oxaloacetate by a reaction that replenishes intermediates of the TCA cycle, and it can be reduced to lactate or transaminated to alanine.

A. Transport of glucose into cells

    1. Glucose travels across the cell membrane on a **transport protein**.

    2. Insulin stimulates glucose transport into **muscle** and **adipose** cells by causing glucose transport proteins (GLUT 4) within cells to move to the cell membrane (Table 5-1).

Table 5-1. Effect of Insulin on Glucose Transport Systems of Various Tissues

Tissues	Insulin Effect on Glucose Transport
Liver	0
Brain	0
Red blood cell	0
Adipose	+
Muscle	+

0 indicates no effect; + indicates stimulation.

3. Insulin does not significantly stimulate the transport of glucose into tissues such as liver, brain, and red blood cells.

B. Reactions of glycolysis (Figure 5-17)

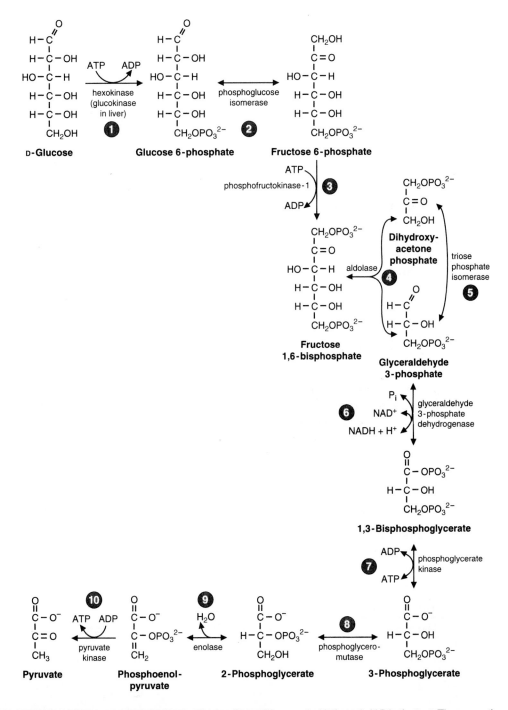

Figure 5-17. The reactions of glycolysis. The numbers correspond with those in V B in the text. These reactions occur in the cytosol.

1. **Glucose** is converted to glucose 6-phosphate in a reaction that uses ATP and produces ADP.
   - Enzymes: **hexokinase** in all tissues and, in the liver, **glucokinase.** Both of these enzymes are subject to regulatory mechanisms.

2. **Glucose 6-phosphate** is isomerized to fructose 6-phosphate.
   - Enzyme: **phosphoglucose isomerase**

3. **Fructose 6-phosphate** is phosphorylated by ATP, forming fructose 1,6-bisphosphate and ADP. This reaction is the first committed step in glycolysis.
   - Enzyme: **phosphofructokinase 1** (PFK1)
   - PFK1 is regulated by a number of effectors.

4. **Fructose 1,6-bisphosphate** is cleaved to form the triose phosphates, glyceraldehyde 3-phosphate and dihydroxyacetone phosphate (DHAP).
   - Enzyme: **aldolase**

5. **Dihydroxyacetone phosphate** is isomerized to glyceraldehyde 3-phosphate.
   - Enzyme: **triose phosphate isomerase**
   Note: *The net result of reactions 1 through 5 is that two moles of glyceraldehyde 3-phosphate are formed from one mole of glucose.*

6. **Glyceraldehyde 3-phosphate** is oxidized by NAD^+ and reacts with inorganic phosphate (P_i) to form 1,3-bisphosphoglycerate and $NADH + H^+$.
   - Enzyme: **glyceraldehyde 3-phosphate dehydrogenase**
   - The aldehyde group of glyceraldehyde 3-phosphate is oxidized to a carboxylic acid, which forms a high-energy anhydride with inorganic phosphate.

7. **1,3-Bisphosphoglycerate** reacts with ADP to produce 3-phosphoglycerate and **ATP.**
   - Enzyme: **phosphoglycerate kinase**

8. **3-Phosphoglycerate** is converted to 2-phosphoglycerate by transfer of the phosphate group from carbon 3 to carbon 2.
   - Enzyme: **phosphoglyceromutase**

9. **2-Phosphoglycerate** is dehydrated to phosphoenolpyruvate (PEP), which contains a high-energy enol phosphate.
   - Enzyme: **enolase**

10. **Phosphoenolpyruvate** reacts with ADP to form **pyruvate** and **ATP** in the last reaction of glycolysis.
    - Enzyme: **pyruvate kinase.** Pyruvate kinase is more active in the fed state than in the fasting state.

C. **Special reactions in red blood cells**

1. In red blood cells, 1,3-bisphosphoglycerate can be converted to **2,3-bisphosphoglycerate** (BPG), a compound that decreases the affinity of hemoglobin for oxygen.

2. 2,3-Bisphosphoglycerate is dephosphorylated to form inorganic phosphate and 3-phosphoglycerate, an intermediate that reenters the glycolytic pathway.

D. Regulatory enzymes of glycolysis (Figure 5-18)

1. **Hexokinase** is found in most tissues and is geared to provide glucose 6-phosphate for ATP production even when blood glucose is low.

   a. Hexokinase has a **low K_m** for glucose (about 0.1 mM). Therefore, it is working near its maximum rate (V_{max}), even at fasting blood glucose levels (about 5 mM).

   b. Hexokinase is **inhibited** by its product, **glucose 6-phosphate**. Therefore, it is most active when glucose 6-phosphate is being rapidly utilized.

2. **Glucokinase** is found in the **liver** and functions at a significant rate only after a meal.

   a. Glucokinase has a **high K_m** for glucose (about 6 mM). Therefore, it is very **active after a meal** when glucose levels in the hepatic portal vein are high, and it is relatively inactive during fasting when glucose levels are low.

   b. Glucokinase is **induced** when insulin levels are high.

   c. Glucokinase is not inhibited by its product, glucose 6-phosphate, at physiologic concentrations.

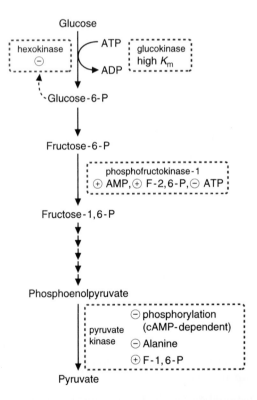

Figure 5-18. Regulation of glycolysis. In muscle, PFK1 is the key enzyme. It is activated (⊕) by AMP and inhibited (⊖) by ATP and citrate. In liver, glucokinase, PFK1 (activated by fructose 2,6-bisphosphate [F-2,6-P]), and pyruvate kinase are the key enzymes.

3. **Phosphofructokinase 1 (PFK1)** is regulated by several factors. It functions at a rapid rate in the liver when blood glucose is high or in cells such as muscle when there is a need for ATP.

   a. PFK1 is **activated by fructose 2,6-bisphosphate,** an important regulatory mechanism in the liver (Figure 5-19).

      (1) After a meal, fructose 2,6-bisphosphate (F-2,6-P) is formed from fructose 6-phosphate by **phosphofructokinase 2 (PFK2)**.

      (2) F-2,6-P activates PFK1, and **glycolysis is stimulated.** The liver is using glycolysis to produce fatty acids for triacylglycerol synthesis.

      (3) In the fasting state (when glucagon is elevated), **PFK2** is phosphorylated by **protein kinase A,** which is activated by cAMP.

      (4) Phosphorylated PFK2 converts fructose 2,6-bisphosphate to fructose 6-phosphate. Fructose 2,6-bisphosphate levels fall, and **PFK1** is **less active**.

      (5) In the fed state, insulin causes **phosphatases** to be stimulated. A phosphatase dephosphorylates PFK2, causing it to become more active in forming fructose 2,6-bisphosphate from fructose 6-phosphate. Fructose 2,6-bisphosphate levels rise, and **PFK1** is **more active**.

      (6) Thus, **PFK2** acts as a **kinase** (in the **fed state** when it is dephosphorylated) and as a **phosphatase** (in the **fasting state** when it is phosphorylated). PFK2 catalyzes two different reactions.

   b. PFK1 is **activated by AMP,** an important regulatory mechanism in **muscle** (see Figure 5-18).

      (1) In muscle during **exercise,** AMP levels are high and ATP levels are low.

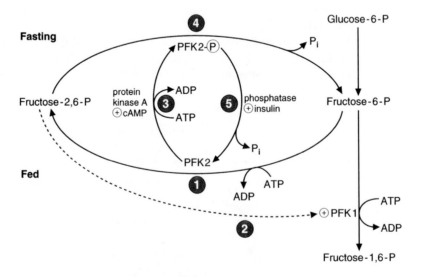

Figure 5-19. Regulation of fructose 2,6-bisphosphate levels in the liver. Fructose-2,6-P is an activator of phosphofructokinase 1 (*PFK1*), which converts fructose 6-phosphate to fructose 1,6- bisphosphate. Phosphofructokinase 2 *(PFK2)* acts as a kinase in the fed state and as a phosphatase during fasting. It regulates the cellular levels of fructose 2,6-phosphate. The *circled numbers* correspond with (1) to (5) under V D 3 a in the text.

(2) Glycolysis is promoted by a more active PFK1, and ATP is generated.

  c. PFK1 is **inhibited** by **ATP** and **citrate,** important regulatory mechanisms in **muscle.**

    (1) When ATP is high, the cell does not need ATP, and glycolysis is inhibited.

    (2) High levels of citrate indicate that adequate amounts of substrate are entering the TCA cycle. Therefore, glycolysis slows down.

  4. Pyruvate kinase

    a. Pyruvate kinase is **activated** by **fructose 1,6-bisphosphate** and **inhibited** by **alanine** and by **phosphorylation** in the liver **during fasting** when glucagon levels are high (see Figure 5-18).

      (1) Glucagon via cAMP activates **protein kinase A**, which phosphorylates and inactivates pyruvate kinase.

      (2) The inhibition of pyruvate kinase promotes gluconeogenesis.

    b. Pyruvate kinase is **activated in the fed state.**

      – Insulin stimulates phosphatases that dephosphorylate and activate pyruvate kinase.

E. The fate of pyruvate (Figure 5-20)

  1. Conversion to lactate

    – Pyruvate can be reduced in the cytosol by NADH, forming **lactate,** and regenerating NAD^+.

    a. NADH, which is produced by glycolysis, must be reconverted to NAD^+ so that carbons of glucose can continue to flow through glycolysis.

    b. Lactate dehydrogenase (**LDH**) converts pyruvate to lactate. LDH consists of four subunits that can be either of the muscle (M) or the heart (H) type.

      (1) Five isozymes occur (MMMM, MMMH, MMHH, MHHH, and HHHH), which can be separated by electrophoresis.

      (2) Different tissues have different mixtures of these isozymes.

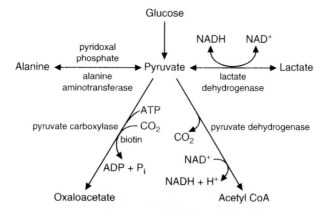

Figure 5-20. The fate of pyruvate.

c. Lactate is released by tissues (e.g., red blood cells or exercising muscle) and is used by the liver for gluconeogenesis or by tissues such as the heart and kidney where it is converted to pyruvate and oxidized for energy.

d. The **LDH** reaction is **reversible.**

2. Conversion to acetyl CoA

– Pyruvate can enter mitochondria and be converted by **pyruvate dehydrogenase** to acetyl CoA, which can enter the TCA cycle.

3. Conversion to oxaloacetate

– Pyruvate can be converted to oxaloacetate by **pyruvate carboxylase,** an enzyme found in tissues such as the liver and brain, but not in muscle.
– This reaction serves to replenish intermediates of the TCA cycle.

4. Conversion to alanine

– Pyruvate can be transaminated to form the amino acid **alanine.**

F. Generation of ATP by glycolysis

1. Production of ATP and NADH in the glycolytic pathway

– Overall, when 1 mole of glucose is converted to 2 moles of pyruvate, 2 moles of ATP are used in the process, and 4 moles of ATP are produced, for a net yield of 2 moles of ATP. In addition, 2 moles of cytosolic NADH are generated

2. Energy generated by conversion of glucose to lactate (Figure 5-21)

– If the NADH generated by glycolysis is used to reduce pyruvate to lactate, the net yield is 2 moles of ATP per mole of glucose converted to lactate.

3. Energy generated by conversion of glucose to CO_2 and H_2O (Figure 5-22)

– When glucose is oxidized completely to CO_2 and H_2O, approximately 36 or 38 moles of ATP are generated.

a. Two moles of ATP and 2 moles of NADH are generated from the conversion of 1 mole of glucose to 2 moles of pyruvate.

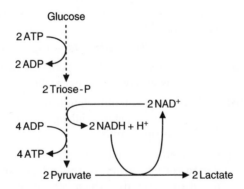

Figure 5-21. Conversion of one molecule of glucose to lactate produces two molecules of adenosine triphosphate (ATP) (net). The NADH produced by glycolysis is used to convert pyruvate to lactate.

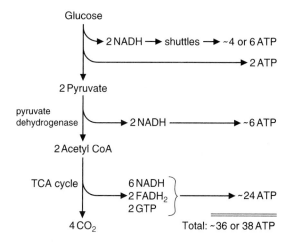

Figure 5-22. Adenosine triphosphate (ATP) produced by conversion of glucose to CO_2. The ATP produced by oxidative phosphorylation is approximate (indicated by ~).

b. The 2 moles of pyruvate enter the mitochondria and are converted to 2 moles of acetyl CoA, producing 2 moles of NADH, which generate approximately 6 moles of ATP by oxidative phosphorylation.

c. The 2 moles of acetyl CoA are oxidized in the TCA cycle, generating approximately 24 moles of ATP.

d. NADH, produced in the cytosol by glycolysis, cannot directly cross the mitochondrial membrane. Therefore, the electrons are passed to the mitochondrial electron transport chain by two shuttle systems.

(1) Glycerol phosphate shuttle (Figure 5-23, *left side*)

    (a) Cytosolic DHAP is reduced to glycerol-3-phosphate by NADH.

    (b) Glycerol-3-phosphate reacts with an FAD-linked dehydrogenase in the inner mitochondrial membrane. DHAP is regenerated and re-enters the cytosol.

    (c) Each mole of $FADH_2$ that is produced generates approximately 2 moles of ATP via oxidative phosphorylation.

    (d) Because glycolysis produces 2 moles of NADH per mole of glucose, approximately **4 moles of ATP are produced by this shuttle.**

(2) Malate aspartate shuttle (see Figure 5-23, *right side*)

    (a) Cytosolic oxaloacetate is reduced to malate by NADH. The reaction is catalyzed by cytosolic malate dehydrogenase.

    (b) Malate enters the mitochondrion and is re-oxidized to oxaloacetate by the mitochondrial malate dehydrogenase, generating NADH in the matrix.

    (c) Oxaloacetate cannot cross the mitochondrial membrane. In order to return carbon to the cytosol, oxaloacetate is transaminated to aspartate, which can be transported into the cytosol and reconverted to oxaloacetate by another transamination reaction.

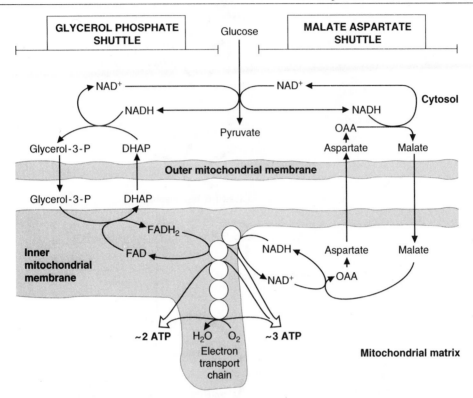

Figure 5-23. The glycerol phosphate and malate aspartate shuttles. *Left,* the glycerol phosphate shuttle produces $FADH_2$, each of which generates approximately 2 ATP by oxidative phosphorylation. *Right,* the malate aspartate shuttle produces NADH, each of which generates approximately 3 ATP. *DHAP* = dihydroxyacetone phosphate; *OAA* = oxaloacetate.

    (d) In the mitochondrial matrix, each mole of NADH generates approximately 3 moles of ATP via oxidative phosphorylation.

    (e) Because glycolysis produces 2 moles of NADH per mole of glucose, approximately **6 moles of ATP are produced by this shuttle.**

  c. Maximal ATP production

    – Overall, when 1 mole of glucose is oxidized to CO_2 and H_2O, approximately 36 moles of ATP are produced if the glycerol phosphate shuttle is used, or 38 moles if the malate aspartate shuttle is used.

VI. Gluconeogenesis (Figure 5-24)

- Gluconeogenesis, which occurs mainly in the liver, is the synthesis of glucose from compounds that are not carbohydrates.
- The major precursors for gluconeogenesis are lactate, amino acids (which form pyruvate or TCA cycle intermediates), and glycerol (which forms dihydroxyacetone phosphate). Even-chain fatty acids do not produce any net glucose.
- Gluconeogenesis involves several enzymatic steps that do not occur in glycolysis; thus glucose is not generated by a simple reversal of glycolysis.

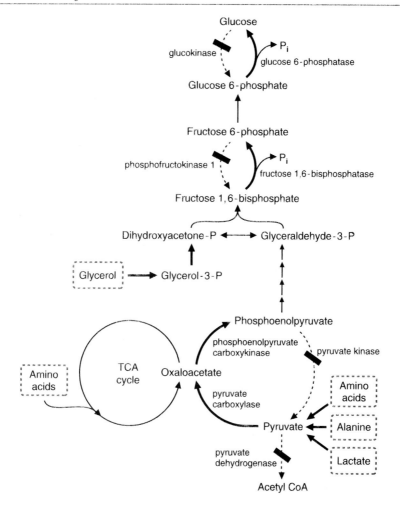

Figure 5-24. The key reactions of gluconeogenesis from the precursors alanine, lactate, and glycerol. *Heavy arrows* indicate steps that differ from those of glycolysis. *Broken arrows* are reactions that are inhibited (∎) under conditions in which gluconeogenesis is occurring.

- Pyruvate carboxylase converts pyruvate to oxaloacetate in the mitochondrion. Oxaloacetate is converted to malate or aspartate, which travels to the cytosol and is reconverted to oxaloacetate.
- Phosphoenolpyruvate carboxykinase converts oxaloacetate to phosphoenolpyruvate. Phosphoenolpyruvate forms fructose 1,6-bisphosphate by reversal of the steps of glycolysis.
- Fructose 1,6-bisphosphatase converts fructose 1,6-bisphosphate to fructose 6-phosphate, which is converted to glucose 6-phosphate.
- Glucose 6-phosphatase converts glucose 6-phosphate to free glucose, which is released into the blood.
- Gluconeogenesis occurs under conditions in which pyruvate dehydrogenase, pyruvate kinase, phosphofructokinase 1, and glucokinase are relatively inactive. The low activity of these enzymes prevents futile cycles from occurring and ensures that, overall, pyruvate is converted to glucose.

- The synthesis of 1 mole of glucose from 2 moles of pyruvate requires energy equivalent to about 6 moles of ATP.

A. Reactions of gluconeogenesis

1. Conversion of pyruvate to phosphoenolpyruvate (Figure 5-25)

– In the liver, pyruvate is converted to phosphoenolpyruvate.

a. Pyruvate (produced from lactate, alanine, and other amino acids) is first converted to oxaloacetate (OAA) by **pyruvate carboxylase**, a mitochondrial enzyme that requires biotin and ATP.

– Oxaloacetate cannot directly cross the inner mitochondrial membrane. Therefore, it is converted to malate or to aspartate, which can cross the mitochondrial membrane and be reconverted to OAA in the cytosol.

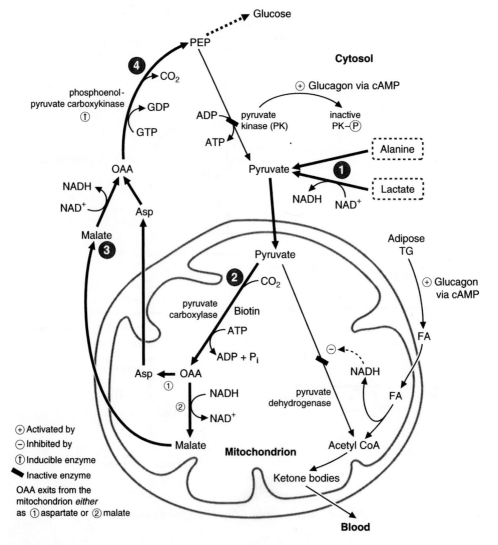

Figure 5-25. The conversion of pyruvate to phosphoenolpyruvate (PEP). Follow the diagram by starting with the precursors alanine and lactate. *FA* = fatty acid; *OAA* = oxaloacetate; *TG* = triacylglycerol.

    b. Oxaloacetate is decarboxylated by **phosphoenolpyruvate car-boxykinase** to form phosphoenolpyruvate. This reaction requires GTP.

    c. Phosphoenolpyruvate is converted to fructose 1,6-bisphosphate by reversal of the glycolytic reactions (Figure 5-26).

2. Conversion of fructose 1,6-bisphosphate to fructose 6-phosphate (see Figure 5-26)

    a. Fructose 1,6-bisphosphate is converted to fructose 6-phosphate in a reaction that releases inorganic phosphate and is catalyzed by fructose **1,6-bisphosphatase**.

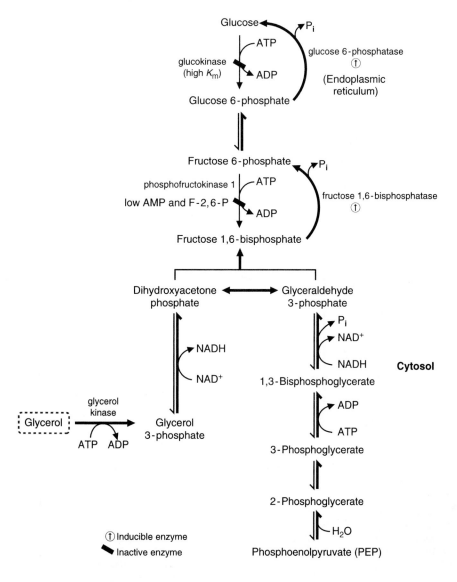

Figure 5-26. The conversion of phosphoenolpyruvate and glycerol to glucose. *Heavy arrows* indicate the pathway. *F-2,6-P* = fructose-2,6-bisphosphate.

    b. Fructose 6-phosphate is converted to glucose 6- phosphate by the same isomerase used in glycolysis.

  3. Conversion of glucose 6-phosphate to glucose

    a. Glucose 6-phosphate releases inorganic phosphate, which produces free glucose that enters the blood. The enzyme is **glucose 6-phosphatase**.

    b. Glucose 6-phosphatase is involved both in **gluconeogenesis and glycogenolysis** (see Figure 5-15).

B. Regulatory enzymes of gluconeogenesis

  – Under fasting conditions, **glucagon** is elevated and stimulates gluconeogenesis. Because of changes in the activity of certain enzymes, futile cycles are prevented from occurring, and the overall flow of carbon is from pyruvate to glucose (see Figures 5-25 and 5-26).

  – A futile cycle is the continuous recycling of substrates and products with the net consumption of energy and no useful result.

  1. Pyruvate dehydrogenase (see Figure 5-25)

    a. Decreased insulin and increased glucagon stimulate the **release of fatty acids** from adipose tissue.

    b. Fatty acids travel to the liver and **are oxidized,** producing acetyl CoA, NADH, and ATP, which cause inactivation of pyruvate dehydrogenase.

    c. Because **pyruvate dehydrogenase** is relatively **inactive,** pyruvate is converted to oxaloacetate, not to acetyl CoA.

  2. Pyruvate carboxylase

    a. Pyruvate carboxylase, which converts pyruvate to oxaloacetate, is **activated by acetyl CoA.**

    b. Note that pyruvate carboxylase is active in both the fed and fasting states.

  3. Phosphoenolpyruvate carboxykinase (PEPCK)

    a. PEPCK is an **inducible** enzyme.

    b. Transcription of the gene encoding PEPCK is stimulated by binding of proteins that are phosphorylated in response to cAMP and by binding of glucocorticoid-protein complexes to regulatory elements in the gene.

    c. Increased production of PEPCK mRNA leads to increased translation, resulting in higher PEPCK levels in the cell.

  4. Pyruvate kinase

    a. Glucagon, via cAMP and protein kinase A, causes pyruvate kinase to be phosphorylated and **inactivated.**

    b. Because pyruvate kinase is relatively inactive, phosphoenolpyruvate formed from oxaloacetate is not reconverted to pyruvate but, in a series of steps, forms fructose 1,6-bisphosphate, which is converted to fructose 6-phosphate.

5. **Phosphofructokinase 1** (see Figure 5-26)

   – Phosphofructokinase 1 is relatively **inactive** because the concentrations of its activators, AMP and fructose 2,6-bisphosphate, are low and its inhibitor, ATP, is relatively high.

6. **Fructose 1,6-bisphosphatase**

   a. The level of **fructose 2,6-bisphosphate,** an inhibitor of fructose 1,6-bisphosphatase, is **low** during fasting. Therefore, fructose 1,6- bisphosphatase is **more active.**

   b. Fructose 1,6-bisphosphatase is also **induced** in the fasting state.

7. **Glucokinase**

   – **Glucokinase** is relatively **inactive** because it has a **high K_m** for glucose, and under conditions that favor gluconeogenesis, the glucose concentration is low. Therefore, free glucose is not reconverted to glucose 6-phosphate

C. **Precursors for gluconeogenesis**

   – Lactate, amino acids, and glycerol are the major precursors for gluconeogenesis in humans.

   1. **Lactate** is oxidized by NAD^+ in a reaction catalyzed by lactate dehydrogenase to form pyruvate, which can be converted to glucose (see Figure 5-25).
      – Sources of lactate include red blood cells and exercising muscle.

   2. **Amino acids** for gluconeogenesis come from degradation of muscle protein.

      a. Amino acids are released directly into the blood from muscle, or carbons from amino acids are converted to alanine and glutamine and released.
         – **Alanine** is also formed by transamination of pyruvate that is derived by oxidation of glucose.
         – **Glutamine** is converted to alanine by tissues such as gut and kidney.

      b. Amino acids travel to the liver and provide carbon for gluconeogenesis. Quantitatively, **alanine is the major gluconeogenic amino acid**.

      c. Amino acid **nitrogen** is converted to **urea**.

   3. **Glycerol,** which is derived from **adipose** triacylglycerols, reacts with ATP to form glycerol 3-phosphate, which is oxidized to dihydroxyacetone phosphate and converted to glucose (see Figure 5-26).

D. **Role of fatty acids in gluconeogenesis**

   1. **Even-chain fatty acids**

      a. Fatty acids are oxidized to acetyl CoA, which enters the TCA cycle.

      b. For every two carbons of acetyl CoA that enter the TCA cycle, two carbons are released as CO_2. Therefore, there is **no net synthesis of glucose from acetyl CoA.**

      c. The pyruvate dehydrogenase reaction is irreversible, thus acetyl CoA cannot be converted to pyruvate.

    d. Although even-chain fatty acids do not provide carbons for gluconeogenesis, β-oxidation of fatty acids provides **ATP** that drives gluconeogenesis.

  2. Odd-chain fatty acids

    – The three carbons at the ω-end of an odd-chain fatty acid are converted to propionate. **Propionate** enters the TCA cycle as succinyl CoA, which forms **malate,** an intermediate in glucose formation (see Figure 5-25).

E. Energy requirements for gluconeogenesis

  1. From pyruvate (see Figures 5-25 and 5-26)

    a. Conversion of pyruvate to oxaloacetate by pyruvate carboxylase requires one ATP.

    b. Conversion of oxaloacetate to phosphoenolpyruvate by phosphoenolpyruvate carboxykinase requires one GTP (the equivalent of one ATP).

    c. Conversion of 3-phosphoglycerate to 1,3- bisphosphoglycerate by phosphoglycerate kinase requires one ATP.

    d. Since 2 moles of pyruvate are required to form 1 mole of glucose, **6 moles of high-energy phosphate are required for synthesis of 1 mole of glucose.**

  2. From glycerol (see Figure 5-26)

    – Glycerol enters the gluconeogenic pathway at the dihydroxyacetone phosphate (DHAP) level.

    a. Conversion of glycerol to glycerol 3-phosphate, which is oxidized to DHAP, requires one ATP.

    b. Since 2 moles of glycerol are required to form 1 mole of glucose, 2 moles of high-energy phosphate are required for synthesis of 1 mole of glucose.

VII. Fructose and Galactose Metabolism

- Although glucose is the most abundant monosaccharide derived from the diet, fructose and galactose are usually obtained in significant quantities, mainly from sucrose and lactose.
- After fructose and galactose enter cells, they are phosphorylated on carbon 1 and converted to intermediates in pathways of glucose metabolism.
- Fructose is metabolized mainly in the liver, where it is converted to fructose 1-phosphate and cleaved to produce dihydroxyacetone phosphate and glyceraldehyde, which is phosphorylated to glyceraldehyde 3-phosphate. These two triose phosphates are intermediates of glycolysis.
- Fructose can be produced from sorbitol, which is generated from glucose.
- Galactose is phosphorylated to galactose 1-phosphate, which reacts with UDP-glucose. The products are glucose 1-phosphate and UDP-galactose, which is epimerized to UDP-glucose. The net result is that galactose is converted to the glucose moieties of UDP-glucose and glucose 1-phosphate, intermediates in pathways of glucose metabolism.
  - UDP-galactose is used in the synthesis of glycoproteins, glycolipids, and proteoglycans.
  - UDP-galactose reacts with glucose in the mammary gland to form the milk sugar lactose.

- Galactose can be reduced to galactitol.

A. Metabolism of fructose

- The major dietary source of fructose is the disaccharide sucrose in table sugar and fruit, but it is also present as the monosaccharide in corn syrup, which is used as a sweetener.

1. **Conversion of fructose to glycolytic intermediates** (Figure 5-27)

   a. **Fructose** is metabolized mainly in the **liver** where it is converted to pyruvate or, under fasting conditions, to glucose.

      (1) Fructose is phosphorylated by ATP to form fructose 1-phosphate. The enzyme is **fructokinase.**

      (2) Fructose 1-phosphate is cleaved by **aldolase B** to form dihydroxyacetone phosphate (DHAP) and glyceraldehyde, which is phosphorylated by ATP to form glyceraldehyde 3-phosphate. DHAP and glyceraldehyde 3-phosphate are intermediates of glycolysis. (Aldolase B is the same liver enzyme that cleaves fructose 1,6-bisphosphate in glycolysis.)

   b. In tissues other than liver, the major fate of fructose is phosphorylation by hexokinase to form fructose 6-phosphate, which enters glycolysis. Hexokinase has an affinity for fructose about one-twentieth of that for glucose.

2. **Production of fructose from glucose**

   a. **Glucose** is reduced to sorbitol by **aldose reductase**, which reduces the aldehyde group to an alcohol (Figure 5-28).

   b. **Sorbitol** is then reoxidized at carbon 2 by sorbitol dehydrogenase to form fructose.

   c. **Fructose,** derived from glucose in seminal vesicles, is the major energy source for sperm cells.

B. Metabolism of galactose

- The disaccharide **lactose**, found in milk or milk products, is the major dietary source of galactose.

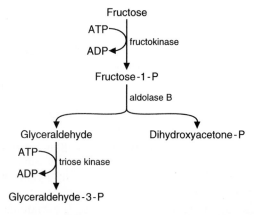

Figure 5-27. Conversion of fructose to intermediates of glycolysis.

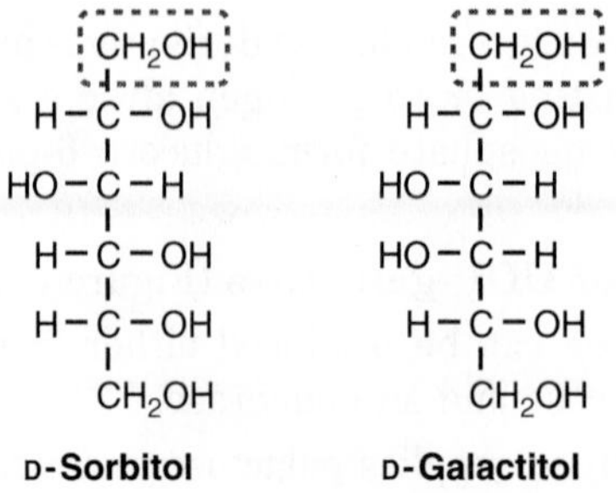

```
        CH2OH              CH2OH
      H - C - OH         H - C - OH
     HO - C - H         HO - C - H
      H - C - OH        HO - C - H
      H - C - OH         H - C - OH
        CH2OH              CH2OH
      D-Sorbitol         D-Galactitol
```

Figure 5-28. Reduced forms of sugars. Sorbitol is produced by reduction of glucose and can be reoxidized at carbon 2 to form fructose. Galactitol is produced by reduction of galactose.

1. **Conversion of galactose** to intermediates of glucose pathways (Figure 5-29)

   a. **Galactose** is phosphorylated by ATP to galactose 1-phosphate. The enzyme is **galactokinase.**

   b. **Galactose 1-phosphate** reacts with UDP-glucose and forms glucose 1-phosphate and UDP-galactose. The enzyme is **galactose 1-phosphate uridyl transferase.**

   c. **UDP-galactose** is epimerized to UDP-glucose in a reaction that is readily reversible. The enzyme is **UDP-glucose epimerase.**

   d. Repetition of reactions a–c results in conversion of galactose to **UDP-glucose** and **glucose 1-phosphate**.

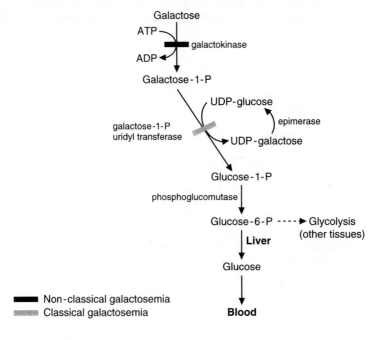

Figure 5-29. Conversion of galactose to intermediates of glucose metabolism. Galactose 1-phosphate uridyl transferase is deficient in classic galactosemia.

– In the **liver**, these glucose derivatives are converted to blood glucose during fasting or to glycogen after a meal. In various tissues, the glucose 1-phosphate forms glucose 6-phosphate and feeds into glycolysis.

2. Other fates of UDP-galactose (Figure 5-30)

– UDP-galactose can be produced either from galactose or from glucose via UDP-glucose and an epimerase.

a. UDP-galactose supplies galactose moieties for the synthesis of **glycoproteins, glycolipids,** and **proteoglycans**.

– The enzyme that adds galactose units to growing polysaccharide chains is **galactosyl transferase**.

b. UDP-galactose reacts with glucose in the **lactating mammary gland** to produce the milk sugar **lactose**.

– The modifier protein, **α-lactalbumin,** reacts with galactosyl transferase, lowering its K_m for glucose so that glucose adds to galactose (from UDP-galactose), forming lactose.

3. Conversion of galactose to galactitol

– Aldose reductase reduces the aldehyde of galactose to an alcohol, forming galactitol (see Figure 5-28).

VIII. Pentose Phosphate Pathway

- In the irreversible oxidative reactions of the pathway, one carbon of glucose 6-phosphate is released as CO_2; NADPH is generated; and ribulose 5-phosphate is produced (Figure 5-31).

– NADPH is used for reductive biosynthesis (particularly of fatty acids) and for protection against oxidative damage (e.g., by reduction of glutathione).

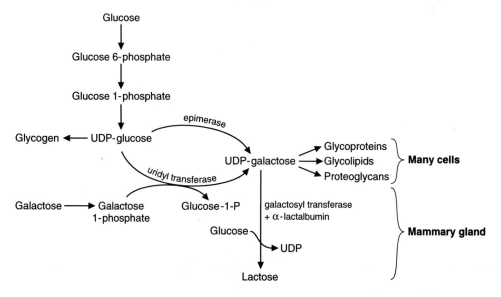

Figure 5-30. Metabolism of uridine diphosphate galactose (UDP-galactose). UDP-galactose can be produced from dietary glucose or galactose.

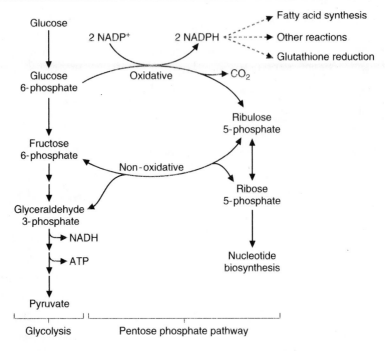

Figure 5-31. Overview of the pentose phosphate pathway.

- Ribulose 5-phosphate provides ribose 5-phosphate for nucleotide biosynthesis or generates pentose phosphates, which enter the nonoxidative portion of the pathway.
- In the reversible nonoxidative reactions, pentose phosphates produced from ribulose 5-phosphate, are converted to the glycolytic intermediates fructose 6-phosphate and glyceraldehyde 3-phosphate.
- Because the nonoxidative reactions are reversible, they can be used to generate ribose 5-phosphate for nucleotide synthesis from intermediates of glycolysis.

A. Reactions of the pentose phosphate pathway

1. The oxidative reactions (Figure 5-32)

a. **Glucose 6-phosphate** is converted to 6- phosphogluconolactone, and $NADP^+$ is reduced to $NADPH + H^+$.
   – Enzyme: **glucose 6-phosphate dehydrogenase**

b. **6-Phosphogluconolactone** is hydrolyzed to 6-phosphogluconate.
   – Enzyme: **gluconolactonase**

c. **6-Phosphogluconate** is oxidatively decarboxylated. CO_2 is released, and a second $NADPH + H^+$ is generated from $NADP^+$. The remaining carbons form ribulose 5-phosphate.
   – Enzyme: **6-phosphogluconate dehydrogenase**

2. The nonoxidative reactions (see Figure 5-31)

a. **Ribulose 5-phosphate** is isomerized to ribose 5- phosphate or epimerized to xylulose 5-phosphate.

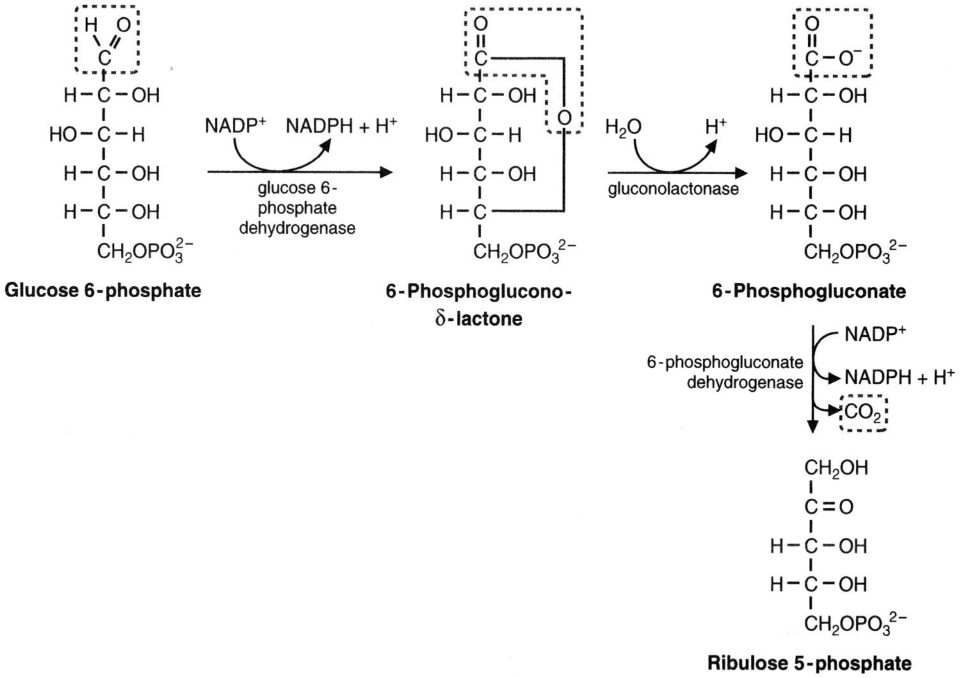

Figure 5-32. The oxidative reactions of the pentose phosphate pathway. These reactions are irreversible. Deficiency of glucose 6-phosphate dehydrogenase can result in hemolytic anemia.

    b. Ribose 5-phosphate and **xylulose 5-phosphate** undergo reactions, catalyzed by **transketolase** and **transaldolase**, that transfer carbon units, ultimately forming fructose 6-phosphate and glyceraldehyde 3-phosphate.

        (1) Transketolase, which requires **thiamine pyrophosphate**, transfers two-carbon units (Figure 5-33).

        (2) Transaldolase transfers three-carbon units.

    3. Overall reactions of the pentose phosphate pathway (Figure 5-34)

$$3 \text{ glucose-6-P} + 6 \text{ NADP}^+ \rightarrow 3 \text{ ribulose-5-P} + 3 \text{ CO}_2 + 6 \text{ NADPH}$$
$$3 \text{ ribulose-5-P} \rightarrow 2 \text{ xylulose-5-P} + \text{ribose-5-P}$$
$$2 \text{ xylulose-5-P} + \text{ribose-5-P} \rightarrow 2 \text{ fructose-6-P} + \text{glyceraldehyde-3-P}$$

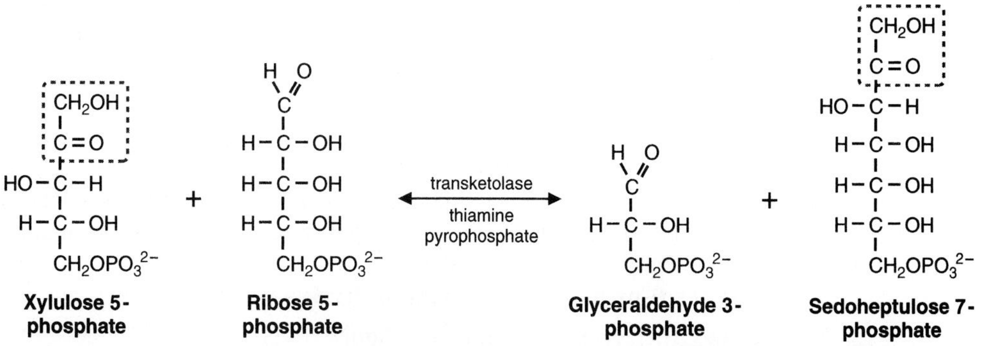

Figure 5-33. A two-carbon unit transferred by transketolase. Thiamine pyrophosphate is a cofactor for this enzyme.

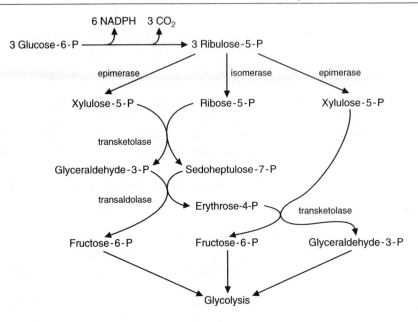

Figure 5-34. The reactions of the pentose phosphate pathway.

B. Functions of NADPH (see Figure 5-31)

1. The pentose phosphate pathway produces NADPH for **fatty acid synthesis.** Under these conditions, the fructose 6-phosphate and glyceraldehyde 3-phosphate generated in the pathway re-enter glycolysis.

2. NADPH is also used to **reduce glutathione** (γ-glutamylcysteinylglycine).
   – Glutathione helps to prevent oxidative damage to cells by reducing hydrogen peroxide (H_2O_2).
   – Glutathione is also used to transport amino acids across the membranes of certain cells by the γ-glutamyl cycle.

C. Generation of ribose 5-phosphate (see Figure 5-31)

1. When **NADPH levels are low,** the oxidative reactions of the pathway can be used to generate ribose 5-phosphate for nucleotide biosynthesis.

2. When **NADPH levels are high,** the reversible nonoxidative portion of the pathway can be used to generate ribose 5-phosphate for nucleotide biosynthesis from fructose 6-phosphate and glyceraldehyde 3-phosphate.

IX. Maintenance of Blood Glucose Levels

- Blood glucose levels are maintained within a very narrow range, although the nature of the diet varies widely and the normal person eats periodically during the day and fasts between meals and at night. Even under circumstances when a person does not eat for extended periods of time, blood glucose levels decrease only slowly.
- The major hormones that regulate blood glucose are insulin and glucagon.
- After a meal, blood glucose is supplied by dietary carbohydrate.
- During fasting, the liver maintains blood glucose levels by the processes of glycogenolysis and gluconeogenesis.

– Within the first few hours of fasting, glycogenolysis is primarily responsible for maintaining blood glucose levels.
– As a fast progresses and glycogen stores decrease, gluconeogenesis becomes an important additional source of blood glucose.
– After about 30 hours, when liver glycogen stores are depleted, gluconeogenesis becomes the only source of blood glucose.

● All cells use glucose for energy; however, the production of glucose during fasting is particularly important for tissues such as the brain and red blood cells.

● During exercise, blood glucose is also maintained by liver glycogenolysis and gluconeogenesis.

A. Blood glucose levels in the fed state

1. Changes in insulin and glucagon levels (Figure 5-35)

   a. Blood insulin levels increase as a meal is digested, following the rise in blood glucose.

     – Increases of blood glucose and of certain amino acids (particularly arginine and leucine) cause the release of insulin from β cells of the **pancreas**.

   b. Blood glucagon levels change depending on the content of the meal. A high-carbohydrate meal causes glucagon levels to decrease. A high-protein meal causes glucagon to increase (see Figure 5-35).

     – On a normal mixed diet, glucagon will remain relatively constant after a meal while insulin increases.

2. Fate of dietary glucose in the liver

   – Glucose is **oxidized** for energy. Excess glucose is converted to **glycogen** and to the **triacylglycerols** of very low density lipoprotein (**VLDL**).

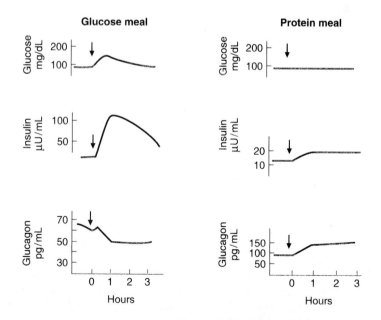

Figure 5-35. Changes in blood glucose, insulin, and glucagon levels in response to a glucose or a protein meal.

a. The enzyme **glucokinase** has a **high K_m** for glucose (about 6 mM), thus its velocity increases after a meal when glucose levels are elevated. On a high-carbohydrate diet, glucokinase is **induced**.

b. **Glycogen synthesis** is promoted by insulin, which stimulates the phosphatase that dephosphorylates and activates glycogen synthase.

c. **Synthesis of triacylglycerols** is also stimulated. The triacylglycerols are converted to VLDL and released into the blood.

3. **Fate of dietary glucose in peripheral tissues**
   – **All cells oxidize glucose** for energy.

   a. **Insulin** stimulates the **transport** of glucose into **adipose** and **muscle** cells.

   b. In **muscle,** insulin stimulates the synthesis of **glycogen**.

   c. **Adipose** cells convert glucose to the **glycerol** moiety for synthesis of triacylglycerols.

4. **Return of blood glucose to fasting levels**

   a. The **uptake of dietary glucose** by tissues (particularly liver, adipose, and muscle) causes blood glucose to decrease.

   b. **By 2 hours after a meal,** blood glucose has returned to the fasting level of 5 mM or 80–100 mg/dL.

B. **Blood glucose levels in the fasting state** (Figure 5-36)

1. **Changes in insulin and glucagon levels**

   a. During fasting, insulin levels decrease and glucagon levels increase.

   b. These hormonal changes promote **glycogenolysis** and **gluconeogenesis** in the liver so that blood glucose levels are maintained.

2. **Stimulation of glycogenolysis**
   – Within a few hours after a meal, as **glucagon** levels increase, glycogenolysis is stimulated and begins to supply glucose to the blood (see Figure 5-15).

3. **Stimulation of gluconeogenesis**

   a. **By 4 hours after a meal,** the liver is supplying glucose to the blood via gluconeogenesis and glycogenolysis (Figure 5-37).

   b. Regulatory mechanisms prevent futile cycles from occurring and promote the conversion of gluconeogenic precursors to glucose (see Figures 5-25 and 5-26).

4. **Stimulation of lipolysis** (see Figure 5-36)

   a. During fasting, the **breakdown of adipose triacylglycerols** is stimulated, and fatty acids and glycerol are released into the blood.

   b. **Fatty acids** are **oxidized** by certain tissues and converted to **ketone bodies** by the liver. The ATP and NADH produced by β-oxidation of fatty acids promotes gluconeogenesis.

   c. **Glycerol** is a source of carbon for gluconeogenesis in the liver.

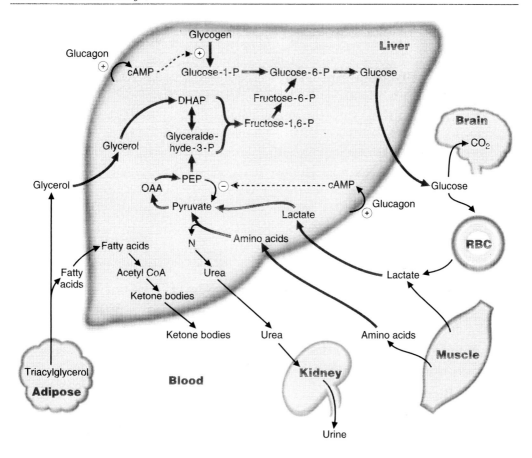

Figure 5-36. Tissue interrelationships in glucose production during fasting. Trace the precursors lactate, amino acids, and glycerol to blood glucose.

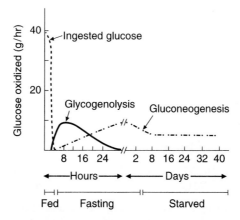

Figure 5-37. Sources of blood glucose in fed, fasting, and starved states. Note that the scale changes from hours to days. (Modified from Hanson RW and Mehlman MA [eds]: *Gluconeogenesis: Its Regulation in Mammalian Species.* p 518. Copyright © 1976 by John Wiley & Sons, Inc. Reprinted by permission of John Wiley & Sons, Inc.)

5. Relative roles of glycogenolysis and gluconeogenesis in maintaining blood glucose (see Figure 5-37)

  a. Glycogenolysis is stimulated as blood glucose falls to the fasting level after a meal. It is the main source of blood glucose for the next 8–12 hours.

  b. Gluconeogenesis is stimulated within a few (4) hours after a meal and supplies an increasingly larger share of blood glucose as the fasting state persists.

  c. By 16 hours of fasting, **gluconeogenesis and glycogenolysis** are approximately **equal** as sources of blood glucose.

  d. As liver glycogen stores become depleted, **gluconeogenesis predominates.**

  e. By about 30 hours of fasting, liver glycogen is depleted, and thereafter, **gluconeogenesis** is the **only source** of blood glucose.

C. Blood glucose levels during prolonged fasting (starvation)

  – Even after 5–6 weeks of starvation, blood glucose levels are still in the range of 65 mg/dL.

  – Changes in fuel utilization by various tissues prevent blood glucose levels from decreasing abruptly during prolonged fasting.

  1. The levels of ketone bodies rise in the blood, and the **brain uses ketone bodies** for energy, decreasing its utilization of blood glucose.

  2. The rate of **gluconeogenesis** and, therefore, of **urea** production by the liver **decreases.**

  3. Muscle protein is spared. Less muscle protein is used to provide amino acids for gluconeogenesis.

D. Blood glucose levels during exercise

  – During exercise, blood glucose is maintained by essentially the same mechanisms that are used during fasting.

  1. Use of endogenous fuels

    a. As the exercising muscle contracts, **ATP** is utilized.

    b. ATP is regenerated initially from **creatine phosphate**.

    c. Muscle glycogen is oxidized to produce ATP. AMP activates phosphorylase *b*, and Ca^{2+}-calmodulin activates phosphorylase kinase. The hormone epinephrine causes the production of cAMP, which stimulates glycogen breakdown. (see Figure 5-15).

  2. Use of fuels from the blood

    a. As blood flow to the exercising muscle increases, **blood glucose** and **fatty acids** are taken up and **oxidized by muscle.**

    b. As blood glucose levels begin to decrease, the **liver,** by the processes of **glycogenolysis** and **gluconeogenesis**, acts to maintain blood glucose levels.

X. Clinical Correlations

A. Common problems associated with carbohydrate metabolism

1. Intestinal lactase deficiency

Intestinal lactase deficiency is a common condition in which **lactose cannot be digested** and is oxidized by bacteria in the gut, which produce gas, and cause bloating and watery diarrhea.

2. Hypoglycemia

Low blood sugar is caused by the inability of the liver to maintain blood glucose levels. It can result from excessive insulin, excessive cellular uptake of glucose, or an impairment of glycogenolysis or gluconeogenesis. Hypoglycemia is caused by liver disease, insulin-secreting tumors, and administration of inappropriately high doses of insulin or sulfonylureas. **Excessive alcohol ingestion** also can cause hypoglycemia. Metabolism of alcohol increases levels of NADH in the liver, which inhibit gluconeogenesis.

3. Lactic acidosis

An increase of lactate levels in the blood causes an **acidosis.** This condition can result from **hypoxia** or **alcohol ingestion.** Lack of oxygen slows the electron transport chain, resulting in increased NADH levels. High NADH levels cause more than normal amounts of pyruvate to be converted to lactate. High NADH levels from alcohol metabolism also cause increased conversion of pyruvate to lactate.

Thiamine deficiency, which is common in alcoholics, decreases pyruvate dehydrogenase activity, causing pyruvate to accumulate and form lactate. Thiamine deficiency also slows the TCA cycle at the α- ketoglutarate dehydrogenase step. This and other conditions that slow the TCA cycle can also produce a lactic acidosis.

4. Glucose 6-phosphate dehydrogenase deficiency

A deficiency of glucose 6-phosphate dehydrogenase causes insufficient amounts of NADPH to be produced under certain conditions (e.g., when antimalarial drugs are being used). As a result, glutathione is not adequately reduced and, in turn, is not available to reduce compounds that are produced by the metabolism of these drugs. Red blood cells lyse, and a **hemolytic anemia** can occur.

5. Diabetes mellitus

High blood glucose levels occur because of either a deficiency of insulin [Type 1, formerly insulin-dependent diabetes mellitus (IDDM)] or decreased secretion or an inability of tissues to respond to insulin [Type 2, formerly noninsulin-dependent diabetes mellitus (NIDDM)]. If diabetes mellitus is untreated, the body responds as if it is starving. Fuel stores are degraded in the face of high blood glucose, and, **ketoacidosis** may occur, particularly in Type 1. Many metabolic pathways are affected. Exposure of red blood cells to glucose results in glycosylation of hemoglobin. An increase in the **HbA$_{1c}$** fraction above 6% of the total hemoglobin is an indication that a diabetic patient's blood glucose has been elevated during the last 6 to 8 weeks.

B. Rare problems associated with carbohydrate metabolism

1. Glycogen storage diseases

In the glycogen storage diseases, **glycogen accumulates** primarily in the liver or muscle, or both. Enzyme deficiencies occur mainly in glycogen degradation or conversion to glucose. Because different forms of the enzymes (isozymes) occur in the liver and muscle, one tissue may be affected, but not the other. In the **liver,** glycogen storage diseases result in hepatomegaly and conditions ranging from mild hypoglycemia to liver failure. In **muscle,** they cause problems ranging from difficulty in performing strenuous exercise to cardiorespiratory failure (Table 5-2).

2. Pyruvate kinase deficiency

Deficiency of pyruvate kinase causes decreased production of ATP from glycolysis. Red blood cells have insufficient ATP for their membrane pumps, and a **hemolytic anemia** results.

3. Essential fructosuria

Fructokinase is deficient in essential fructosuria; therefore, fructose cannot be metabolized as rapidly as normal. Blood fructose levels rise, and fructose appears in the urine. The condition is **benign.**

4. Fructose intolerance

Aldolase B is the liver isozyme of the glycolytic enzyme aldolase. When defective because of a genetic mutation, aldolase B still functions normally in glycolysis but not in fructose metabolism. Fructose 1-phosphate accumulates and inhibits glucose production, causing severe **hypoglycemia** if fructose is ingested. Dietary fructose (found mainly in sucrose) must be avoided.

5. Galactosemia

The appearance of high concentrations of galactose in the blood after lactose ingestion may be due to a **galactokinase deficiency** or to a **uridyl transferase deficiency.** In both conditions, galactose accumulates and is reduced to **galactitol,** which causes **cataracts. Uridyl transferase deficiency** is more severe, causing elevation of galactose 1-phosphate, which inhibits phosphoglucomutase, interfering with glycogen synthesis

Table 5-2. Glycogen Storage Diseases

Type	Enzyme Affected	Primary Organ Involved
I	Glucose-6-phosphatase (von Gierke's disease)	Liver
II	Lysosomal α-glucosidase (Pompe's disease)	All organs with lysosomes
III	Amylo 1,6-glucosidase (debrancher)	Liver, skeletal muscle, heart
IV	Amylo 4,6-glucosidase (branching enzyme)	Liver
V	Muscle glycogen phosphorylase (McArdle's disease)	Skeletal muscle
VI	Liver glycogen phosphorylase	Liver
VII	Phosphofructokinase	Muscle, red blood cells
IX	Phosphorylase kinase	Liver
X	Protein kinase A (cAMP dependent)	Liver

and degradation. **Hypoglycemia** can occur after ingestion of galactose. Dietary galactose (found mainly in milk and milk products, but also in "artificial sweeteners" and as a "filler" in some medications) must be avoided.

6. **Mucopolysaccharidoses and gangliosidoses (or sphingolipidoses)**

   A **deficiency of lysosomal enzymes** results in the inability to degrade the carbohydrate portions of proteoglycans and sphingolipids. Partially digested products accumulate in lysosomes. Tissues become engorged with these "residual bodies," and their function is impaired. These diseases, which include Hunter's and Hurler's mucopolysaccharidoses and Tay-Sachs' and Gaucher's gangliosidoses, are often **fatal.**

Review Test

Directions: Each of the numbered items or incomplete statements in this section is followed by answers or by completions of the statement. Select the **one** lettered answer or completion that is **best** in each case.

1. The enzyme that interconverts UDP-galactose and UDP-glucose is called an epimerase. This name is appropriate because glucose and galactose are epimers, which means that they are

(A) mirror images of each other
(B) ketoses rather than aldolases
(C) hexoses of the L configuration
(D) monosaccharides that differ only in the position of one hydroxyl group
(E) disaccharides that contain a β-1,4-glycosidic bond

2. The sugar shown below

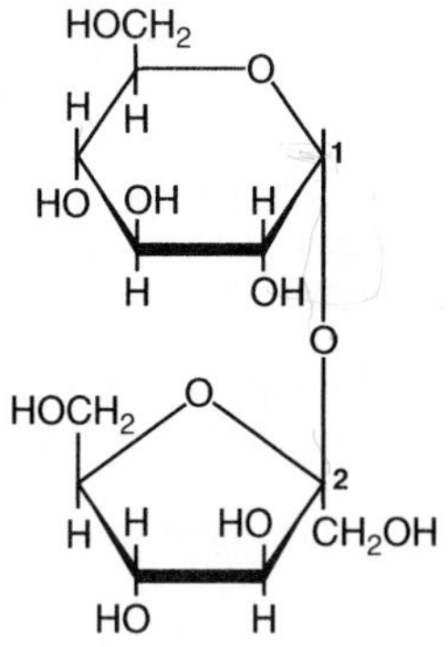

Sucrose
(Glucose-α(1→2)-fructose)

(A) contains a β-1,4 glycosidic bond
(B) is cleaved by lactase
(C) undergoes mutarotation
(D) contains a pentose sugar
(E) is sucrose (table sugar)

3. Which of the following statements concerning glycosaminoglycans is TRUE?

(A) They contain repeating disaccharides
(B) They are usually positively charged
(C) They contain short oligosaccharide chains
(D) They rarely contain sulfate groups
(E) They contain branches of *N*-acetylneuraminic acid

4. Which of the following statements concerning glycoproteins is TRUE?

(A) They are usually positively charged
(B) They never contain branched oligosaccharide chains
(C) They contain oligosaccharides that are synthesized on dolichol phosphate and transferred to serine residues
(D) They are degraded by lysosomal enzymes
(E) They are all secreted into the blood

5. The mucopolysaccharidoses are caused by deficiencies of enzymes involved in the degradation of

(A) fructose
(B) galactose
(C) glycosaminoglycans
(D) glycoproteins
(E) glycogen

6. After digestion of a piece of cake that contains flour, milk, and sucrose as its primary ingredients, the major carbohydrate products entering the blood are

(A) glucose
(B) fructose and galactose
(C) galactose and glucose
(D) fructose and glucose
(E) glucose, fructose, and galactose

7. A patient has a genetic defect that causes intestinal epithelial cells to produce disaccharidases of much lower activity than normal. Compared with a normal person, after eating a bowl of milk and oatmeal sweetened with table sugar, this patient will have higher levels of

(A) maltose, sucrose, and lactose in the stool
(B) starch in the stool
(C) galactose and fructose in the blood
(D) glycogen in the muscles
(E) insulin in the blood

8. A young infant, who was nourished by a synthetic formula, had a sugar in the blood and urine. This compound gave a positive reducing sugar test but was negative when measured with glucose oxidase. Treatment of blood and urine with acid (which cleaves glycosidic bonds) did not increase the amount of reducing sugar measured. Which of the following compounds is most likely to be present in this infant's blood and urine?

(A) glucose
(B) fructose
(C) sorbitol
(D) maltose
(E) lactose

9. The degradation of glycogen normally produces

(A) more glucose than glucose 1-phosphate
(B) more glucose 1-phosphate than glucose
(C) equal amounts of glucose and glucose 1-phosphate
(D) neither glucose nor glucose 1-phosphate
(E) only glucose 1-phosphate

10. Which of the following statements about liver phosphorylase kinase is TRUE?

(A) It is present in an inactive form when epinephrine is elevated
(B) It phosphorylates phosphorylase to an inactive form
(C) It catalyzes a reaction that requires ATP
(D) It is phosphorylated in response to elevated insulin
(E) It is not affected by cAMP

11. A patient had large deposits of liver glycogen, which, after an overnight fast, had shorter than normal branches. This abnormality could be caused by a defective

(A) glycogen phosphorylase
(B) glucagon receptor
(C) glycogenin
(D) amylo-1,6-glucosidase (α-glucosidase)
(E) amylo-4,6-transferase (4:6 transferase)

12. An adolescent patient with a deficiency of muscle phosphorylase was examined while exercising her forearm by squeezing a rubber ball. Compared with a normal person performing the same exercise, this patient

(A) could exercise for a longer period of time without fatigue
(B) had increased glucose levels in blood drawn from her forearm
(C) had decreased lactate levels in blood drawn from her forearm
(D) had lower levels of glycogen in biopsies of her forearm muscle

13. In which compartment of the cell does glycolysis occur?
(A) Mitochondrion
(B) Nucleus
(C) Soluble cytoplasm (cytosol)
(D) Rough endoplasmic reticulum
(E) Smooth endoplasmic reticulum

14. What type of bond is formed between phosphate and carbon 1 of 1,3-bisphosphoglycerate?

(A) Anhydride
(B) Ester
(C) Phosphodiester
(D) Amide
(E) Ether

15. During glycolysis, the conversion of compound I to compound II

$CH_2OPO_3^{2-}$	COO^-
$\mid$	$\mid$
$C = O$	$C = O$
$\mid$	$\mid$
$CH_2 - OH$	CH_3
Compound I	**Compound II**

(A) requires a dehydrogenase
(B) releases inorganic phosphate
(C) produces one molecule of ATP per molecule of product
(D) is catalyzed by a phosphatase
(E) requires two molecules of NADH

16. Which of the following statements about glycolysis is TRUE?

(A) Glucokinase catalyzes the conversion of glucose to glucose 6-phosphate in the liver
(B) Phosphofructokinase 1 catalyzes the conversion of fructose 1,6-bisphosphate to dihydroxyacetone phosphate
(C) When one molecule of glucose is converted to pyruvate via glycolysis, one molecule of NAD^+ is reduced
(D) When one molecule of glucose is converted to pyruvate via glycolysis, one carbon is lost as CO_2
(E) Hexokinase catalyzes the conversion of fructose 6-phosphate to fructose 1,6-bisphosphate

17. In an embryo with a complete deficiency of pyruvate kinase, how many net moles of ATP are generated in the conversion of one mole of glucose to one mole of pyruvate?

(A) 0
(B) 1
(C) 2
(D) 3
(E) 4

18. A positive allosteric activator of phosphofructokinase 1 in the liver is

(A) ADP
(B) acetyl CoA
(C) fructose 2,6-bisphosphate
(D) ATP
(E) citrate

19. Which of the following is a regulatory mechanism of glycolysis?

(A) Inhibition of phosphofructokinase 1 by AMP
(B) Inhibition of hexokinase by its product
(C) Activation of pyruvate kinase when glucagon levels are elevated
(D) Inhibition of aldolase by fructose 1,6-bisphosphate
(E) Inhibition of glucokinase by fructose 2,6-bisphosphate

20. An alcoholic went on a weekend binge. The metabolism of ethanol produces NADH, mainly in the liver. As a result of high NADH levels, pyruvate is converted to

(A) oxaloacetate
(B) acetyl CoA
(C) phosphoenolpyruvate
(D) lactate

21. Caffeine inhibits 3′,5′-cAMP phosphodiesterase, which converts cAMP to AMP. Which of the following effects would be observed if cells were treated with caffeine?

(A) Decreased activity of liver protein kinase A
(B) Decreased activity of muscle protein kinase A
(C) Increased activity of liver pyruvate kinase
(D) Decreased activity of liver glycogen synthase

22. Which of the following glycolytic enzymes is used in gluconeogenesis?

(A) Glucokinase
(B) Phosphofructokinase 1
(C) Pyruvate kinase
(D) Aldolase B

23. In the conversion of pyruvate to glucose during gluconeogenesis,

(A) biotin is required
(B) CO_2, added in one reaction, appears in the final product
(C) energy is utilized only in the form of GTP
(D) all of the reactions occur in the cytosol

24. In gluconeogenesis, both alanine and lactate are converted in a single step to

(A) oxaloacetate
(B) acetyl CoA
(C) phosphoenolpyruvate
(D) pyruvate
(E) aspartate

25. A common intermediate in the conversion of glycerol and lactate to glucose is

(A) pyruvate
(B) oxaloacetate
(C) malate
(D) glucose 6-phosphate
(E) phosphoenolpyruvate

26. In which of the following compounds do carbons derived from pyruvate leave the mitochondria for the synthesis of glucose during fasting?

(A) Malate
(B) Acetyl CoA
(C) Oxaloacetate
(D) Lactate
(E) Glutamine

27. An alcoholic who went on a weekend binge without eating any food was found to have severe hypoglycemia. Hypoglycemia occurred because the metabolism of ethanol prevented the production of blood glucose from

(A) glycogen
(B) lactate
(C) glycerol
(D) alanine
(E) lactate, glycerol, and alanine

28. Dietary fructose is phosphorylated in the liver and cleaved to form

(A) two molecules of dihydroxyacetone phosphate
(B) one molecule each of dihydroxyacetone phosphate and glyceraldehyde
(C) one molecule each of dihydroxyacetone phosphate and glyceraldehyde 3-phosphate
(D) one molecule each of dihydroxyacetone and glyceraldehyde 3-phosphate
(E) two molecules of glyceraldehyde 3-phosphate

29. In fructose intolerance, aldolase B is defective in the liver. It is still active in glycolysis, but not in the metabolism of dietary fructose. Which of the following is most likely to be found in a patient with fructose intolerance when compared with a normal person on a similar diet that includes sucrose?

(A) decreased levels of fructose in the blood
(B) elevated levels of glyceraldehyde in liver cells
(C) high levels of sucrose in the stool
(D) elevated levels of fructose 1-phosphate in liver cells
(E) decreased levels of fructose in the urine

30. A patient was found to have elevated levels of galactose and galactitol in the blood, but low cellular levels of galactose 1-phosphate. Which of the following enzymes is most likely defective?

(A) galactokinase
(B) UDP-glucose epimerase
(C) phosphoglucomutase
(D) galactose 1-phosphate uridyl transferase
(E) hexokinase

31. Which of the following statements concerning lactose synthesis is TRUE?

(A) The reactions occur in most tissues
(B) α-Lactalbumin acts as a modifier of galactosyl transferase
(C) UDP-glucose reacts with galactose
(D) UDP-galactose requires dietary galactose for its synthesis

32. A pregnant woman who has a lactase deficiency and cannot tolerate milk in her diet is concerned that she will not be able to produce milk of sufficient caloric value to nourish her baby. She should be advised that

(A) she must eat pure galactose in order to produce the galactose moiety of lactose
(B) she will not be able to breast-feed her baby because she cannot produce lactose
(C) the production of lactose by the mammary gland does not require the ingestion of milk or milk products
(D) she can produce lactose by degrading α-lactalbumin.

33. A mother with a deficiency of galactose 1-phosphate uridyl transferase

(A) can convert galactose to UDP-galactose for lactose synthesis during lactation
(B) can form galactose 1-phosphate from galactose
(C) can convert galactose to blood glucose
(D) can convert galactose to liver glycogen
(E) will have lower than normal blood galactose levels after ingestion of milk

34. The pentose phosphate pathway generates

(A) NADH, which may be used for fatty acid synthesis
(B) ribose 5-phosphate, which may be used for the biosynthesis of ATP
(C) pyruvate and fructose 1,6-bisphosphate by the transaldolase and transketolase reactions
(D) xylulose 5-phosphate by one of the oxidative reactions
(E) glucose from ribose 5-phosphate and CO_2

35. In an alcoholic with a thiamine deficiency, which enzyme of the pentose phosphate pathway would be less active than normal?

(A) The epimerase
(B) Transaldolase
(C) The isomerase
(D) Transketolase
(E) Glucose 6-phosphate dehydrogenase

36. In patients with Type 1 or Type 2 diabetes mellitus, the transport of glucose across cell membranes is diminished in

(A) brain
(B) liver
(C) red blood cells
(D) skeletal muscle

37. In an individual at rest who has fasted for 12 hours,

(A) gluconeogenesis is the major process by which blood glucose is maintained
(B) adenylate cyclase is inactivated in liver
(C) liver glycogen stores are depleted
(D) phosphorylase, pyruvate kinase, and glycogen synthetase are phosphorylated in liver

38. In a glucose tolerance test, an individual in the basal metabolic state ingests a large amount of glucose. If the individual is normal, this ingestion results in

(A) enhanced glycogen synthase activity in liver
(B) an increased ratio of phosphorylase a to phosphorylase b in the liver
(C) an increased rate of lactate formation by erythrocytes
(D) inhibition of glycogen synthase phosphatase activity in the liver

39. An infant with an enlarged liver has a glucose 6-phosphatase deficiency. This infant

(A) cannot maintain blood glucose levels either by glycogenolysis or by gluconeogenesis
(B) can use liver glycogen to maintain blood glucose levels
(C) can use muscle glycogen to maintain blood glucose levels
(D) can convert both alanine and glycerol to glucose to maintain blood glucose levels

40. A 16-year-old patient with Type 1 diabetes mellitus was admitted to the hospital with a blood glucose level of 400 mg/dL. (The reference range for blood glucose is 80–100 mg/dL.) One hour after an insulin infusion was begun, her blood glucose level had decreased to 320 mg/dL. One hour later, it was 230 mg/dL. The patient's glucose level decreased because insulin

(A) stimulates the transport of glucose across the cell membranes of the liver and brain
(B) stimulates the conversion of glucose to glycogen and triacylglycerol in the liver
(C) inhibits the synthesis of ketone bodies from blood glucose
(D) stimulates glycogenolysis in the liver
(E) inhibits the conversion of muscle glycogen to blood glucose

Questions 41–43

A patient presented with a bacterial infection that produced an endotoxin that inhibits phosphoenolpyruvate carboxykinase.

41. In this patient, inhibition of phosphoenolpyruvate carboxykinase would cause inhibition of glucose production from

(A) alanine
(B) glycerol
(C) even-chain fatty acids
(D) phosphoenolpyruvate

42. Administration of a high dose of glucagon to this patient 2–3 hours after a high-carbohydrate meal would

(A) result in a substantial increase in blood glucose levels
(B) decrease blood glucose levels
(C) have little effect on blood glucose levels

43. Administration of a high dose of glucagon to this patient 30 hours after a high-carbohydrate meal would

(A) result in a substantial increase in blood glucose levels
(B) decrease blood glucose levels
(C) have little effect on blood glucose levels

44. Mary Smith, a patient with Type 1 diabetes mellitus, has a fasting blood glucose level of 160 mg/dL and a HbA$_{1c}$ of 10%. These tests indicate that her current glycemic control is

(A) good, and has been good during the past 6 weeks
(B) poor, and has been poor during the past 6 weeks
(C) good, but has been poor during the past 6 weeks
(D) poor, but has been good during the past 6 weeks

Directions: Each group of items in this section consists of lettered options followed by a set of numbered items. For each item, select the **one** lettered option that is most closely associated with it. Each lettered option may be selected once, more than once, or not at all.

Questions 45–48

(A) Protein kinase A
(B) Phosphorylase kinase
(C) Glucagon receptor
(D) Phosphodiesterase

Match each enzyme below with the protein that most directly alters its activity.

45. Phosphorylase b

46. Glycogen synthase

47. Adenylate cyclase

48. Phosphorylase kinase

Questions 49–51

(A) Glucose 6-phosphate dehydrogenase
(B) 6-Phosphogluconate dehydrogenase
(C) Transaldolase
(D) Transketolase

Match the products below with the enzyme that catalyzes their formation.

49. NADPH and a lactone

50. CO_2

51. Glyceraldehyde 3-phosphate in a reaction requiring thiamine pyrophosphate

Questions 52–58

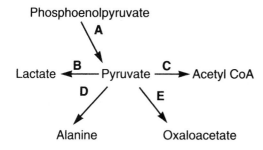

Match each description below with the most appropriate enzyme (A–E) indicated in the diagram above.

52. Inhibited by NADH and acetyl CoA

53. Requires thiamine pyrophosphate

54. Activated by acetyl CoA

55. Requires biotin

56. Requires pyridoxal phosphate

57. Phosphorylated and inactivated by protein kinase A

58. Forms product (as indicated by the arrow) when NADH levels are elevated

Questions 59–62

(A) Dietary glucose
(B) Glucose produced by glycogenolysis
(C) Glucose produced by gluconeogenesis

For each time period below, choose the major source of glucose that is being oxidized by cells.

59. 1 hour after a meal

60. 4 hours after a meal

61. 2 days after a meal

62. after 6 weeks of fasting

Questions 63–68

(A) Galactosemia
(B) A hemolytic anemia
(C) Fructose intolerance
(D) Lactose intolerance
(E) McArdle's disease

For each enzyme below, choose the condition above that would result from a deficiency of that enzyme.

63. Lactase

64. Glucose 6-phosphate dehydrogenase

65. Galactokinase

66. Aldolase B

67. Muscle glycogen phosphorylase

68. Uridyl transferase

Answers and Explanations

1–D. Glucose and galactose are not mirror images (enantiomers). They differ only in that they contain hydroxyl groups on different sides of carbon 4 (i.e., they are epimers). They are aldoses, not ketoses. They are hexoses (containing six carbons) in the D configuration. They are monosaccharides.

2–E. This sugar is sucrose. It contains glucose and fructose (two hexoses) joined by their anomeric carbons, thus it is not a reducing sugar and does not mutarotate.

3–A. Glycosaminoglycans are long, linear carbohydrate chains that contain repeating disaccharide units, which usually contain a hexosamine and a uronic acid. They often contain sulfate groups. The uronic acid and sulfate residues cause them to be negatively charged. They are unbranched and do not contain N-acetylneuraminic acid.

4–D. Glycoproteins contain branched oligosaccharide chains. These chains may be synthesized by addition of sugars to serine or threonine residues of the protein, or they may be synthesized on dolichol phosphate and transferred to asparagine residues on the protein. They are not positively charged. They are synthesized in the RER and Golgi and may be secreted from cells, anchored in the cell membrane, or segregated into lysosomes. They are internalized by endocytosis and degraded by lysosomal enzymes.

5–C. Glycosaminoglycans (formerly called mucopolysaccharides) are the long, linear polysaccharide chains of proteoglycans. They are synthesized and secreted by cells. Ultimately, they are taken up by cells via endocytosis and degraded by lysosomal enzymes. A deficiency of any one of these lysosomal enzymes can result in a mucopolysaccharidosis (e.g., Hurler's, Hunter's).

6–E. The cake contains starch, lactose (milk sugar), and sucrose (table sugar). Digestion of starch produces glucose. Lactase cleaves lactose to galactose and glucose, and sucrase cleaves sucrose to fructose and glucose.

7–A. In this patient, starch will be digested by salivary and pancreatic α-amylases to small oligosaccharides and maltose, but a lower than normal amount of glucose will be produced because of the deficiency of the brush border disaccharidases, which have maltase, isomaltase, sucrase, and lactase activity. Sucrose and lactose will not be cleaved. There will be more maltose, sucrose, and lactose in the stool and less monosaccharides in the blood and tissues. Insulin levels will be lower than normal.

8–B. Fructose gives a positive result in a reducing sugar test and a negative result in a glucose oxidase test. It is a monosaccharide, and, so, is not cleaved by acid. Glucose gives a positive test result with the enzyme glucose oxidase. Sorbitol has no aldehyde or ketone group, and, thus, cannot be oxidized in the reducing sugar test. Maltose and lactose are disaccharides that undergo acid hydrolysis, which doubles the amount of reducing sugar. This infant probably has benign fructosuria or the more dangerous condition, fructose intolerance. A galactose oxidase test would rule out the possibility that the sugar was galactose.

9–B. Phosphorylase produces glucose 1-phosphate from glucose residues linked α-1,4. Free glucose is produced from α-1,6-linked residues at branch points by an α-1,6-glucosidase. Degradation of glycogen produces glucose 1-phosphate and glucose in about a 10:1 ratio.

10–C. Glucagon in the liver and epinephrine in both the liver and muscle cause cAMP levels to rise, activating protein kinase A. Protein kinase A phosphorylates and activates phosphorylase kinase, which in turn phosphorylates and activates phosphorylase. These phosphorylation reactions require ATP.

11–D. If, after fasting, the branches were shorter than normal, phosphorylase must be functional and capable of being activated by glucagon. The branching enzyme (the 4:6 transferase) must be normal because branches are present. The protein glycogenin must be present in order for large amounts of glycogen to be synthesized and deposited. The defect has to be in the debranching enzyme (which contains an α-1,6-glucosidase). If the debrancher is defective, phosphorylase would break the glycogen down to the branch points, but complete degradation would not occur. Therefore, short branches would be present in the glycogen. If the short branches contain only one glucose unit, the defect is in the α-1,6-glucosidase activity of the debrancher. If they contained four glucose units, the defect would be in the 4:4 transferase activity of the debrancher.

12–C. This patient has McArdle's disease, a glycogen storage disease caused by a deficiency of muscle glycogen phosphorylase. Because she cannot degrade glycogen to produce energy for muscle contraction, she becomes fatigued more readily than a normal person, the glycogen levels in her muscle will be higher than normal, and her blood lactate levels will be lower. She will use more blood glucose, thus her blood glucose levels will be decreased.

13–C. All of the reactions of glycolysis occur in the cytosol.

14–A. The carboxylic acid (carbon 1) reacts with phosphoric acid, splitting out H_2O and forming an anhydride. Cleavage of this bond in the next step of glycolysis generates enough energy to produce one ATP from ADP and P_i.

15–A. Dihydroxyacetone phosphate (compound I) is isomerized to glyceraldehyde 3-phosphate and converted in a series of steps to pyruvate (compound II). One of the reactions requires glyceraldehyde 3-phosphate dehydrogenase, which uses one molecule of inorganic phosphate for each molecule of NADH it produces. In the conversion of one molecule of 1,3-bisphosphoglycerate to one molecule of pyruvate, two molecules of ATP are produced. A phosphatase is not required.

16–A. Glucokinase, a liver enzyme, converts glucose to glucose 6-phosphate. Phosphofructokinase 1 converts fructose 6-phosphate to fructose 1,6-bisphosphate. In glycolysis, one molecule of glucose is converted to two molecules of pyruvate and two molecules of NADH are produced. No carbons are lost as CO_2.

17–A. Normally, one mole of ATP is used to convert one mole of glucose to one mole of glucose 6-phosphate and a second to convert one mole of fructose 6-phosphate to the bisphosphate. Two triose phosphates are produced by cleavage of fructose 1,6-bisphosphate. As the two triose phosphates are converted to pyruvate, four ATPs are generated; two by phosphoglycerate kinase and two by pyruvate kinase. Net, two ATPs are produced. If pyruvate kinase is completely deficient, two less ATPs will be produced, thus net ATP production will be zero. It is unlikely that the embryo would survive with a complete deficiency of this enzyme.

18–C. Phosphofructokinase 1 is activated by AMP and fructose 2,6-bisphosphate. It is inhibited by ATP and citrate and not directly affected by acetyl CoA or ADP. In the liver, fructose 2,6-bisphosphate is the major activator.

19–B. Hexokinase is inhibited by its product, glucose 6-phosphate. PFK1 is activated by AMP and fructose 2,6-bisphosphate (F-2,6-P). F-2,6-P does not inhibit glucokinase. Aldolase is not inhibited by its substrate, fructose-1,6-P. Pyruvate kinase is inactivated by glucagon-mediated phosphorylation.

20–D. All of these compounds can be produced from pyruvate, but when NADH levels are elevated (and, thus, NAD^+ levels are low), pyruvate is converted to lactate by lactate dehydrogenase. The binging alcoholic could develop a lactic acidosis.

21–D. If the phosphodiesterase that degrades cAMP were inhibited, cAMP levels would be elevated. Protein kinase A would become more active in the liver and muscle; pyruvate kinase would become less active; and glycogen synthase activity would be decreased.

22–D. During gluconeogenesis, glucokinase, phosphofructokinase 1, and pyruvate kinase are not active, and, thus, futile cycles do not occur. Aldolase B, the liver isozyme, is used both in glycolysis and gluconeogenesis.

23–A. In the mitochondria, CO_2 is added to pyruvate to form oxaloacetate (OAA). The enzyme is pyruvate carboxylase, which requires biotin and ATP. OAA leaves the mitochondrion as malate or aspartate and is regenerated in the cytosol. OAA is converted to phosphoenolpyruvate by a reaction that utilizes GTP and releases the same CO_2 that was added in the mitochondrion. The remainder of the reactions occur in the cytosol.

24–D. Alanine is transaminated and lactate is oxidized by NAD^+ to form pyruvate. The other compounds are not produced in a single step from alanine or lactate.

25–D. The only intermediate included on the list that glycerol has in common with lactate is glucose 6-phosphate. Glycerol enters gluconeogenesis as dihydroxyacetone phosphate. Therefore, it bypasses the other compounds.

26–A. Pyruvate is converted in the mitochondria to malate, which can cross the mitochondrial membrane. Oxaloacetate and acetyl CoA cannot. Lactate is produced from pyruvate in the cytosol. The reverse reaction is involved in gluconeogenesis. Glutamine is not derived from pyruvate during gluconeogenesis.

27–E. Ethanol metabolism (which produces high NADH levels) does not prevent glycogen degradation. In fact, glycogen stores would be rapidly depleted under these conditions because of decreased gluconeogenesis. Alanine is transaminated to pyruvate. The pyruvate/lactate equilibrium greatly favors lactate when NADH is high. Thus, alanine and lactate are prevented from producing glucose. Lactate levels are elevated, and a lactic acidosis can result. Glycerol normally enters gluconeogenesis by forming glycerol 3-P, which is oxidized to dihydroxyacetone phosphate. High NADH levels prevent this oxidation. Thus, the three major gluconeogenic precursors (alanine, glycerol, and lactate) do not form glucose because of the high NADH, and as glycogen stores are depleted, hypoglycemia results.

28–B. Fructose 1-phosphate is cleaved by aldolase B to dihydroxyacetone phosphate and glyceraldehyde.

29–D. Sucrose would still be cleaved by sucrase, thus it would not increase in the stool. Fructose would not be metabolized normally, therefore it would be elevated in the blood and urine. Aldolase B would not cleave fructose-1-P, thus its levels would be elevated and the product, glyceraldehyde, would not be produced.

30–A. Galactose is phosphorylated by galactokinase to galactose-1-P, which reacts with UDP-glucose in a reaction catalyzed by uridyl transferase to form UDP-galactose and glucose-1-P. An epimerase converts UDP-galactose to UDP-glucose. Phosphoglucomutase interconverts glucose-1-P and glucose-6-P. Hexokinase converts glucose to glucose-6-P. If galactose-1-P levels are low, but galactose (and galactitol) levels are elevated, the defect is in galactokinase.

31–B. UDP-galactose reacts with glucose to form lactose only in the mammary gland. α-Lactalbumin acts as a modifier of the enzyme galactosyl transferase, lowering its K_m for glucose. Glucose can be converted to UDP-glucose and epimerized to form the UDP-galactose used in lactose synthesis; therefore, dietary galactose is not required.

32–C. She will be able to breast-feed her baby because she can produce lactose. However, she does not have to eat pure galactose or even lactose. Glucose can be converted to UDP-galactose (Glucose → glucose 6-phosphate → glucose 1-phosphate → UDP-glucose → UDP- galactose). UDP-galactose reacts with glucose to form lactose. α-Lactalbumin is a protein that serves as the modifier of galactosyl transferase, which catalyzes this reaction.

33–B. A person with a uridyl transferase deficiency (classic galactosemia) can phosphorylate galactose but will not be able to react the galactose 1-phosphate with UDP-glucose to form UDP-galactose and glucose 1-phosphate. Therefore, she will not be able to convert galactose to UDP-galactose, liver glycogen, or blood glucose. Cellular galactose 1-phosphate and blood galactose levels will be elevated if she consumes galactose or lactose.

34–B. In the first three reactions of the pentose phosphate pathway, glucose is converted to ribulose 5-phosphate and CO_2, with the production of NADPH. These reactions are not reversible. Ribose 5-phosphate and xylulose 5-phosphate are formed from ribulose 5-phosphate by two of the nonoxidative reactions of the pathway. Ribose 5-phosphate is used for biosynthesis of nucleotides such as ATP. A series of reactions catalyzed by transketolase and transaldolase produce the glycolytic intermediates fructose 6-phosphate and glyceraldehyde 3-phosphate. Glucose is produced by gluconeogenesis in humans.

35–D. Transketolase would be less active because it requires thiamine pyrophosphate as a cofactor. Other enzymes do not require cofactors except for the two dehydrogenases, which require $NADP^+$.

36–D. Insulin stimulates glucose transport into muscle and adipose cells. There is no significant stimulation in brain, liver, and red blood cells.

37–D. After 12 hours of fasting, liver glycogen stores are still substantial. Glycogenolysis is stimulated by glucagon, which activates adenylate cyclase. cAMP activates protein kinase A, which phosphorylates phosphorylase kinase, pyruvate kinase, and glycogen synthase. As a result, phosphorylase is activated, whereas glycogen synthase and pyruvate kinase are inactivated. Gluconeogenesis does not become the major process for maintaining blood glucose until 18–20 hours of fasting. After about 30 hours, liver glycogen is depleted.

38–A. After ingestion of glucose, glycogen synthase is activated by a phosphatase. The ratio of phosphorylase a to phosphorylase b is decreased by a phosphatase, thus glycogen degradation decreases. Red blood cells continue to use glucose and form lactate at their normal rate.

39–A. Glucose 6-phosphatase deficiency results in a glycogen storage disease (von Gierke's disease) in which neither liver glycogen nor gluconeogenic precursors (e.g., alanine and glycerol) can be used to maintain normal blood glucose levels. The last step (conversion of glucose 6-phosphate to glucose) is deficient for both glycogenolysis and gluconeogenesis. Muscle glycogen cannot be used to maintain blood glucose because muscle does not contain glucose 6-phosphatase.

40–B. Blood glucose decreases because insulin stimulates the transport of glucose into muscle and adipose cells and stimulates the conversion of glucose to glycogen and triacylglycerols in the liver. Ketone bodies are not made from blood glucose. During fasting, when the liver is producing ketone bodies, it is also synthesizing glucose. Carbon for ketone body synthesis comes from fatty acids. Insulin stimulates glycogen synthesis, not glycogenolysis. Muscle glycogen is not converted to blood glucose.

41–A. Phosphoenolpyruvate carboxykinase converts oxaloacetate to phosphoenolpyruvate. It is a gluconeogenic enzyme required for the conversion of alanine and lactate (but not phosphoenolpyruvate or glycerol) to glucose. Acetyl CoA from oxidation of fatty acids is not converted to glucose.

42–A. By 2–3 hours after a high-carbohydrate meal, the patient's glycogen stores would be filled. Glucagon would stimulate glycogenolysis, and blood glucose levels would rise.

43–C. Thirty hours after a meal, liver glycogen is normally depleted, and blood glucose is maintained solely by gluconeogenesis after this time. However, in this case, a key gluconeogenic enzyme is inhibited by an endotoxin. Therefore, gluconeogenesis will not occur at a normal rate and glycogen stores will be depleted more rapidly than normal. Blood glucose levels will not change significantly if glucagon is administered after 30 hours of fasting.

44–B. Mary Smith's blood glucose is currently above the range for normal fasting blood glucose (80–100 mg/dL). Her HbA_{1c} is also above the normal 6%. Therefore, her glycemic control is poor at present and has been poor over the last 6 weeks.

45–B. Phosphorylase kinase phosphorylates phosphorylase b, converting it to the more active phosphorylase a, which releases glucose-1-P from glycogen.

46–A. Glycogen synthase is phosphorylated and inactivated by a cAMP- dependent protein kinase (protein kinase A).

47–C. Glucagon combines with its membrane receptor, and the complex stimulates G proteins that activate adenylate cyclase in the cell membrane, causing the conversion of ATP to cAMP.

48–A. A cAMP-dependent protein kinase (protein kinase A) phosphorylates phosphorylase kinase, causing it to become active.

49–A. Both A and B produce NADPH, but only A produces 6-phosphogluconolactone.

50–B. 6-Phosphogluconate is decarboxylated to form ribulose 5-phosphate, NADPH, and CO_2.

51–D. Both transaldolase and transketolase produce glyceraldehyde 3-phosphate, but only transketolase requires thiamine pyrophosphate.

52–C. Pyruvate dehydrogenase is inhibited by NADH and acetyl CoA.

53–C. Pyruvate dehydrogenase requires thiamine pyrophosphate.

54–E. Pyruvate carboxylase is activated by acetyl CoA.

55–E. Pyruvate carboxylase requires biotin, CO_2, and ATP.

56–D. Alanine aminotransferase (transaminase) requires pyridoxal phosphate.

57–A. Pyruvate kinase is inactivated by protein kinase A. Pyruvate dehydrogenase is inactivated by a kinase that is a subunit of the enzyme complex.

58–B. Lactate dehydrogenase produces lactate from pyruvate when NADH levels are high.

59–A. Dietary glucose is the source of blood glucose for about 2 hours after a meal.

60–B. By 4 hours after a meal, digestion and absorption of carbohydrates have been completed, and liver glycogen is supplying glucose to the blood.

61–C. By 2 days after a meal, liver glycogen stores have been depleted, and gluconeogenesis is the only source of blood glucose.

62–C. After 6 weeks of fasting, gluconeogenesis is still the major process for production of blood glucose.

63–D. A lactase deficiency results in lactose intolerance, which is characterized by gas, bloating, and watery diarrhea following lactose ingestion.

64–B. A glucose 6-phosphate dehydrogenase deficiency results in a hemolytic anemia because adequate levels of NADPH are not produced by the pentose phosphate pathway. NADPH is required for the reduction of glutathione, which helps to prevent oxidative damage to cells.

65–A. Non-classical galactosemia is caused by a deficiency of galactokinase. Galactose accumulates and forms galactitol. Cataracts occur.

66–C. A deficiency of aldolase B results in fructose intolerance. Fructose 1-phosphate accumulates because it is not cleaved. Hypoglycemia results. The glycolytic reaction catalyzed by aldolase B is not affected.

67–E. In McArdle's disease, muscle glycogen phosphorylase is deficient. Strenuous exercise cannot be tolerated because muscle glycogen cannot be degraded.

68–A. In classical galactosemia, the uridyl transferase is deficient. Galactose, galactitol, and galactose 1-phosphate accumulate when galactose is ingested. Cataracts and hypoglycemia result.

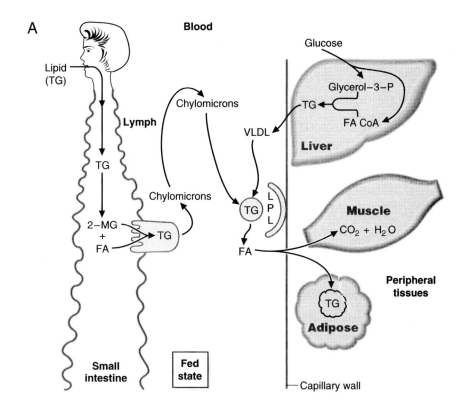

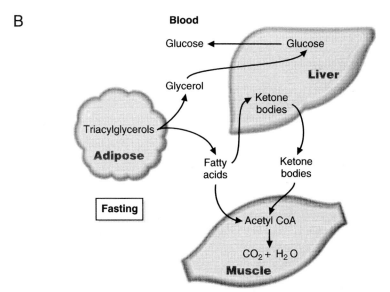

Figure 6-1. *A,* Overview of lipid metabolism in the fed state. *FA* = fatty acid; *HDL* = high-density lipoprotein; *LPL* = lipoprotein lipase; *2-MG* = 2-monoacylglycerol; *TG* = triacylglycerol; *circled TG* = triacylglycerols of VLDL and chylomicrons; *VLDL* = very low density lipoprotein. *B,* Overview of lipid metabolism in the fasting state.

6

Lipid Metabolism

Overview

- Lipids are a diverse group of compounds that are related by their insolubility in water.
- Membranes contain lipids, particularly phosphoglycerides, sphingolipids, and cholesterol.
- Triacylglycerols, which provide the body with its major source of energy, are obtained from the diet or synthesized mainly in the liver. They are transported in the blood as lipoproteins and are stored in adipose tissue (Figure 6-1A).
- The major classes of blood lipoproteins include chylomicrons, very low density lipoprotein (VLDL), intermediate-density lipoprotein (IDL), low-density lipoprotein (LDL), and high-density lipoprotein (HDL).
- Chylomicrons are produced in intestinal cells from dietary lipid, and VLDL is produced in the liver, mainly from dietary carbohydrate.
- The triacylglycerols of chylomicrons and VLDL are hydrolyzed in the blood by lipoprotein lipase to fatty acids and glycerol. In adipose cells, the fatty acids are converted to triacylglycerols and stored.
  - IDL consists of the remains of VLDL after digestion of some of the triacylglycerols. IDL can either be endocytosed by liver cells and digested by lysosomal enzymes or converted to LDL by further digestion of triacylglycerols.
  - LDL undergoes endocytosis and lysosomal digestion, both in the liver and in the peripheral tissues.
  - Chylomicron remnants are endocytosed by the liver.
- Cholesterol travels through the blood as a component of the blood lipoproteins. Cholesterol is synthesized in most cells of the body. The key regulatory enzyme is HMG CoA reductase. Cholesterol is a component of cell membranes. In the liver, cholesterol is converted to bile salts, and it forms steroid hormones in endocrine tissues.
- HDL transfers proteins (including an activator of lipoprotein lipase, apoC$_{II}$) to chylomicrons and VLDL. HDL also picks up cholesterol from peripheral tissues and from other blood lipoproteins. This cholesterol ultimately returns to the liver.
- During fasting, fatty acids (derived from adipose triacylglycerol stores) are oxidized by various tissues to produce energy (see Figure 6-1B). In the liver, fatty acids are converted to ketone bodies, which are oxidized by tissues such as muscle and kidney.
- Eicosanoids (prostaglandins, thromboxanes, and leukotrienes) are derived from polyunsaturated fatty acids.

I. Lipid Structure

- Lipids have diverse structures but are similar in that they are insoluble in water.

A. Fatty acids exist free or esterified to glycerol (Figure 6-2).

1. In humans, fatty acids usually have an **even number** of carbon atoms, are **16 to 20 carbon atoms** in length, and may be **saturated** or **unsaturated** (contain double bonds). They are described by the number of carbons and the positions of the double bonds (e.g., arachidonic acid, which has 20 carbons and 4 double bonds, is $20:4, \Delta^{5,8,11,14}$).

2. **Polyunsaturated fatty acids** are often classified according to the position of the first double bond from the ω-end (the carbon furthest from the carboxyl group; e.g., ω-3 or ω-6).

B. Monoacylglycerols (monoglycerides), **diacylglycerols** (diglycerides), and **triacylglycerols** (triglycerides) contain one, two, and three fatty acids esterified to glycerol, respectively.

C. Phosphoglycerides contain fatty acids esterified to positions 1 and 2 of the glycerol moiety and a phosphoryl group at position 3 (e.g., phosphocholine).

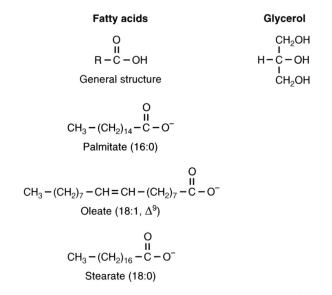

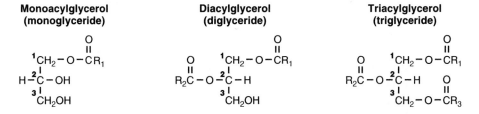

Figure 6-2. The structures of fatty acids, glycerol, and the acylglycerols. *R* indicates a linear aliphatic chain. Fatty acids are identified by the number of carbons and the number of double bonds and their positions (e.g., $18:1, \Delta^9$).

D. Sphingolipids contain ceramide with a variety of groups attached.

    1. Sphingomyelin contains phosphocholine.

    2. Cerebrosides contain a sugar residue.

    3. Gangliosides contain a number of sugar residues.

E. Cholesterol contains four rings and an aliphatic side chain (see Figure 6-9).

    – Bile salts and steroid hormones are derived from cholesterol (see Figure 6-10).

F. Prostaglandins and **leukotrienes** are derived from polyunsaturated fatty acids such as arachidonic acid (see Figure 6-18).

G. The **fat-soluble vitamins** include vitamins A, D, E, and K (see Figure 4-10).

II. Membranes

- The cell (plasma) membrane is a fluid mosaic of lipids and proteins.
- The proteins serve as transporters, enzymes, receptors, and mediators that allow extracellular compounds, such as hormones, to exert intracellular effects.

A. Membrane structure

    1. Membranes are composed mainly of lipids and proteins (Figure 6-3).

    2. Phosphoglycerides are the major membrane lipids, but sphingolipids and cholesterol are also present.

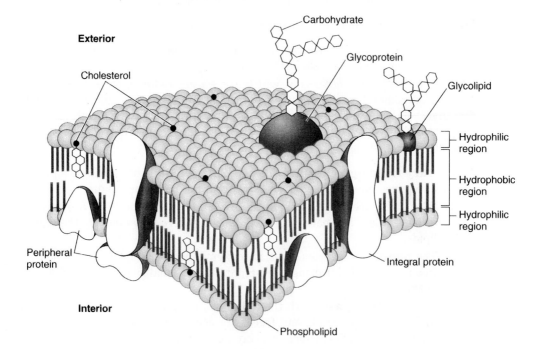

Figure 6-3. The structure of the cell membrane.

– **Phospholipids** form a bilayer, with their hydrophilic head groups interacting with water on both the extracellular and intracellular surfaces, and their hydrophobic fatty acyl chains in the central portion of the membrane.

3. **Peripheral proteins** are embedded at the periphery; **integral proteins** span from one side to the other.

4. **Carbohydrates** are attached to proteins and lipids on the exterior side of the cell membrane. They extend into the extracellular space.

5. **Lipids and proteins** can **diffuse laterally** within the plane of the membrane. Therefore, the membrane is a fluid mosaic.

B. Membrane function

1. Membranes serve as **barriers** that separate the contents of a cell from the external environment or the contents of organelles from the remainder of the cell.

2. The **proteins** in the cell membrane have many functions.

    a. Some are involved in the **transport** of substances across the membrane.

    b. Some are **enzymes** that catalyze biochemical reactions.

    c. Those on the exterior surface can function as **receptors** that bind external ligands such as hormones or growth factors.

    d. Others are **mediators** that aid the ligand-receptor complex in triggering a sequence of events (e.g., G proteins); as a consequence, **second messengers** (e.g., cAMP) that alter metabolism are produced inside the cell. Therefore, an external agent, such as a hormone, can elicit intracellular effects without entering the cell.

III. Digestion of Dietary Triacylglycerol

- The major dietary fat is triacylglycerol, which is obtained from the fat stores of the plants and animals in the food supply.
- The dietary triacylglycerols, which are water-insoluble, are emulsified by bile salts and digested in the small intestine to fatty acids and 2-monoacylglycerols. These digestive products are resynthesized to triacylglycerols in intestinal epithelial cells and are secreted in chylomicrons via the lymph into the blood.

A. Dietary triacylglycerols are digested in the **small intestine** by a process that requires bile salts and secretions from the pancreas (Figure 6-4).

1. **Bile salts** are synthesized in the liver from cholesterol and are secreted into the bile. They pass into the intestine, where they emulsify the dietary lipids.

2. The **pancreas** secretes digestive enzymes and bicarbonate, which neutralizes stomach acid, raising the pH into the optimal range for the digestive enzymes.

3. **Pancreatic lipase,** with the aid of colipase, digests the triacylglycerols to 2-monoacylglycerols and free fatty acids, which are packaged into micelles. The micelles, which are tiny microdroplets emulsified by bile salts, also contain other dietary lipids such as cholesterol and the fat-soluble vitamins.

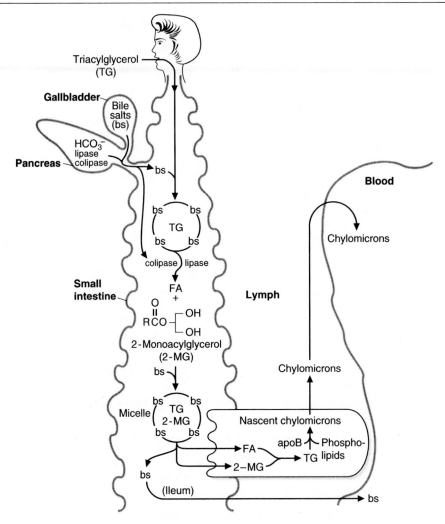

Figure 6-4. Digestion of triacylglycerols. *bs* = bile salts; *FA* = fatty acid; *2-MG* = 2-monoacylglycerol; *TG* = triacylglycerols.

4. The **micelles** travel to the microvilli of the intestinal epithelial cells, which absorb the fatty acids, 2-monoacylglycerols, and other dietary lipids.

5. The **bile salts are resorbed,** recycled by the liver, and secreted into the gut during subsequent digestive cycles.

B. Synthesis of chylomicrons

1. In intestinal epithelial cells, the **fatty acids** from micelles are **activated** by fatty acyl CoA synthetase (thiokinase) to form fatty acyl CoA.

2. A **fatty acyl CoA** reacts with a 2-monoacylglycerol to form a **diacylglycerol.** Then another fatty acyl CoA reacts with the diacylglycerol to form a **triacylglycerol.**

3. The triacylglycerols pass into the lymph packaged in **nascent (newborn) chylomicrons,** which eventually enter the blood.

IV. Fatty Acid and Triacylglycerol Synthesis

- Lipogenesis, the synthesis of fatty acids and their esterification to glycerol to form triacylglycerols, occurs mainly in the liver in humans, with dietary carbohydrate as the major source of carbon.
- The de novo synthesis of fatty acids from acetyl CoA occurs in the cytosol on the fatty acid synthase complex.
- Acetyl CoA, derived mainly from glucose, is converted by acetyl CoA carboxylase to malonyl CoA.
- The growing fatty acyl chain on the fatty acid synthase complex is elongated, two carbons at a time, by the addition of the three-carbon compound, malonyl CoA, which is subsequently decarboxylated. With each two-carbon addition, the growing chain, which initially contains a β-keto group, is reduced in a series of steps that require NADPH.
  - NADPH is produced by the pentose phosphate pathway and by the reaction catalyzed by the malic enzyme.
- Palmitate, the product released by the fatty acid synthase complex, is converted to a series of other fatty acyl CoAs by elongation and desaturation reactions.
- Fatty acyl CoA combines with glycerol 3-phosphate in the liver to form triacylglycerols by a pathway in which phosphatidic acid serves as an intermediate.
- The triacylglycerols, packaged in VLDL, are secreted into the blood.

A. Conversion of glucose to acetyl CoA for fatty acid synthesis (Figure 6-5)

1. **Glucose** enters liver cells and is converted via glycolysis to pyruvate, which enters mitochondria.

2. **Pyruvate** is converted to acetyl CoA by pyruvate dehydrogenase and to **oxaloacetate** by pyruvate carboxylase.

3. Because acetyl CoA cannot directly cross the mitochondrial membrane and enter the cytosol to be used for the process of fatty acid synthesis, acetyl CoA and oxaloacetate condense to form **citrate,** which can cross the mitochondrial membrane.

4. In the cytosol, **citrate is cleaved** to oxaloacetate and acetyl CoA by citrate lyase, an enzyme that requires ATP and is induced by insulin.

   a. **Oxaloacetate** from the citrate lyase reaction is reduced in the cytosol by NADH, producing NAD^+ and **malate**. The enzyme is cytosolic malate dehydrogenase.

   b. In a subsequent reaction, **malate** is converted to pyruvate, NADPH is produced, and CO_2 is released. The enzyme is the **malic enzyme** (also known as decarboxylating malate dehydrogenase or $NADP^+$-dependent malate dehydrogenase).

   (1) **Pyruvate** re-enters the mitochondrion and is reutilized.

   (2) **NADPH** supplies reducing equivalents for reactions that occur on the fatty acid synthase complex.

   - **NADPH** is produced not only by the **malic enzyme** but also by the **pentose phosphate pathway.**

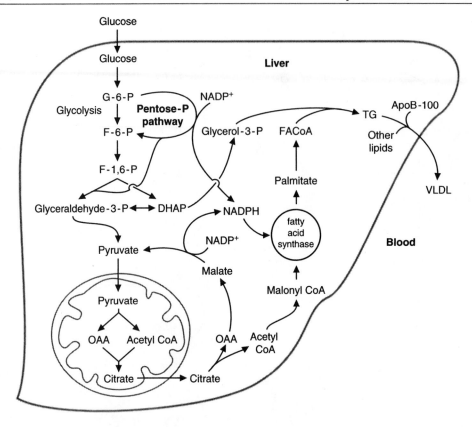

Figure 6-5. Synthesis of fatty acids and triacylglycerols from glucose. *DHAP* = dihydroxyacetone phosphate; *F-6-P* = fructose 6-phosphate; *F-1,6-P* = fructose-1,6-bisphosphate; *G-6-P* = glucose 6-phosphate; *OAA* = oxaloacetate; *VLDL* = very low density lipoprotein.

    5. Acetyl CoA (from the citrate lyase reaction or from other sources) supplies carbons for fatty acid synthesis in the cytosol.

B. Synthesis of fatty acids by the fatty acid synthase complex (Figure 6-6)

    – **Fatty acid synthase** is a multienzyme complex located in the cytosol. It has two identical subunits with seven catalytic activities.

    – This enzyme contains a **phosphopantetheine residue,** derived from the vitamin pantothenic acid, and a **cysteine residue;** both contain sulfhydryl groups that can form thioesters with acyl groups. The growing fatty acyl chain moves from one to the other of these sulfhydryl residues as it is elongated.

1. Addition of two-carbon units

    a. Initially, **acetyl CoA** reacts with the phosphopantetheinyl residue and then the acetyl group is transferred to the cysteinyl residue. This acetyl group provides the **ω-carbon** of the fatty acid produced by the fatty acid synthase complex.

    b. A malonyl group from **malonyl CoA** forms a **thioester** with the phosphopantetheinyl sulfhydryl group.

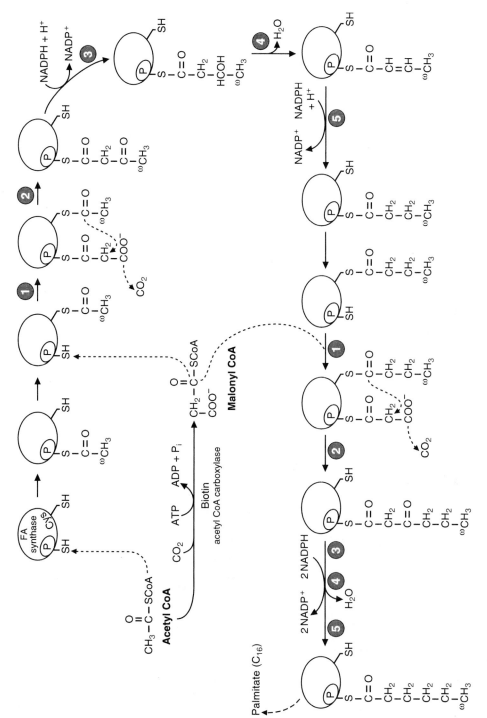

Figure 6-6. Fatty acid synthesis. Malonyl CoA provides the 2-carbon units that are added to the growing fatty acyl chain. The addition and reduction steps (1–5) are repeated until palmitic acid is produced. *Cys-SH* = a cysteinyl residue; *P* = a phosphopantetheinyl group attached to the fatty acid synthase complex.

(1) Malonyl CoA is formed from acetyl CoA by a carboxylation reaction that requires **biotin** and ATP.

(2) The enzyme is **acetyl CoA carboxylase,** a regulatory enzyme that is inhibited by phosphorylation, activated by dephosphorylation and by citrate, and induced by insulin.

c. The **acetyl group** on the fatty acid synthase complex condenses with the malonyl group; the CO_2 that was added to the malonyl group by acetyl CoA carboxylase is released; and a **β-ketoacyl group,** containing four carbons, is produced.

2. Reduction of the β-ketoacyl group

a. The β-keto group is **reduced** by NADPH to a β-hydroxy group.

b. Then **dehydration** occurs, producing an **enoyl group** with the double bond between carbons 2 and 3.

c. Finally, the double bond is reduced by NADPH, and a **four-carbon acyl group** is generated.

– The **NADPH** for these reactions is produced by the **pentose phosphate pathway** and by the **malic enzyme.**

3. Elongation of the growing fatty acyl chain

a. The acyl group is transferred to the cysteinyl sulfhydryl group, and **malonyl CoA** reacts with the phosphopantetheinyl group. Condensation of the acyl and malonyl groups occurs with the release of CO_2, followed by the three reactions that reduce the β-keto group. The chain is now longer by two carbons.

b. This sequence of reactions repeats until the growing chain is 16 carbons in length.

c. Palmitate, a 16-carbon saturated fatty acid, is the final product released by hydrolysis from the fatty acid synthase complex.

C. Elongation and desaturation of fatty acids

– **Palmitate** can be elongated and desaturated to form a **series of fatty acids.**

1. Elongation of long-chain fatty acids occurs on the endoplasmic reticulum, by reactions similar, but not identical, to those that occur on the fatty acid synthase complex.

a. Malonyl CoA provides the two-carbon units that add to palmitoyl CoA or to longer-chain fatty acyl CoAs.

b. Malonyl CoA condenses with the carbonyl group of the fatty acyl residue and CO_2 is released.

c. The β-keto group is reduced by NADPH to a β-hydroxy group, dehydration occurs; and a double bond is formed, which is reduced by NADPH.

2. Desaturation of fatty acids is a complex process that requires O_2, NADPH, and cytochrome b_5.

– In humans, desaturases may add double bonds at the 9-10 position of a fatty acyl CoA and at intervals between carbon 9 and the carboxyl group.

a. Plants can introduce double bonds between carbon 9 and the ω-carbon, but animals cannot. Therefore, certain unsaturated fatty acids from plants are required in the human diet.

b. **Linoleate** ($18:2,\Delta^{9,12}$) and **α-linolenate** ($18:3,\Delta^{9,12,15}$) are the major sources of the essential fatty acids required in the human diet. They are used for synthesis of **arachidonic acid** and other polyunsaturated fatty acids from which eicosanoids (e.g., prostaglandins) are produced.

D. Synthesis of triacylglycerols (Figure 6-7)

1. In intestinal epithelial cells, triacylglycerol synthesis occurs by a different pathway than in other tissues (see III B). This triacylglycerol becomes a component of chylomicrons. Ultimately, the fatty acyl groups are stored in adipose triacylglycerols.

2. In the liver and adipose tissue, glycerol 3-phosphate provides the glycerol moiety that reacts with two fatty acyl CoAs to form **phosphatidic acid.** The phosphate group is cleaved to form a diacylglycerol, which reacts with another fatty acyl CoA to form a triacylglycerol.

a. The liver can use glycerol to produce glycerol 3-phosphate by a reaction that requires ATP and is catalyzed by glycerol kinase.

b. Adipose tissue, which **lacks glycerol kinase,** cannot generate glycerol 3-phosphate from glycerol.

c. Both liver and adipose tissue can convert glucose, through glycolysis, to dihydroxyacetone phosphate (**DHAP**), which is reduced by NADH to glycerol 3-phosphate.

d. Triacylglycerol is **stored in adipose tissue.**

e. In the **liver,** triacylglycerol is incorporated into **VLDL,** which enters the blood. Ultimately, the fatty acyl groups are stored in adipose triacylglycerols.

E. Regulation of triacylglycerol synthesis from carbohydrate

1. Synthesis of triacylglycerols from carbohydrate occurs in the liver in the **fed state.**

2. Key regulatory enzymes in the pathway are activated, and a high-carbohydrate diet causes their induction.

a. The glycolytic enzymes **glucokinase, phosphofructokinase 1,** and **pyruvate kinase** are active (see Chapter 5 for mechanisms).

b. Pyruvate dehydrogenase is dephosphorylated and active.

c. Pyruvate carboxylase is activated by acetyl CoA.

d. Citrate lyase is inducible.

e. Acetyl CoA carboxylase is induced, activated by citrate, and converted to its active, dephosphorylated state by a phosphatase that is stimulated by insulin.

f. The **fatty acid synthase complex** is inducible.

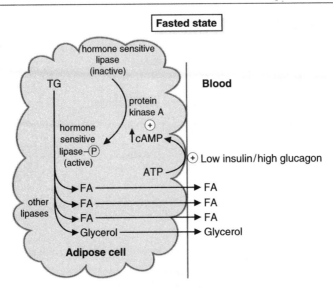

Figure 6-13. Mobilization of triacylglycerols from adipose cells in the fasted state. *FA* = fatty acid; *TG* = triacylglycerols; ⊕ = stimulated by.

    b. In the **liver,** fatty acids are converted to **ketone bodies** that are oxidized by tissues such as muscle and kidney. During starvation (after fasting has lasted about 3 or more days), the brain uses ketone bodies for energy.

  2. **Glycerol** is used by the liver as a source of carbon for **gluconeogenesis,** which produces glucose for tissues such as the brain and red blood cells.

IX. Fatty Acid Oxidation

- Fatty acids, which are the major source of energy in the human, are oxidized mainly by β-oxidation.
- Prior to oxidation, long-chain fatty acids are activated, forming fatty acyl CoA, which is transported into mitochondria by a carnitine carrier system.
- The process of β-oxidation occurs in mitochondria. In four steps that produce $FADH_2$ and NADH, two carbons are cleaved from a fatty acyl CoA and are released as acetyl CoA. This series of steps is repeated until an even-chain fatty acid is completely converted to acetyl CoA.
- ATP is obtained when $FADH_2$ and NADH interact with the electron transport chain or when acetyl CoA is oxidized further.
- In tissues such as skeletal and heart muscle, acetyl CoA enters the TCA cycle and is oxidized to CO_2 and H_2O. In the liver, acetyl CoA is converted to ketone bodies.
- β-Oxidation is regulated by the mechanisms that control oxidative phosphorylation (i.e., by the demand for ATP).
- Fatty acids also undergo α- and ω-oxidation and peroxisomal oxidation.

A. Activation of fatty acids

  1. In the cytosol of the cell, long-chain fatty acids are activated by **ATP** and **coenzyme A,** and **fatty acyl CoA** is formed (Figure 6-14). Short-chain fatty acids are activated in mitochondria.

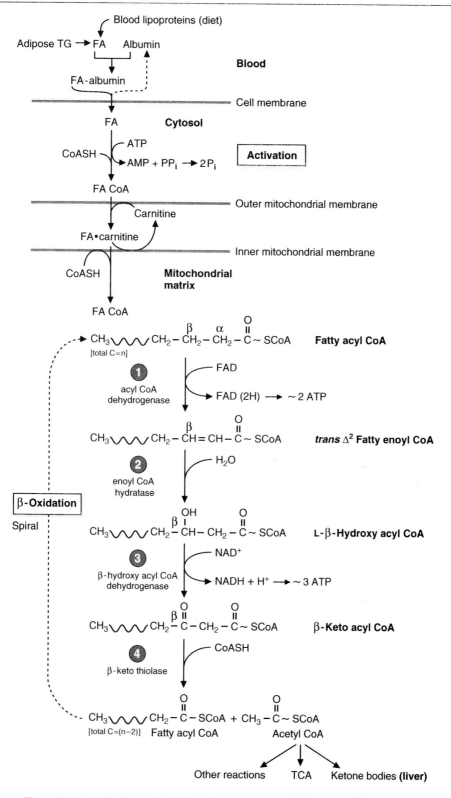

Figure 6-14. Activation and oxidation of fatty acids. *FA* = fatty acid; *TG* = triacylglycerol.

2. The **ATP** is converted to **AMP and pyrophosphate** (PP_i), which is cleaved by pyrophosphatase to two inorganic phosphates (2 P_i). Because two high-energy phosphate bonds are cleaved, the equivalent of two molecules of ATP are used for fatty acid activation.

B. Transport of fatty acyl CoA from the cytosol into mitochondria

1. **Fatty acyl CoA** from the cytosol reacts with **carnitine** in the outer mitochondrial membrane, forming fatty acyl carnitine. The enzyme is **carnitine acyl transferase I** (CATI), which is also called carnitine palmitoyl transferase I (CPTI). **Fatty acyl carnitine** passes to the inner membrane, where it **re-forms fatty acyl CoA,** which enters the matrix. The second enzyme is carnitine acyl transferase II (CAT II).

2. **Carnitine acyltransferase I,** which catalyzes the transfer of acyl groups from coenzyme A to carnitine, is **inhibited by malonyl CoA,** an intermediate in fatty acid synthesis. Therefore, when fatty acids are being synthesized in the cytosol, malonyl CoA inhibits their transport into mitochondria and, thus, prevents a futile cycle (synthesis followed by immediate degradation).

3. Inside the mitochondrion, fatty acyl CoA undergoes **β-oxidation.**

C. β-Oxidation of even-chain fatty acids

– **β-Oxidation** (in which all reactions involve the β-carbon of a fatty acyl CoA) is a spiral consisting of four sequential steps, the first three of which are similar to those in the TCA cycle between succinate and oxaloacetate. These steps are repeated until all the carbons of an even-chain fatty acyl CoA are converted to acetyl CoA (see Figure 6-14).

1. **FAD accepts hydrogens** from a fatty acyl CoA in the first step. A double bond is produced between the α- and β-carbons, and an enoyl CoA is formed. The $FADH_2$ that is produced interacts with the electron transport chain, generating ATP.
   – Enzyme: **acyl CoA dehydrogenase**

2. **H_2O adds across the double bond**, and a β-hydroxyacyl CoA is formed.
   – Enzyme: **enoyl CoA hydratase**

3. **β–Hydroxyacyl CoA is oxidized** by NAD^+ to a β-ketoacyl CoA. The NADH that is produced interacts with the electron transport chain, generating ATP.
   – Enzyme: **L-3-hydroxyacyl CoA dehydrogenase** (which is specific for the L-isomer of the β-hydroxyacyl CoA)

4. The **bond between the α- and β-carbons** of the β-ketoacyl CoA is cleaved by a **thiolase** that requires coenzyme A. Acetyl CoA is produced from the two carbons at the carboxyl end of the original fatty acyl CoA, and the remaining carbons form a fatty acyl CoA that is two carbons shorter than the original.
   – Enzyme: **β-ketothiolase**

5. The shortened **fatty acyl CoA repeats** these four steps. Repetitions continue until all the carbons of the original fatty acyl CoA are converted to acetyl CoA.

    a. The 16-carbon palmitoyl CoA undergoes seven repetitions.

    b. In the last repetition, a four-carbon fatty acyl CoA (butyryl CoA) is cleaved to two acetyl CoAs.

6. Energy is generated from the products of β-oxidation.

    a. When one palmitoyl CoA is oxidized, seven $FADH_2$, seven NADH, and eight acetyl CoA are formed.

        (1) The 7 $FADH_2$ each generate approximately 2 ATP, for a total of about 14 ATP.

        (2) The 7 NADH each generate about 3 ATP, for a total of about 21 ATP.

        (3) The 8 acetyl CoA can enter the TCA cycle, each producing about 12 ATP, for a total of about 96 ATP.

        (4) From the oxidation of palmitoyl CoA to CO_2 and H_2O, a total of about 131 ATP are produced.

    b. The **net ATP** produced from palmitate that enters the cell from the blood is about 129 because palmitate must undergo activation (a process that requires the equivalent of 2 ATP) before it can be oxidized (131 ATP – 2 ATP = 129 ATP).

    c. Oxidation of other fatty acids will yield different amounts of ATP.

D. Oxidation of odd-chain and unsaturated fatty acids

    1. Odd-chain fatty acids produce acetyl CoA and propionyl CoA.

        a. These fatty acids repeat the four steps of the β-oxidation spiral, producing **acetyl CoA** until the last cleavage when the three remaining carbons are released as propionyl CoA.

        b. Propionyl CoA, but not acetyl CoA, can be converted to glucose. (See Chapter 5 VI D2 and Figure 7-10.)

    2. Unsaturated fatty acids, which comprise about half the fatty acid residues in human lipids, require enzymes in addition to the four that catalyze the repetitive steps of the β-oxidation spiral.

        a. β-Oxidation occurs until a double bond of the unsaturated fatty acid is near the carboxyl end of the fatty acyl chain.

        b. If the double bond is not between the α and β carbons in a trans configuration, it is moved so that it is α–β trans. The normal steps of β-oxidation can then proceed.

E. ω-Oxidation of fatty acids

    1. The ω (omega)-**carbon** (the methyl carbon) of fatty acids is oxidized to a carboxyl group in the endoplasmic reticulum.

    2. β-Oxidation can then occur in mitochondria at this end of the fatty acid as well as from the original carboxyl end. **Dicarboxylic acids** are produced.

F. Oxidation of very long chain fatty acids in peroxisomes

    1. The process differs from β-oxidation in that **molecular O_2** is used, **hydrogen peroxide** (H_2O_2) is formed, and **no ATP** is generated.

2. The shorter-chain fatty acids that are produced travel to mitochondria, where they undergo β-oxidation, generating ATP.

G. α-Oxidation of fatty acids

1. **Very long chain fatty acids** are oxidized at the α-carbon (mainly in brain and other nervous tissue), and the carboxyl carbon is released as CO_2.

2. The fatty acid is thus degraded one carbon at a time.

X. Ketone Body Synthesis and Utilization

- The ketone bodies, acetoacetate and β-hydroxybutyrate, serve as a source of fuel. They are synthesized mainly in liver mitochondria whenever fatty acid levels are high in the blood.
- Fatty acids are activated in liver cells and converted to acetyl CoA, generating ATP. As NADH and ATP levels rise, acetyl CoA accumulates.
- Acetyl CoA reacts with acetoacetyl CoA to form HMG CoA, which is cleaved to form acetoacetate.
- Acetoacetate can be reduced to a second ketone body, 3-hydroxybutyrate (β-hydroxybutyrate), by NADH.
- Acetone is produced by spontaneous (nonenzymatic) decarboxylation of acetoacetate.
- The liver cannot use ketone bodies because it lacks the thiotransferase enzyme that activates acetoacetate.
- Ketone bodies are used as fuels by tissues such as muscle and kidney. During starvation (after about 3-5 days of fasting), the brain also oxidizes ketone bodies.
- Ketone bodies enter cells, where 3-hydroxybutyrate is oxidized to form acetoacetate in a reaction that produces NADH.
- Acetoacetate, obtained directly from the blood or produced from 3-hydroxybutyrate, is activated to acetoacetyl CoA by reacting with succinyl CoA. Acetoacetyl CoA is cleaved by β-ketothiolase to 2 acetyl CoAs, which enter the TCA cycle and are oxidized to CO_2 and H_2O, generating ATP.

A. Synthesis of ketone bodies (Figure 6-15) occurs in **liver mitochondria** when fatty acids are in high concentration in the blood (during fasting, starvation, or as a result of a high-fat diet).

– **β-Oxidation** produces NADH and ATP and results in the accumulation of acetyl CoA. The liver is producing glucose, using oxaloacetate (OAA), so there is decreased condensation of acetyl CoA with OAA to form citrate.

1. **Two molecules of acetyl CoA** condense to produce acetoacetyl CoA. This reaction is catalyzed by thiolase or an isoenzyme of **thiolase**.

2. Acetoacetyl CoA and acetyl CoA form HMG CoA in a reaction catalyzed by HMG CoA synthetase.

3. **HMG CoA** is cleaved by HMG CoA lyase to form acetyl CoA and acetoacetate.

4. **Acetoacetate** can be reduced by an NAD-requiring dehydrogenase (3-hydroxybutyrate dehydrogenase) to **3-hydroxybutyrate.** This is a reversible reaction.

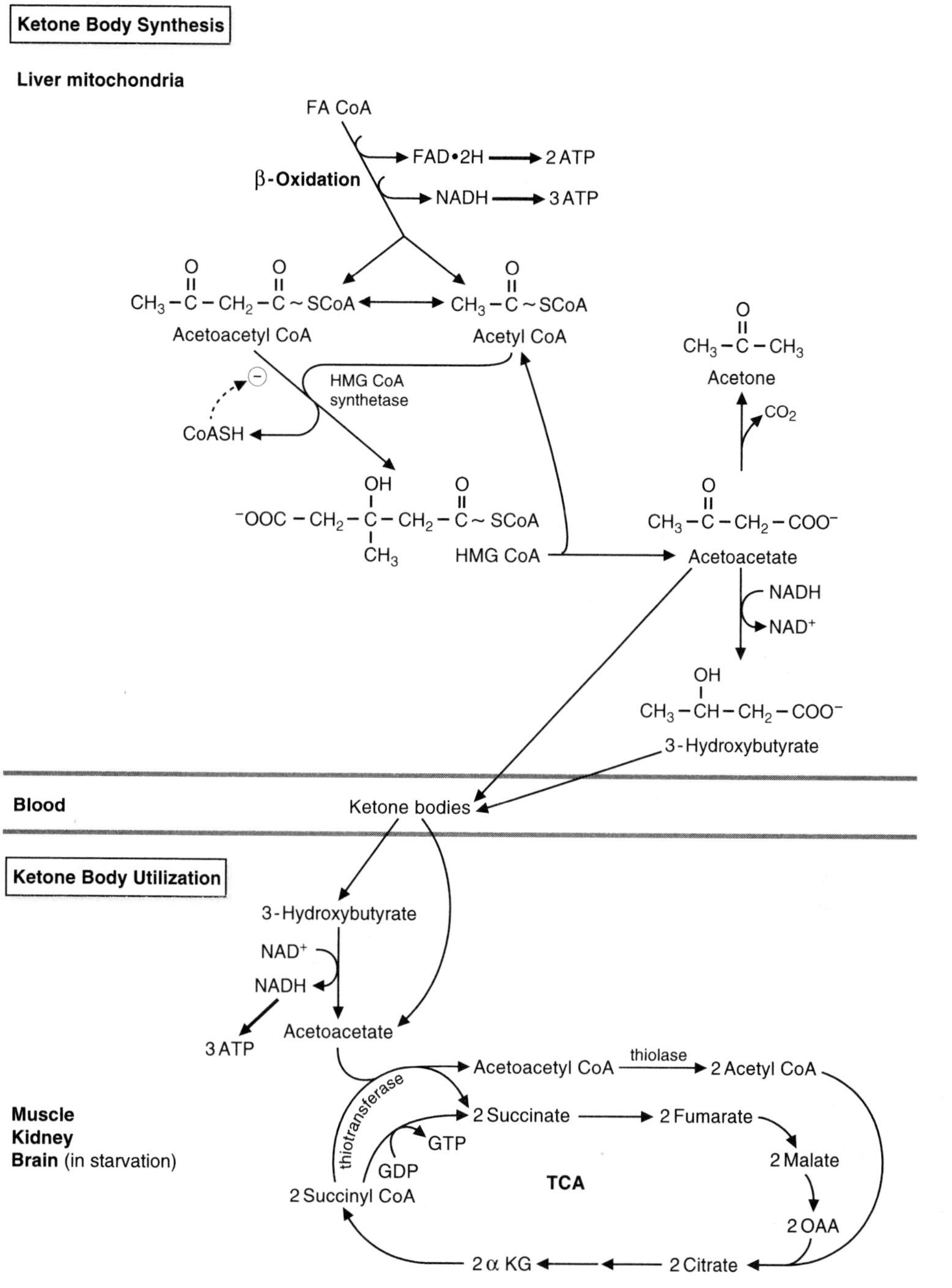

Ketone Body Synthesis

Liver mitochondria

FA CoA

β-Oxidation

FAD•2H ⟶ 2 ATP

NADH ⟶ 3 ATP

$CH_3 - \overset{O}{\overset{\|}{C}} - CH_2 - \overset{O}{\overset{\|}{C}} \sim SCoA$ ⟵ $CH_3 - \overset{O}{\overset{\|}{C}} \sim SCoA$

Acetoacetyl CoA   Acetyl CoA

$CH_3 - \overset{O}{\overset{\|}{C}} - CH_3$

Acetone

CO_2

HMG CoA synthetase

CoASH

$^-OOC - CH_2 - \overset{OH}{\underset{CH_3}{\overset{|}{C}}} - CH_2 - \overset{O}{\overset{\|}{C}} \sim SCoA$ $CH_3 - \overset{O}{\overset{\|}{C}} - CH_2 - COO^-$

HMG CoA ⟶ Acetoacetate

NADH

NAD^+

$CH_3 - \overset{OH}{\overset{|}{CH}} - CH_2 - COO^-$

3-Hydroxybutyrate

Blood

Ketone bodies

Ketone Body Utilization

3-Hydroxybutyrate

NAD^+

NADH

3 ATP   Acetoacetate

Acetoacetyl CoA ⟶ thiolase ⟶ 2 Acetyl CoA

thiotransferase

Muscle
Kidney
Brain (in starvation)

2 Succinate ⟶ 2 Fumarate

GTP

GDP

2 Succinyl CoA

TCA

2 Malate

2 OAA

2 α KG ⟵ ⟵ 2 Citrate ⟵

Figure 6-15. Ketone body synthesis and utilization. *FA* = fatty acid; α*KG* = α-ketoglutarate; *HMG CoA* = hydroxymethylglutaryl CoA; *OAA* = oxaloacetate. The thiotransferase is succinyl CoA- acetoacetate-CoA transferase.

5. Acetoacetate is also spontaneously **decarboxylated,** in a nonenzymatic reaction, forming **acetone** (the source of the odor on the breath of ketotic diabetics).

6. The **liver** lacks succinyl CoA-acetoacetate-CoA transferase (a thiotransferase) so it **cannot use ketone bodies.** Therefore, acetoacetate and 3-hydroxybutyrate are released into the blood by the liver.

B. Utilization of ketone bodies (see Figure 6-15)

1. When ketone bodies are released from the liver into the blood, they are taken up by peripheral tissues such as **muscle and kidney,** where they are oxidized for energy.

– During **starvation,** ketone bodies in the blood increase to a level that permits entry into **brain** cells, where they are oxidized.

2. Acetoacetate can enter cells directly, or it can be produced from the oxidation of 3-hydroxybutyrate by 3-hydroxybutyrate dehydrogenase. NADH is produced by this reaction and can generate ATP.

3. Acetoacetate is activated by reacting with succinyl CoA to form **acetoacetyl CoA** and succinate. The enzyme is succinyl CoA-acetoacetate-CoA transferase (a thiotransferase).

4. Acetoacetyl CoA is cleaved by **thiolase** to form two acetyl CoAs, which enter the TCA cycle and are oxidized to CO_2 and H_2O.

5. Energy is produced from the oxidation of ketone bodies.

a. One acetoacetate produces 2 acetyl CoAs, each of which can generate about 12 ATP, or a total of about 24 ATP via the TCA cycle.

b. However, activation of acetoacetate results in the generation of one less ATP because GTP, the equivalent of ATP, is not produced when succinyl CoA is used to activate acetoacetate. (In the TCA cycle, when succinyl CoA forms succinate, GTP is generated.) Therefore, the oxidation of acetoacetate produces a net yield of only 23 ATP.

c. When **3-hydroxybutyrate** is oxidized, three additional ATP are formed because the oxidation of 3-hydroxybutyrate to acetoacetate produces NADH.

XI. Phospholipid and Sphingolipid Metabolism

- Phospholipids and sphingolipids are major components of cell membranes. They are amphipathic molecules; that is, one portion of the molecule is hydrophilic and associates with H_2O, and another portion contains the hydrocarbon chains derived from fatty acids, which are hydrophobic and associate with lipids (see Figure 6-3).
- Phosphoglycerides (the major phospholipids) contain glycerol, fatty acids, and phosphate. The phosphate is esterified to choline, serine, ethanolamine, or inositol.
- The phosphoglycerides are synthesized via a number of pathways.
- Degradation of phosphoglycerides involves phospholipases, which are each specific for one of the ester linkages of the phosphodiester bonds.

- The sphingolipids include sphingomyelin (which contains phosphocholine) and the cerebrosides and gangliosides (which contain sugar residues). These compounds are major components of cell membranes in nervous tissue.
- The sphingolipids are synthesized from ceramide, which is produced from serine and palmitoyl CoA.
- During degradation, the phosphocholine and sugar units of the sphingolipids are removed by lysosomal enzymes.

A. Synthesis and degradation of phosphoglycerides

- The phosphoglycerides are synthesized by a process similar in its initial steps to triacylglycerol synthesis (glycerol 3-phosphate combines with two fatty acyl CoAs to form **phosphatidic acid**).

1. Synthesis of phosphatidylinositol

a. Phosphatidic acid reacts with CTP to form CDP-diacylglycerol, which reacts with inositol to form phosphatidylinositol.

b. Phosphatidylinositol can be further phosphorylated to form phosphatidylinositol 4,5-bisphosphate, which is cleaved in response to various stimuli to form the compounds inositol 1,4,5-trisphosphate (IP_3) and diacylglycerol (DAG), which serve as second messengers (see Chapter 8).

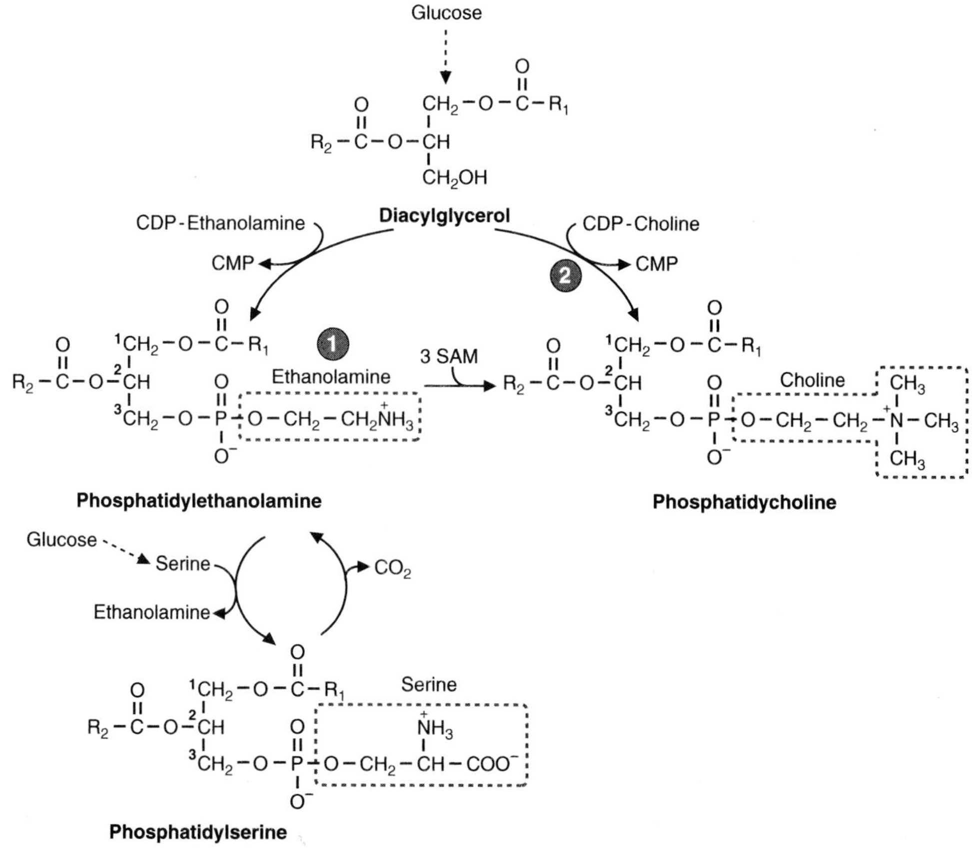

Figure 6-16. Synthesis of phospholipids. *SAM* = *S*-adenosylmethionine. ❶ and ❷ are two different pathways for synthesis of phosphatidylcholine.

2. **Synthesis of phosphatidylethanolamine, phosphatidylcholine, and phosphatidylserine** (Figure 6-16)

   – **Phosphatidic acid** releases inorganic phosphate, and diacylglycerol is produced. **Diacylglycerol** reacts with compounds containing cytosine nucleotides to form **phosphatidylethanolamine** and **phosphatidylcholine**.

   a. **Phosphatidylethanolamine**

      (1) Diacylglycerol reacts with CDP-ethanolamine to form phosphatidylethanolamine.

      (2) Phosphatidylethanolamine can also be formed by decarboxylation of phosphatidylserine.

   b. **Phosphatidylcholine**

      (1) Diacylglycerol reacts with CDP-choline to form **phosphatidylcholine (lecithin)**.

      (2) Phosphatidylcholine can also be formed by methylation of phosphatidylethanolamine. *S*-Adenosylmethionine (SAM) provides the methyl groups.

         – In addition to being an important component of cell membranes and the blood lipoproteins, phosphatidylcholine provides the fatty acid for the synthesis of cholesterol esters in HDL by the **LCAT reaction** and, as the dipalmitoyl derivative, serves as **lung surfactant**. If choline is deficient in the diet, phosphatidylcholine can be synthesized de novo from glucose (see Figure 6-16).

   c. **Phosphatidylserine**

      – Phosphatidylserine is formed when phosphatidylethanolamine reacts with serine, which replaces the ethanolamine moiety (see Figure 6-16).

3. **Degradation of phosphoglycerides**

   a. Phosphoglycerides are hydrolyzed by **phospholipases.**

   b. Phospholipase A_1 releases the fatty acid at position 1 of the glycerol moiety; phospholipase A_2 releases the fatty acid at position 2; phospholipase C releases the phosphorylated base (e.g., choline) at position 3; and phospholipase D releases the free base.

B. **Synthesis and degradation of sphingolipids** (Figure 6-17)

   – Sphingolipids are derived from **serine** rather than glycerol.

   1. **Serine** condenses with **palmitoyl CoA** in a reaction in which the serine is decarboxylated by a pyridoxal phosphate-requiring enzyme.

   2. The product is converted to a derivative of **sphingosine.**

   3. A fatty acyl CoA forms an amide with the nitrogen, and the resulting compound is **ceramide.**

   4. The hydroxymethyl moiety of ceramide combines with various compounds to form **sphingolipids.**

      a. **Phosphatidylcholine** reacts with ceramide to form **sphingomyelin.**

      b. **UDP-galactose,** or **UDP-glucose,** reacts with ceramide to form **galactocerebrosides** or **glucocerebrosides.**

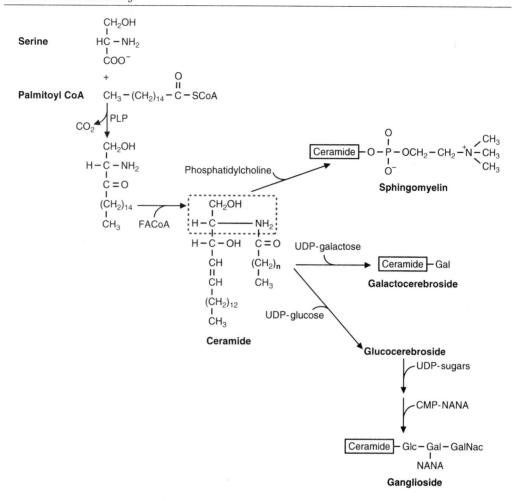

Figure 6-17. Synthesis of sphingolipids. *FA* = fatty acyl groups derived from fatty acids; *Gal* = galactose; *GalNAc* = N-acetylgalactosamine; *Glc* = glucose; *NANA* = N-acetylneuraminic acid; *PLP* = pyridoxal phosphate. The *dashed box* contains the portion of ceramide derived from serine.

    c. A series of sugars can add to ceramide, UDP-sugars serving as precursors. **CMP-NANA** (N-acetylneuraminic acid, a sialic acid) can form branches from the carbohydrate chain. These ceramide-oligosaccharide compounds are **gangliosides.**

  5. Sphingolipids are degraded by **lysosomal enzymes.**

XII. Metabolism of the Eicosanoids

- The eicosanoids (prostaglandins, thromboxanes, and leukotrienes) are synthesized from polyunsaturated fatty acids (e.g., arachidonic acid). These fatty acids are released from membrane phospholipids by phospholipase A_2, which is inhibited by glucocorticoids and other steroidal anti-inflammatory agents.

- For prostaglandin synthesis, the polyunsaturated fatty acid is cyclized and oxidized by a cyclooxygenase, which is inhibited by aspirin and the nonsteroidal anti-inflammatory agents. Further oxidations and rearrangements occur that produce a series of prostaglandins, including the prostacyclins.
- Thromboxanes are produced from certain prostaglandins.
- Leukotrienes are produced from arachidonic acid by a pathway that differs from that for prostaglandin synthesis.

A. Prostaglandins, prostacyclins, and thromboxanes (Figure 6-18)

1. **Polyunsaturated fatty acids** containing 20 carbons and three to five double bonds (e.g., arachidonic acid) are usually esterified to position 2 of the glycerol moiety of phospholipids in cell membranes. These fatty acids require **essential fatty acids** such as dietary linoleic acid ($18:2, \Delta^{9,12}$) for their synthesis.

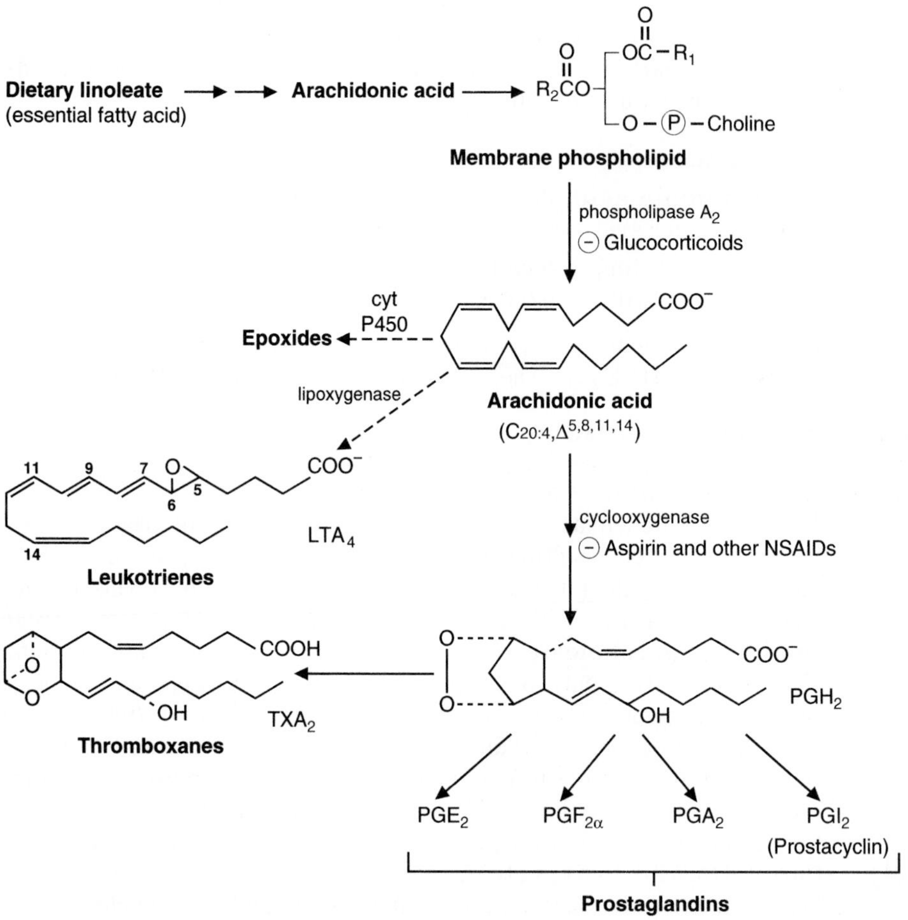

Figure 6-18. Prostaglandins, thromboxanes, and leukotrienes. *LT* = leukotriene; *PG* = prostaglandin; *TX* = thromboxane. For each of the classes of prostaglandins (H, E, F, A), the *ring* contains hydroxyl and keto groups at different positions and the subscript refers to the number of double bonds in the non-ring portion. The class with two double bonds is derived from arachidonate. Other classes (with one or three double bonds) are derived from other polyunsaturated fatty acids.

2. The polyunsaturated fatty acid is cleaved from the membrane phospholipid by **phospholipase A_2,** which is inhibited by the steroidal anti-inflammatory agents.

3. Oxygen is added and a 5-carbon ring is formed by a **cyclooxygenase** that produces the initial prostaglandin, which is converted to other classes of **prostaglandins** and to the **thromboxanes**.

– **Aspirin, acetaminophen**, and other nonsteroidal anti-inflammatory agents **inhibit** this cyclooxygenase.

a. The **prostaglandins** have a multitude of effects that differ from one tissue to another and include inflammation, pain, fever, and aspects of reproduction. These compounds are known as **autocoids** because they exert their effects primarily in the tissue in which they are produced.

b. Certain **prostacyclins** (PGI_2), produced by vascular endothelial cells, **inhibit platelet aggregation**, while certain **thromboxanes** (TXA_2) **promote platelet aggregation**.

4. Inactivation of the prostaglandins occurs when the molecule is oxidized from the carboxyl and ω-methyl ends to form **dicarboxylic acids** that are excreted in the urine.

B. Leukotrienes

– **Arachidonic acid,** derived from membrane phospholipids, is the major precursor for synthesis of the leukotrienes.

1. In the first step, oxygen is added by lipoxygenases, and a family of linear molecules, hydroperoxyeicosatetraenoic acids (**HPETEs**), is formed.

2. A series of compounds, comprising the family of leukotrienes, is produced from these HPETEs. The leukotrienes are involved in **allergic reactions.**

XIII. Clinical Correlations

A. Hyperlipidemias

In the hyperlipidemias, the blood levels of cholesterol or triacylglycerols, or both, are elevated resulting from overproduction of lipoproteins or defects in various stages of their degradation. Elevations of blood lipid levels (particularly LDL) are associated with a high incidence of heart attacks and strokes. In **familial hypercholesterolemia,** cellular receptors for LDL are defective. Therefore, LDL is not taken up at a normal rate by cells and degraded by lysosomal enzymes. The consequent increase of blood LDL (which contains a large amount of cholesterol and cholesterol ester) is associated with **xanthomas** (lipid deposits often found under the skin) and **coronary artery disease.** Treatment may involve diets low in saturated fat and cholesterol, HMG CoA reductase inhibitors (e.g., lovastatin), bile-acid binding resins, and nicotinic acid (niacin). In **hypertriglyceridemia** due to deficiencies in lipoprotein lipase (LPL) or apo C_{II} (the lipoprotein lipase activator), triacylglycerol levels rise markedly because of decreased degradation of VLDL and chylomicrons. These deficiencies are associated with characteristic xanthomas and an intolerance to fatty foods. Low-fat diets may be effective. In **diabetes mellitus (DM)**, VLDL levels are often elevated, which results in high blood triacylglycerol levels. Cholesterol may also be elevated. In diabetes, elevated VLDL

levels result from deranged carbohydrate and lipid metabolism caused by decreased insulin levels (Type 1 DM) or insulin resistance (Type 2 DM).

B. Atherosclerosis

Atherosclerosis involves the formation of **lipid-rich plaques** in the intima of arteries. The plaques begin as fatty streaks containing foam cells, which initially are macrophages filled with oxidized LDL. These early lesions develop into fibrous plaques that can occlude an artery and cause a **myocardial infarct** or a **cerebral infarct.** Formation of these plaques is often associated with abnormalities in plasma lipoprotein metabolism. In contrast to the other lipoproteins, HDL has a protective effect.

C. Diabetic ketoacidosis

If a Type 1 **diabetic** who has failed to take insulin is suffering from an illness or is subjected to stress, blood glucose may rise markedly. Decreased insulin and elevated glucagon levels cause adipose tissue to release increased amounts of fatty acids, which are converted to ketone bodies by the liver. Decarboxylation of acetoacetate produces acetone, which gives a characteristic odor to the patient's breath. Ketone body levels can become extremely high, causing a **metabolic acidosis** that, if not treated rapidly and effectively, can lead to **coma and death.**

D. Fatty liver related to alcoholism

Oxidation of ingested alcohol produces acetaldehyde, acetate, and NADH. A high NADH/NAD$^+$ ratio slows the TCA cycle and promotes the synthesis of glycerol 3-phosphate from dihydroxyacetone phosphate. Fatty acid synthesis is stimulated and, because of the effects of ethanol on mitochondria, fatty acid oxidation is decreased. The net result is that fatty acids react with glycerol 3-phosphate to form triacylglycerols, which accumulate in the liver. Impairment of protein synthesis due to **chronic liver dysfunction** results in an inability to produce and secrete VLDL and adds to the hepatic buildup of fats (**fatty liver**).

E. Malabsorption of fats

Blockage of the bile duct caused by problems such as cholesterol-containing gallstones or duodenal or pancreatic tumors can lead to an inadequate concentration of bile salts in the intestine. Digestion and absorption of dietary lipids are diminished. Diseases that affect the pancreas, such as cystic fibrosis and alcoholism, can lead to a decrease in bicarbonate and digestive enzymes in the intestinal lumen. (Bicarbonate is required to raise the intestinal pH so that bile salts and digestive enzymes can function.) If dietary fats are not adequately digested, **steatorrhea** can result. Malabsorption of fats can lead to **caloric deficiencies** and **lack of fat-soluble vitamins** and **essential fatty acids**.

F. Use of nonsteroidal anti-inflammatory drugs (NSAIDs)

NSAIDs, such as aspirin, acetaminophen, and ibuprofen, inhibit the cyclooxygenase involved in prostaglandin synthesis. These drugs reduce pain, inflammation, and fever associated with the action of the prostaglandins. Aspirin irreversibly acetylates the enzyme in platelets, inhibiting thromboxane (TXA$_2$) formation, thus reducing platelet aggregation for the lifespan of the platelet. Because platelets turn over rapidly, the daily ingestion of small doses of aspirin

is often recommended to inhibit the platelet aggregation (thrombus formation) that, in conjunction with atherosclerotic plaques, often precipitates heart attacks.

G. Sphingolipidoses

Sphingolipids are normally degraded by lysosomal enzymes. If these enzymes are deficient, partially degraded sphingolipids accumulate in cells, compromising cell function. Death may result. An α-galactosidase is deficient in **Fabry's disease,** a β-glucosidase in **Gaucher's disease,** a sphingomyelinase in **Neimann-Pick disease,** and a hexosaminidase in **Tay-Sachs disease.**

H. Respiratory distress syndrome in the newborn

Dipalmitoylphosphatidylcholine serves as the major component of lung surfactant in adults, allowing the lungs to function normally. This phospholipid develops in the fetus after week 30 of gestation. Premature infants do not have an adequate amount of this phospholipid. As a result, **acute respiratory distress syndrome** can occur.

I. Jamaican vomiting sickness

Jamaican vomiting sickness is caused by a toxin (hypoglycin) from the unripe fruit of the akee tree. This toxin inhibits an acyl CoA dehydrogenase of β-oxidation; consequently, more glucose must be oxidized to compensate for the decreased ability to use fatty acids as a fuel, and severe **hypoglycemia** can occur. ω-Oxidation of fatty acids is increased, and dicarboxylic acids are excreted in the urine. Unwary children are usually the victims of this frequently fatal disease.

J. MCAD deficiency

A genetic deficiency of the medium-chain acyl CoA dehydrogenase (MCAD) of β-oxidation prevents the normal use of fatty acids as fuels. Hypoglycemia results, and dicarboxylic acids, produced by ω-oxidation, are excreted in the urine.

Review Test

Directions: Each of the numbered items or incomplete statements in this section is followed by answers or by completions of the statement. Select the **one** lettered answer or completion that is **best** in each case.

1. The process by which dietary lipids are digested and absorbed requires the

(A) production of very low density lipoprotein in the intestine
(B) synthesis of bile salts in the gallbladder
(C) hydrolysis of ester bonds in triacylglycerols
(D) presence of glycerol 3-phosphate in intestinal epithelial cells

2. A deficiency of pancreatic exocrine secretion can result in

(A) increased pH in the intestinal lumen
(B) increased absorption of fat-soluble vitamins
(C) decreased formation of bile salt micelles
(D) increased levels of blood chylomicrons
(E) decreased amounts of fat in the stool

3. Which one of the following statements about acetyl CoA carboxylase is correct?

(A) It requires thiamine for the carboxylation of acetyl CoA
(B) It utilizes citrate as a substrate
(C) It produces malonyl CoA, which is subsequently decarboxylated
(D) It is located mainly in the matrix of liver mitochondria

4. The synthesis of fatty acids from glucose in the liver

(A) occurs in mitochondria
(B) requires a covalently bound derivative of pantothenic acid
(C) utilizes NADPH derived solely from the pentose phosphate pathway
(D) is regulated mainly by isocitrate
(E) does not require biotin

5. The product of the fatty acid synthase complex in the liver can be

(A) elongated to stearic acid
(B) reduced to form oleic acid
(C) oxidized directly to palmitic acid
(D) converted to arachidonic acid
(E) converted into low-density lipoprotein and secreted into the blood

6. In the pathway for triacylglycerol synthesis in the liver,

(A) fatty acids directly react with glycerol 3-phosphate
(B) coenzyme A is not required
(C) phosphatidic acid is an intermediate
(D) a 2-monoacylglycerol is an intermediate

7. For the synthesis of triacylglycerols in adipose tissue

(A) fatty acids are obtained from chylomicrons and very low density lipoprotein
(B) glycerol 3-phosphate is derived from blood glycerol
(C) coenzyme A is not required
(D) a 2-monoacylglycerol is an intermediate
(E) lipoprotein lipase catalyzes the formation of ester bonds

8. Which one of the following sequences places the lipoproteins in the order of most dense to least dense?

(A) HDL/VLDL/chylomicrons/LDL
(B) HDL/LDL/VLDL/chylomicrons
(C) LDL/chylomicrons/HDL/VLDL
(D) VLDL/chylomicrons/LDL/HDL
(E) LDL/chylomicrons/VLDL/HDL

9. The conversion of HMG CoA to mevalonic acid

(A) requires NADH and H^+
(B) is a key reaction in the synthesis of compounds that contain isoprene units
(C) is stimulated by cholesterol
(D) is a step in the synthesis of ketone bodies
(E) is inhibited by insulin

10. A patient with high blood cholesterol levels was treated with lovastatin. This drug lowers blood cholesterol levels because it inhibits

(A) absorption of dietary cholesterol
(B) lipoprotein lipase in adipose tissue
(C) citrate lyase in liver
(D) VLDL excretion by the liver
(E) HMG CoA reductase in liver and peripheral tissues

11. The compound shown below is

(A) a bile salt
(B) cholesterol
(C) a steroid hormone
(D) vitamin D_3
(E) a cholesterol ester

12. In the conversion of cholesterol to bile salts,

(A) carbon 8 is hydroxylated
(B) the side chain is oxidized and can be conjugated with serine or taurine
(C) the double bond is reduced
(D) the hydroxyl group on carbon 3 remains in the β-position

13. If intestinal pH decreases to 3 as a result of a deficiency of pancreatic exocrine secretion, which of the following will be most negatively charged?

(A) Glycocholic acid
(B) Taurocholic acid
(C) Palmitate
(D) Cholic acid
(E) Cholesterol

14. A person with an intestinal infection caused by a proliferation of bacteria in the gut would most likely have an increase in the

(A) synthesis of bile salts in the liver
(B) amount of conjugated bile salts in the intestine
(C) absorption of dietary lipid by intestinal cells
(D) body stores of fat-soluble vitamins

15. A person with a low-density lipoprotein (LDL) receptor deficiency was treated with lovastatin. As a consequence of the action of this drug, the person should have

(A) fewer LDL receptors in cell membranes
(B) increased de novo cholesterol synthesis
(C) increased ACAT activity
(D) lower blood cholesterol levels
(E) higher blood triacylglycerol levels

16. Which of the following is characteristic of high-density lipoprotein?

(A) It is digested by muscle lysosomes
(B) It carries cholesterol that is converted to cholesterol esters in the blood by the lecithin:cholesterol acyltransferase (LCAT) reaction
(C) It carries apoprotein E, an activator of lipoprotein lipase
(D) It is produced by the action of hormone-sensitive lipase on very low density lipoprotein (VLDL)

17. A patient with a hyperlipoproteinemia would be most likely to benefit from a low-carbohydrate diet if the lipoproteins that are elevated in the blood belong to the class of

(A) chylomicrons
(B) VLDL
(C) LDL
(D) HDL

18. A person with a type IIA hyperlipoproteinemia had a blood cholesterol level of 360 mg/dL (recommended level below 200 mg/dL) and blood triglyceride (triacylglycerol) levels of 140 mg/dL (recommended level below 160 mg/dL). This person most likely has

(A) a decreased ability for receptor-mediated endocytosis of LDL
(B) a decreased ability to degrade the triacylglycerols of chylomicrons
(C) an increased ability to produce VLDL
(D) an elevation of HDL in the blood
(E) a decreased ability to convert VLDL to IDL

19. The blood of a person who consumes large amounts of animal fat would most likely contain

(A) increased levels of chylomicrons
(B) increased levels of VLDL
(C) increased levels of HDL
(D) increased levels of LDL
(E) decreased levels of cholesterol

20. During fasting, which of the following statements about lipid metabolism is TRUE?

(A) Hormone-sensitive lipase is inhibited because the glucagon level in blood is increased and insulin is decreased
(B) Glycerol, released from adipose tissue, is utilized for glycogen synthesis in liver
(C) Liver is converting fatty acids, derived from adipose tissue, to ketone bodies
(D) Liver is actively synthesizing VLDL from carbohydrate

21. Which one of the following statements about fatty acids is TRUE?

(A) Fatty acids are very soluble in water and need no carrier in the blood
(B) When fatty acids are activated in the cytosol, ATP is converted to ADP
(C) Fatty acyl groups are covalently linked to carnitine by an enzyme inhibited by malonyl CoA
(D) Fatty acids can be oxidized to CO_2 and H_2O in the mitochondria of red blood cells

22. Which one of the following statements about β-oxidation is true?

(A) FAD is required to form a double bond in fatty acyl CoA
(B) Carbon 2 of the fatty acid is oxidized to form a β-hydroxy compound
(C) NAD^+ removes water from the β-hydroxy fatty acyl CoA intermediate
(D) Thiolase removes one carbon from the β-keto intermediate
(E) Two acetyl CoA molecules are produced in each turn of the β-oxidation spiral

23. If 1 mole of the compound shown below is oxidized to CO_2 and H_2O in muscle mitochondria, what will be the approximate net number of moles of ATP produced?

$$CH_3 - (CH_2)_9 - CH = CH - CH_2 - COOH$$

(A) 95
(B) 97
(C) 110
(D) 114
(E) 119

24. Which one of the following statements about the conversion of fatty acids to ketone bodies is TRUE?

(A) Carnitine transports the fatty acid across the plasma membrane
(B) Activation of the fatty acid is driven by the conversion of ATP to ADP
(C) Thiolase cleaves HMG CoA
(D) Acetoacetate and acetyl CoA are produced by cleavage of HMG CoA
(E) The complete sequence of reactions occurs in all tissues of the body

25. The complete oxidation of

$$CH_3 - \overset{\overset{\displaystyle O}{\|}}{C} - CH_2 - COOH$$

to CO_2 and H_2O in muscle requires

(A) elevated insulin levels
(B) thiamine pyrophosphate
(C) HMG CoA synthetase
(D) biotin
(E) cytosolic ATP for activation of the molecule

26. Approximately how many net moles of ATP are generated when one mole of β-hydroxybutyrate is oxidized to carbon dioxide and water in skeletal muscle?

(A) 23
(B) 24
(C) 25
(D) 26
(E) 27

27. After an overnight fast, the blood levels of which of the following compounds will be higher in a person with a carnitine deficiency than in a normal person?

(A) Glucose
(B) Fatty acids
(C) Acetoacetate
(D) 3-Hydroxybutyrate

28. Newly synthesized fatty acids are not immediately degraded because

(A) tissues that synthesize fatty acids do not contain the enzymes that degrade fatty acids
(B) high NADPH levels inhibit β-oxidation
(C) transport of fatty acids into mitochondria is inhibited under conditions in which fatty acids are being synthesized
(D) in the presence of insulin, the key fatty acid degrading enzyme is not induced
(E) newly synthesized fatty acids cannot be converted to their CoA derivatives

29. Type 1 diabetes mellitus is caused by a decreased ability of the β cells of the pancreas to produce insulin. A person with Type 1 diabetes mellitus who has neglected to take insulin injections will have

(A) increased fatty acid synthesis from glucose in liver
(B) decreased conversion of fatty acids to ketone bodies
(C) increased stores of triacylglycerol in adipose tissue
(D) increased production of acetone

30. Which one of the following characteristics of phospholipids is TRUE?

(A) They always contain choline and glycerol
(B) They are an important source of energy during fasting
(C) They are a major component of membranes
(D) They are not charged in the body
(E) They are not soluble in water

31. A cytosine nucleotide is involved in the biosynthesis of a

(A) galactocerebroside
(B) ceramide
(C) phosphatidic acid
(D) phosphatidylcholine

32. Which one of the following is a characteristic of ceramide?

(A) It is not a precursor of gangliosides
(B) It is converted to sphingomyelin by reacting with a UDP-sugar
(C) It has palmitoyl CoA and serine as precursors
(D) It contains a glycerol moiety

33. The accumulation of the GM_2 ganglioside in Tay-Sachs disease is caused by

(A) an increased synthesis of the ganglioside precursor, ceramide
(B) an increased concentration of the UDP-sugars required for ganglioside synthesis
(C) a genetic deficiency of phospholipase A_2
(D) a deficiency of a lysosomal enzyme that degrades gangliosides

34. Respiratory distress syndrome in premature newborns is caused by deficiency in the lungs of a

(A) sphingomyelin
(B) ganglioside
(C) triacylglycerol
(D) phosphatidylcholine
(E) prostaglandin

35. In the human, prostaglandins can be derived from

(A) glucose
(B) acetyl CoA
(C) arachidonic acid
(D) oleic acid
(E) leukotrienes

36. Which one of the following characteristics correctly describes prostaglandins?

(A) They are derived from fatty acids with 22 carbons
(B) They are linear compounds with no ring structures
(C) They do not contain keto or hydroxy groups
(D) They are synthesized from polyunsaturated fatty acids

37. A cyclooxygenase, which is inhibited by aspirin, is required for the production of

(A) thromboxanes from arachidonic acid
(B) leukotrienes from arachidonic acid
(C) phospholipids from arachidonic acid
(D) arachidonic acid from linoleic acid

Directions: Each group of items in this section consists of lettered options followed by a set of numbered items. For each item, select the **one** lettered option that is most closely associated with it. Each lettered option may be selected once, more than once, or not at all.

Questions 38–41

(A) VLDL
(B) Chylomicron
(C) Fatty acid-albumin complex
(D) Bile salt micelle
(E) LDL

A molecule of palmitic acid, attached to carbon 1 of the glycerol moiety of a triacylglycerol, is ingested and digested. It passes into the blood, is stored in a fat cell, and ultimately is oxidized to CO_2 and H_2O in a muscle cell. Choose the molecular complex in the blood in which the palmitate residue is carried from the first site to the second.

38. From the lumen of the gut to the surface of the gut epithelial cell

39. From the gut epithelial cell to the blood

40. From the intestine through the blood to a fat cell

41. From a fat cell to a muscle cell

Questions 42–45

(A) Palmitate
(B) Acetoacetate
(C) Cholesterol
(D) Bile salts

Match the following descriptions with the appropriate lipid.

42. Oxidized by the brain during prolonged starvation

43. Produced from acetyl CoA by most cells in the body

44. Efficiently recycled by the liver

45. Produced by the liver during fasting

Questions 46–52

(A) Lipoprotein lipase
(B) Pancreatic lipase
(C) Hormone-sensitive lipase
(D) Phospholipase A_2

Match the following descriptions with the appropriate enzyme.

46. Produces 2-monoacylglycerols

47. Degrades the triacylglycerols of chylomicrons in blood capillaries

48. Is activated by protein kinase A

49. Secretion is blocked in cystic fibrosis

50. A deficiency would be most likely to result in morbid obesity

51. Inhibited in an asthmatic patient who is treated with glucocorticoids

52. Less of the active enzyme is present in a patient with Type 1 diabetes mellitus who does not comply with treatment than in a normal person

Answers and Explanations

1–C. Bile salts, synthesized in the liver and secreted by the gallbladder, emulsify dietary triacylglycerols, which contain ester bonds that are hydrolyzed by pancreatic lipase to produce fatty acids and 2-monoacylglycerols. These products are absorbed by intestinal epithelial cells, where they are reconverted to triacylglycerols (by a process that does not require glycerol 3-phosphate) and secreted into the lymph in chylomicrons. (VLDL are produced in the liver.)

2–C. The pancreas produces bicarbonate (which neutralizes stomach acid) and digestive enzymes (including the lipase that degrades dietary lipids). Decreased production of bicarbonate will lead to a decrease of intestinal pH. Lower levels of pancreatic lipase will result in decreased digestion of dietary triacylglycerols, which will lead to formation of fewer bile salt micelles. Intestinal cells will have less substrate for chylomicron formation, and less fat-soluble vitamins will be absorbed. More dietary fat will be excreted in the feces.

3–C. Biotin is required for the acetyl CoA carboxylase reaction in which the substrate, acetyl CoA, is carboxylated by the addition of CO_2 to form malonyl CoA. This reaction occurs in the cytosol. Malonyl CoA provides the 2-carbon units that add to the growing fatty acid chain on the fatty acid synthase complex. As the growing chain is elongated, malonyl CoA is decarboxylated.

4-B. The synthesis of fatty acids from glucose occurs in the cytosol, except for the mitochondrial reactions in which pyruvate is converted to citrate. Biotin is required for the conversion of pyruvate to oxaloacetate, which combines with acetyl CoA to form citrate. Biotin is also required by acetyl CoA carboxylase. Citrate, not isocitrate, is a key regulatory compound for acetyl CoA carboxylase. Pantothenic acid is covalently bound to the fatty acid synthase complex as part of a phosphopantetheinyl residue. During the reduction reactions on the synthase complex, the growing fatty acid chain is attached to this residue. NADPH, produced by the malic enzyme as well as by the pentose phosphate pathway, provides the reducing equivalents.

5–A. The 16-carbon, fully saturated fatty acid, palmitate (16:0), is the product of the fatty acid synthase complex. It can be elongated by two carbons to form stearic acid (18:0), or it can be oxidized to form palmitoleic acid ($16:1,\Delta^9$). Stearate can be oxidized to oleic acid ($18:1,\Delta^9$). Arachidonic acid ($20:4,\Delta^{5,8,11,14}$) can be synthesized from the essential fatty acid linoleate ($18:2,\Delta^{9,12}$). It cannot be produced from palmitate. Fatty acids synthesized in the liver are converted to triacylglycerols, packaged in very low density lipoprotein, and secreted into the blood.

6–C. In the liver, 2 fatty acyl CoAs react with glycerol 3-phosphate to form phosphatidic acid, which releases inorganic phosphate to form a diacylglycerol. The diacylglycerol reacts with fatty acyl CoA to form a triacylglycerol.

7–A. Fatty acids, cleaved from the triacylglycerols of chylomicrons and VLDL by the action of lipoprotein lipase, are taken up by adipose cells and react with coenzyme A to form fatty acyl CoA. Glucose is converted via dihydroxyacetone phosphate to glycerol 3-phosphate, which reacts with fatty acyl CoA to form phosphatidic acid. (Adipose tissue lacks glycerol kinase and cannot use glycerol.) After inorganic phosphate is released from phosphatidic acid, the resultant diacylglycerol reacts with another fatty acyl CoA to form a triacylglycerol, which is stored in the adipose cells. (2-Monoacylglycerol is an intermediate only in intestinal cells.)

8–B. Because chylomicrons contain the most triacylglycerol, they are the least dense of the blood lipoproteins. Because VLDL contains more protein, it is more dense than chylomicrons. Because LDL is produced by degradation of the triacylglycerols of VLDL, LDL is more dense than VLDL. HDL is the most dense of the blood lipoproteins. It has the most protein and the least triacylglycerol.

9–B. In the synthesis of cholesterol, but not of ketone bodies, HMG CoA is reduced by NADPH + H⁺ to mevalonic acid (mevalonate). The enzyme, HMG CoA reductase, is highly regulated (it is inhibited by cholesterol and bile salts and induced by insulin). Mevalonic acid is converted to isopentenyl pyrophosphate, which provides isoprene units for the synthesis of cholesterol (and its derivatives), ubiquinone, dolichol, 1,25-dihydroxycholecalciferol, and compounds that contain geranyl or farnesyl groups.

10–E. The class of drugs known as the statins (e.g., lovastatin) lower blood cholesterol levels by inhibiting HMG CoA reductase, a key regulatory enzyme in cholesterol biosynthesis.

11–A. This compound is the bile salt glycocholic acid. During its synthesis, the ring structure of cholesterol is hydroxylated and reduced, and the side chain is oxidized and conjugated with glycine. Although cholesterol can be converted to steroid hormones, this is not one of them. The cholesterol ring structure opens when vitamin D_3 is formed. When cholesterol is converted to a cholesterol ester, the hydroxyl group at position 3 becomes esterified to a fatty acid.

12–C. During the conversion of cholesterol to bile salts, carbon 7 is hydroxylated. For cholic acid, carbon 12 is also hydroxylated. All hydroxyl groups, including the one on carbon 3, assume an α-configuration. The double bond is reduced, and the side chain is oxidized and conjugated with glycine or taurine.

13–B. Taurocholic acid has the lowest pK (pK = 2) of these compounds. At pH 3, the ratio of negatively charged to uncharged taurocholate molecules would be approximately 10:1.

14–A. Bacteria in the intestine deconjugate and dehydroxylate bile salts, converting them to secondary bile salts. Therefore, the bile salts become less water-soluble and less effective as detergents, less readily absorbed, and more likely to be excreted in the feces than recycled by the liver. Fewer micelles would be produced, so less dietary lipid (including the fat-soluble vitamins) would be absorbed. Because fewer bile salts would return to the liver, more bile salts would be synthesized. Bile salts inhibit the 7α-hydroxylase that is involved in their synthesis. In addition, the person's food intake might decrease which would augment some of the effects noted above.

15–D. HMG CoA reductase inhibitors cause cells to decrease the rate of cholesterol synthesis. Lower cellular levels of cholesterol cause decreased conversion of cholesterol to cholesterol esters (by the ACAT reaction) for storage and increased production of LDL receptors. An increased number of receptors will cause more LDL to be taken up by cells and degraded by lysosomes. Thus, blood cholesterol levels will decrease. Blood triacylglycerol levels will also decrease but not to a great extent because LDL contains only small amounts of triacylglycerol.

16–B. HDL is produced in the liver. It transfers apoprotein C_{II}, which activates lipoprotein lipase, to chylomicrons and VLDL. HDL picks up cholesterol from cell membranes. This cholesterol is converted to cholesterol esters by the LCAT reaction and transferred to other lipoproteins by the cholesterol ester transfer protein (CETP). Ultimately, these lipoproteins and HDL enter liver cells by endocytosis and are digested by lysosomal enzymes. Hormone-sensitive lipase degrades triacylglycerols stored in adipose cells.

17–B. VLDL is produced mainly from dietary carbohydrate, LDL from VLDL, and chylomicrons from dietary triacylglycerol. Elevated HDL levels are desirable and are not considered to be a lipid disorder.

18–A. Of the blood lipoproteins, LDL contains the highest concentration of cholesterol and lowest concentration of triacylglycerols. Elevation of blood LDL levels (the result of decreased endocytosis of LDL) would result in high blood cholesterol levels and relatively normal triacylglycerol levels. A decreased ability to degrade the triacylglycerols of chylomicrons or to convert VLDL to IDL, as well as an increased ability to produce VLDL, would all result in elevated triacylglycerol levels. Because HDL helps to transfer cholesterol from peripheral cells to the liver, high levels are associated with low cholesterol.

19–A. Because chylomicrons are derived from dietary fat, they would be the lipid most likely to be elevated in the blood. VLDL levels would depend on other factors such as the amount of dietary carbohydrate and might or might not be elevated. LDL are derived from VLDL. It is unlikely that a high-fat diet would increase HDL levels. Because cholesterol is present in dietary fat of animal origin, cholesterol levels would most likely be increased.

20–C. During fasting, the hormone-sensitive lipase of adipose tissue is activated by a mechanism involving increased glucagon (and decreased insulin), cAMP, and protein kinase A. Triacylglycerols are degraded, and fatty acids and glycerol are released into the blood. In the liver, glycerol is converted to glucose and fatty acids to ketone bodies. These fuels are released into the blood and supply energy to various tissues. During fasting, the liver does not produce significant quantities of VLDL.

21–C. Fatty acids are very insoluble in water and are transported in the blood by serum albumin. They cross the plasma membrane and are converted to fatty acyl CoA by CoASH and ATP. In the process, ATP is converted to AMP, thus fatty acid activation utilizes the equivalent of 2 ATP. Fatty acids cross the mitochondrial membranes via a carnitine carrier system. A key enzyme in this process, carnitine acyl transferase I, is inhibited during fatty acid synthesis by malonyl CoA. In mitochondria, fatty acids are oxidized to CO_2 and H_2O. They cannot be oxidized in red blood cells, which lack mitochondria.

22–A. During β-oxidation, a double bond is formed between the α and β carbons of a fatty acyl CoA, and FAD is reduced to $FADH_2$. Then water adds across the double bond, and a β-hydroxy compound is formed. The hydroxyl group on carbon 3 (the β-carbon) is oxidized to a keto group by NAD^+, which is converted to NADH + H^+. Finally, a cleavage catalyzed by thiolase releases one acetyl CoA (which contains two carbons in the acetyl group).

23–C. This fatty acid contains 14 carbons. If it were fully saturated, it would undergo six spirals of β-oxidation, which would produce 6 $FADH_2$ and 6 NADH + H^+, which would generate about 2 × 6 and 3 × 6 ATP, respectively, or a total of 30 ATP. Seven acetyl CoA would be produced, which would enter the TCA cycle and generate about 7 x 12, or 84 ATP. Therefore, for a fully saturated, 14-carbon fatty acid, approximately 114 ATP would be produced. However, 2 ATP are required to activate the fatty acid, reducing the ATP yield to 112. Because this fatty acid is unsaturated (it contains one double bond), one fewer $FADH_2$ would be produced (two fewer ATP would be generated), and the net yield of ATP would be approximately 110.

24–D. Ketone bodies are synthesized in the liver from fatty acids derived from the blood. During the cytosolic activation of the fatty acid, ATP is converted to AMP. Carnitine is required to carry the fatty acyl group across the mitochondrial membrane. In the mitochondrion, the fatty acid is oxidized. Acetyl CoA and acetoacetyl CoA are produced and react to form HMG CoA, which is cleaved by HMG CoA lyase to form acetyl CoA and the ketone body acetoacetate.

25–B. This compound is acetoacetate, which is synthesized in the liver during fasting when blood insulin levels are low. HMG CoA synthetase is the key regulatory enzyme for synthesis, not oxidation. Acetoacetate is transported to tissues, such as muscle, where it is activated in the mitochondrion by succinyl CoA (not ATP), cleaved to 2 acetyl CoA, and oxidized via the tricarboxylic acid (TCA) cycle, which requires the vitamin thiamine as thiamine pyrophosphate, a cofactor for α-ketoglutarate dehydrogenase. Biotin is not required.

26–D. This reaction will produce 26 net moles of ATP, as follows: + 3 ATP produced from the NADH generated when β-hydroxybutyrate is oxidized to acetoacetate. - 1 ATP because, when succinyl CoA is converted to succinate via the thiotransferase reaction that converts acetoacetate to acetoacetyl CoA, no GTP is produced. + 24 ATP produced when 2 acetyl CoA are oxidized in the TCA cycle; therefore, + 26 ATP net.

27–B. After an overnight fast, fatty acids, released from adipose tissue, serve as fuel for other tissues. In the liver, β-oxidation supplies acetyl CoA for ketone body (acetoacetate and 3-hydroxybutyrate) synthesis. In a carnitine deficiency, blood levels of fatty acids will be elevated and ketone bodies will be low because carnitine is required to transport the fatty acids into mitochondria for β-oxidation and ketone body synthesis. Consequently, the body will use more glucose for energy, so glucose levels will decrease.

28–C. During fatty acid synthesis (which occurs in the cytosol), malonyl CoA is produced. Malonyl CoA inhibits carnitine acyltransferase I, an enzyme involved in the transport of fatty acids into mitochondria (where β-oxidation occurs).

29–D. Decreased insulin levels cause fatty acid synthesis to decrease and glucagon levels to increase. Adipose triacylglycerols are degraded, and fatty acids are released. They are converted to ketone bodies in liver, and a ketoacidosis can occur. Nonenzymatic decarboxylation of acetoacetate forms acetone, which causes the odor associated with diabetic ketoacidosis.

30–C. Phospholipids are important components of membranes but are also found in blood lipoproteins and in lung surfactant. They are amphipathic molecules that are not involved in storing energy but in interfacing between body lipids and their aqueous environment. They are soluble in water because they contain a phosphate residue that is negatively charged, and they often contain either choline, ethanolamine, or serine residues that have a positive charge at physiologic pH. (A serine residue will contain both a negative charge and a positive charge.)

31–D. CDP-choline reacts with a diacylglycerol to form phosphatidylcholine. UDP-galactose reacts with ceramide to form a galactocerebroside. Cytosine nucleotides are not required for the synthesis of phosphatidic acid or ceramide.

32–C. Palmitoyl CoA and serine react to form a precursor that is converted to ceramide by formation of an amide with a fatty acyl CoA. Ceramide does not contain a glycerol moiety. Ceramide may be converted to sphingomyelin (by addition of a phosphocholine group), to a cerebroside (by a reaction with a UDP-sugar), and to a ganglioside (by reaction with UDP-sugars and CMP-NANA).

33–D. Accumulation of gangliosides is not caused by increased synthesis but rather by decreased degradation in lysosomes. Phospholipase A_2 cleaves fatty acids from position 2 of phospholipids in cell membranes. It is not a lysosomal enzyme.

34–D. Respiratory distress syndrome is caused by a deficiency of lung surfactant, which is composed mainly of dipalmitoylphosphatidylcholine.

35–C. Prostaglandins can be synthesized from arachidonic acid (which requires the essential fatty acid, linoleate, for its synthesis). They cannot be synthesized from glucose, and they cannot be made from acetyl CoA or oleic acid. Although leukotrienes are derived from arachidonic acid, they are not precursors of prostaglandins.

36–D. Prostaglandins are synthesized from 20-carbon polyunsaturated fatty acids with three, four, or five double bonds. A cyclooxygenase converts the fatty acid to a compound that contains a 5-membered ring. In subsequent reactions, a series of prostaglandins is produced that contain various keto and hydroxy groups.

37–A. Arachidonic acid is produced from linoleic acid (an essential fatty acid) by a series of elongation and desaturation reactions. Arachidonic acid is stored in membrane phospholipids, released, and oxidized by a cyclooxygenase (which is inhibited by aspirin) in the first step in the synthesis of prostaglandins, prostacyclins, and thromboxanes. Leukotrienes require a lipoxygenase, rather than a cyclooxygenase, for their synthesis from arachidonic acid.

38–D. A palmitate residue attached to carbon 1 of a dietary triacylglycerol is released by pancreatic lipase and carried from the intestinal lumen to the gut epithelial cell in a bile salt micelle.

39–B. Palmitate is absorbed into the intestinal cell and utilized to synthesize a triacylglycerol, which is packaged in a nascent chylomicron and secreted via the lymph into the blood.

40–B. The chylomicron, containing the palmitate, matures in the blood by accepting proteins from HDL. It travels to a fat cell.

41–C. The chylomicron triacylglycerol is digested by lipoprotein lipase, and the palmitate enters a fat cell and is stored as triacylglycerol. It is released as free palmitate and carried, complexed with albumin, to a muscle cell, where it is oxidized.

42–B. Ketone bodies such as acetoacetate are oxidized by the brain during prolonged starvation.

43–C. Most cells produce cholesterol.

44–D. Ninety-five percent of the bile salts secreted by the liver are returned from the gut to the liver.

45–B. The liver produces ketone bodies such as acetoacetate during fasting.

46–B. Pancreatic lipase produces 2-monoacylglycerols.

47–A. Lipoprotein lipase, which is attached to cell membranes of blood capillary walls, degrades the triacylglycerols of chylomicrons and VLDL.

48–C. Hormone-sensitive lipase is phosphorylated and activated by protein kinase A in response to cAMP.

49–B. Cystic fibrosis, the result of a genetic defect in a chloride channel protein, is characterized by a decreased secretory activity. Pancreatic secretions are blocked. Therefore, food is not adequately digested.

50–C. Deficiencies in pancreatic lipase or lipoprotein lipase would result in decreased fat absorption from the gut and decreased deposition of fat in adipose tissue, respectively. Only a deficiency of hormone-sensitive lipase would result in increased fat stores because of a decreased ability to mobilize triacylglycerols from adipose tissue.

51–D. Glucocortocoids inhibit phospholipase A_2 and thus the release of arachidonic acid for eicosanoid synthesis. Certain leukotrienes cause bronchoconstriction. Inhibition of their synthesis aids asthma sufferers.

52–A. The synthesis of lipoprotein lipase (LPL) by adipose tissue and its secretion into capillaries is stimulated by insulin. In an untreated diabetic who does not produce enough insulin (Type 1 diabetes mellitus) or is resistant to its actions (Type 2 diabetes mellitus), the amount of LPL available to act on chylomicron and VLDL triacylglycerols would be low. Decreased insulin action causes the hormone-sensitive lipase of adipose cells to be active, releasing fatty acids and glycerol, which travel to the liver and form VLDL. Thus, diabetics tend to have high VLDL and chylomicron levels (hyperlipidemia).

7

Nitrogen Metabolism

Overview

- Nitrogen is obtained mainly from protein in the diet, which is digested to amino acids by the combined action of proteases produced by the stomach, pancreas, and intestinal epithelial cells (Figure 7-1).
- Amino acids are absorbed by intestinal epithelial cells, pass into the blood, and are taken up by other cells of the body.
- Amino acids are used by cells for the synthesis of proteins, which is a dynamic process; proteins are constantly being synthesized and degraded.
- After nitrogen is removed from amino acids, the carbon skeletons can be oxidized for energy.
- The nitrogen of amino acids is converted to urea in the liver and ultimately excreted by the kidney.
- Although urea is the major nitrogenous excretory product, nitrogen is also excreted as NH_4^+, uric acid, and creatinine.
- In the fed state, the liver can convert amino acid carbons to fatty acids and glycerol, which form the triacylglycerols of very low density lipoprotein (VLDL).
- During fasting, muscle protein is degraded and supplies amino acids to the blood, and the liver converts amino acid carbons to glucose or ketone bodies.
- The essential amino acids (histidine, isoleucine, leucine, lysine, methionine, phenylalanine, threonine, tryptophan, and valine) are required in the diet. Arginine and increased amounts of histidine are required during periods of growth.
- The nonessential amino acids can be synthesized in the body.
  – The carbons of 10 of the nonessential amino acids can be derived from glucose. However, the synthesis of cysteine requires sulfur from the essential amino acid methionine.
  – Tyrosine, the eleventh nonessential amino acid, is produced by hydroxylation of the essential amino acid phenylalanine.
- Amino acids are used for the synthesis of many nitrogen-containing compounds such as the purine and pyrimidine bases, heme, creatine, nicotinamide, serotonin, thyroxine, epinephrine, melanin, and sphingosine.

I. Protein Digestion and Amino Acid Absorption

- Proteins are converted to amino acids by digestive enzymes.
- Many of the digestive proteases are produced and secreted as inactive zymogens. They are converted to their active forms by removal of a peptide fragment in the lumen of the digestive tract.

237

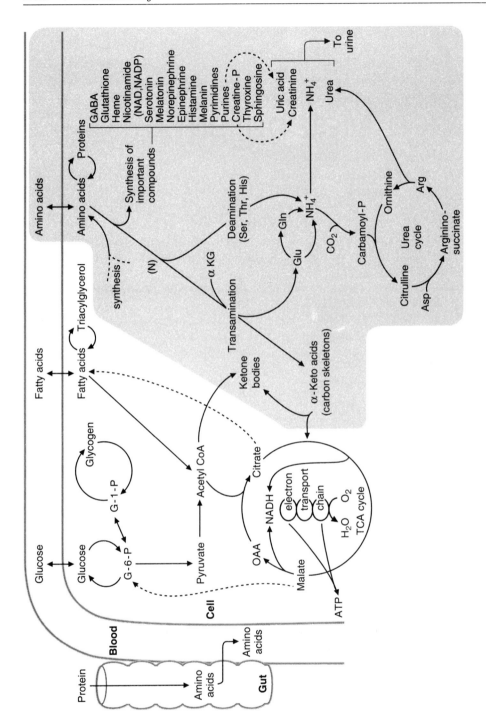

Figure 7-1. Overview of nitrogen metabolism. The metabolism of nitrogen-containing compounds is shown in the *shaded area* on the *right,* and that of glucose and fatty acids is shown on the *left.* ATP = adenosine triphosphate; *G-1-P* = glucose 1-phosphate; *G-6-P* = glucose 6-phosphate; *OAA* = oxaloacetate; *TCA* = tricarboxylic acid; αKG = α-ketoglutarate.

- The digestion of proteins begins in the stomach, where pepsin converts dietary proteins into smaller polypeptides.
- In the lumen of the small intestine, proteolytic enzymes produced by the pancreas (trypsin, chymotrypsin, elastase, and the carboxypeptidases) cleave the polypeptides into oligopeptides and amino acids.
- Digestive enzymes produced by the intestinal epithelial cells (aminopeptidases, dipeptidases, and tripeptidases) cleave the small peptides to amino acids.
- Amino acids, the final products of protein digestion, are absorbed through intestinal epithelial cells and enter the blood.

A. Digestion of proteins (Figure 7-2)

1. The 70–100 g of **protein consumed** each day and an equal or larger amount of protein that enters the digestive tract as **digestive enzymes** or in **sloughed-off cells** from the intestinal epithelium are converted to amino acids by **digestive enzymes.**

2. In the **stomach,** pepsin is the major proteolytic enzyme. It cleaves proteins to smaller polypeptides.

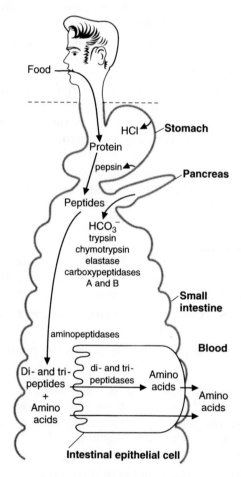

Figure 7-2. Digestion of proteins.

a. Pepsin is produced and secreted by the chief cells of the stomach as the inactive zymogen **pepsinogen.**

b. HCl produced by the parietal cells of the stomach causes a conformational change in pepsinogen that enables it to cleave itself (autocatalysis), forming pepsin.

c. Pepsin has a **broad specificity** but tends to cleave peptide bonds in which the carboxyl group is contributed by the aromatic amino acids or by leucine.

3. In the **intestine,** the partially digested material from the stomach encounters **pancreatic secretions**, which include bicarbonate and a group of proteolytic enzymes.

a. Bicarbonate neutralizes the stomach acid, raising the pH of the contents of the intestinal lumen into the optimal range for the digestive enzymes to act.

b. Endopeptidases from the pancreas cleave peptide bonds within protein chains.

(1) **Trypsin** cleaves peptide bonds in which the carboxyl group is contributed by **arginine** or **lysine.**

– Trypsin is secreted as the inactive zymogen **trypsinogen.**
– Trypsinogen is cleaved to form trypsin by the enzyme **enteropeptidase** (enterokinase), which is produced by intestinal cells. Trypsinogen may also undergo autocatalysis by trypsin.

(2) **Chymotrypsin** usually cleaves peptide bonds in which the carboxyl group is contributed by the **aromatic amino acids** or by **leucine. Chymotrypsinogen,** the inactive zymogen, is cleaved to form chymotrypsin by trypsin.

(3) **Elastase** cleaves at the carboxyl end of amino acid residues with small, uncharged side chains such as alanine, glycine, or serine. **Proelastase,** the inactive zymogen, is cleaved to elastase by trypsin.

c. Exopeptidases from the pancreas (carboxypeptidases A and B) cleave one amino acid at a time from the C-terminal end of the peptide.

(1) The carboxypeptidases are produced as **procarboxypeptidases,** which are cleaved to the active form by trypsin.

(2) **Carboxypeptidase A** cleaves **aromatic** amino acids from the C-terminal end of peptides.

(3) **Carboxypeptidase B** cleaves the **basic** amino acids, lysine and arginine, from the C-terminal end of peptides.

d. Proteases produced by **intestinal epithelial cells** complete the conversion of dietary proteins to amino acids.

(1) **Aminopeptidases** are exopeptidases produced by intestinal cells that cleave one amino acid at a time from the *N*-terminal end of peptides.

(2) **Dipeptidases** and **tripeptidases** associated with the intestinal cells produce amino acids from dipeptides and tripeptides.

B. Transport of amino acids from the intestinal lumen into the blood
 – Amino acids are absorbed by intestinal epithelial cells and released into the blood by two types of transport systems.
 – At least seven different carrier proteins transport different groups of amino acids.

1. Sodium-amino acid carrier system

 a. The major transport system involves the uptake by the cell of a **sodium ion** and an **amino acid** by the same carrier protein on the luminal surface.

 b. The **sodium ion** is pumped from the cell into the blood by the Na^+-K^+ ATPase, while the **amino acid** travels down its concentration gradient into the blood.
  – Thus, the transport of amino acids from the intestinal lumen to the blood is driven by the hydrolysis of ATP (secondary active transport).

2. γ-Glutamyl cycle

 a. An amino acid in the lumen reacts with **glutathionine** (γ-glutamyl-cysteinyl-glycine) in the cell membrane, forming a γ-glutamyl amino acid and the dipeptide cysteinyl-glycine.

 b. The amino acid is carried across the cell membrane attached to **γ-glutamate** and released into the cytoplasm. The γ-glutamyl moiety is used in the resynthesis of glutathione.

II. Addition and Removal of Amino Acid Nitrogen

 • When amino acids are synthesized, nitrogen is added to the carbon precursors.
 • When amino acids are oxidized to produce energy, the nitrogen is removed and converted mainly to urea.
 • Nitrogen is transferred from one amino acid to another by transamination reactions, which always involve two different pairs of amino acids and their corresponding α-keto acids.
  – Glutamate and α-ketoglutarate usually serve as one of the pairs.
  – Pyridoxal phosphate is the cofactor.
 • Nitrogen is removed as ammonium ions from glutamate by glutamate dehydrogenase; from glutamine by glutaminase; from histidine by histidase; from serine and threonine by a dehydratase; and from asparagine by asparaginase. Ammonium ions are also removed from amino acids by the purine nucleotide cycle.
 • Glutamate is a pivotal compound in amino acid metabolism.

A. Transamination reactions (Figure 7-3)
 – Transamination involves the **transfer of an amino group** from one amino acid (which is converted to its corresponding α-keto acid) to an α-keto acid (which is converted to its corresponding α-amino acid). Thus, the nitrogen from one amino acid appears in another amino acid.

1. The enzymes that catalyze transamination reactions are known as **transaminases or aminotransferases.**

2. Glutamate and **α-ketoglutarate** are often involved in transamination reactions, serving as one of the amino acid/α-keto acid pairs.

A

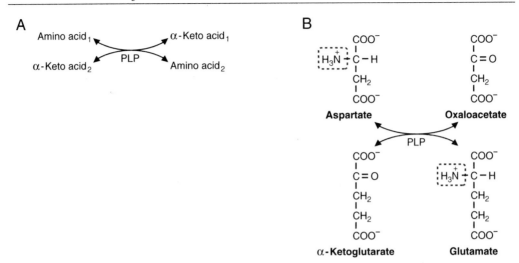

Figure 7-3. Transamination. *PLP* = pyridoxol phosphate

3. Transamination reactions are readily reversible and can be used in the **synthesis** or the **degradation** of amino acids.

4. Most amino acids participate in transamination reactions. **Lysine** is an exception; it **is not transaminated.**

5. **Pyridoxal phosphate (PLP)** serves as the cofactor for transamination reactions. PLP is derived from vitamin B_6.

B. Removal of amino acid nitrogen as ammonia

– A number of amino acids undergo reactions in which their nitrogen is released as ammonia or ammonium ion (NH_4^+).

1. **Glutamate dehydrogenase** catalyzes the oxidative deamination of glutamate (Figure 7-4). Ammonium ion is released, and α-ketoglutarate is formed. The glutamate dehydrogenase reaction, which is readily reversible, requires NAD or NADP.

2. **Histidine** is deaminated by histidase to form NH_4^+ and urocanate.

3. **Serine** and **threonine** are deaminated by serine dehydratase, which requires PLP. Serine is converted to pyruvate, and threonine to α-ketobutyrate; NH_4^+ is released.

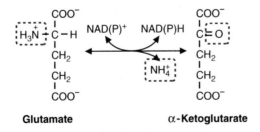

Figure 7-4. The reaction catalyzed by glutamate dehydrogenase. This reaction is readily reversible and can use either NAD or NADP as a cofactor.

4. The amide groups of **glutamine** and **asparagine** are released as ammonium ions by hydrolysis. Glutaminase converts glutamine to glutamate and NH_4^+. Asparaginase converts asparagine to aspartate and NH_4^+.

5. The **purine nucleotide cycle** serves to release NH_4^+ from amino acids, particularly in muscle.
   a. Glutamate collects nitrogen from other amino acids and transfers it to aspartate by a transamination reaction.
   b. Aspartate reacts with inosine monophosphate (IMP) to form AMP and generate fumarate.
   c. NH_4^+ is released from AMP, and IMP is re-formed.

C. The role of glutamate

1. **Glutamate provides nitrogen for synthesis** of many amino acids.
   a. NH_4^+ provides the nitrogen for amino acid synthesis by reacting with α-ketoglutarate to form glutamate in the glutamate dehydrogenase reaction.
   b. Glutamate transfers nitrogen by transamination reactions to α-keto acids to form their corresponding α-amino acids.

2. **Glutamate plays a key role in removing nitrogen** from amino acids.
   a. Glutamate collects nitrogen from other amino acids by means of transamination reactions.
   b. The nitrogen of glutamate is released as NH_4^+ via the glutamate dehydrogenase reaction.
   c. NH_4^+ and aspartate provide nitrogen for urea synthesis via the urea cycle. Aspartate obtains its nitrogen from glutamate by transamination of oxaloacetate.

III. Urea Cycle

- Ammonia, which is very toxic in humans, is converted to urea, which is nontoxic, very soluble, and readily excreted by the kidneys.
- Urea is formed in the urea cycle from NH_4^+, CO_2, and the nitrogen of aspartate. The cycle occurs mainly in the liver.
- NH_4^+, CO_2, and ATP react to form carbamoyl phosphate. The enzyme, carbamoyl phosphate synthetase I, is activated by *N*-acetylglutamate.
- Carbamoyl phosphate reacts with ornithine to form citrulline.
- Citrulline reacts with aspartate to form argininosuccinate, which releases fumarate to form arginine.
- The cleavage of arginine by arginase releases urea and regenerates ornithine.
- The enzymes of the urea cycle are induced if a high-protein diet is consumed for several days.
- When the nitrogen of amino acids is converted to urea in the liver, their carbon skeletons are converted either to glucose (in the fasting state) or to fatty acids (in the fed state).

A. Transport of nitrogen to the liver

– **Ammonia** is **very toxic**, particularly to the central nervous system.

1. The concentration of ammonia and ammonium ions in the blood is normally very low. ($NH_3 + H^+ \leftrightarrow NH_4^+$.)

2. Ammonia travels to the **liver** from other tissues, mainly in the form of **alanine and glutamine.** It is released from amino acids in the liver by a series of transamination and deamination reactions.

3. Ammonia ia also produced **by bacteria in the gut** and travels to the liver via the hepatic portal vein.

B. **Reactions of the urea cycle** (Figure 7-5)

– NH_4^+ and **aspartate** provide the nitrogen that is used to produce **urea,** and CO_2 provides the carbon. Ornithine serves as a carrier that is regenerated by the cycle.

1. **Carbamoyl phosphate** is synthesized in the first reaction from NH_4^+, CO_2, and two ATP. Inorganic phosphate and two ADP are also produced.

   – Enzyme: **carbamoyl phosphate synthetase I,** which is located in mitochondria and is activated by *N*-acetylglutamate.

2. **Ornithine** reacts with carbamoyl phosphate to form citrulline. Inorganic phosphate is released.

   – Enzyme: **ornithine transcarbamoylase,** which is found in mitochondria. The product, citrulline, is transported to the cytosol.

3. **Citrulline** combines with aspartate to form argininosuccinate in a reaction that is driven by the hydrolysis of ATP to AMP and inorganic pyrophosphate.

   – Enzyme: **argininosuccinate synthetase**

4. **Argininosuccinate** is cleaved to form arginine and fumarate.

   – Enzyme: **argininosuccinase.** This reaction occurs in the cytosol.

   a. The carbons of fumarate, which are derived from the aspartate added in reaction 3, can be converted to malate.

   b. In the fasting state in the liver, malate can be converted to glucose or to oxaloacetate, which is transaminated to regenerate the aspartate required for reaction 3.

5. **Arginine** is cleaved to form urea and regenerate ornithine.

   – Enzyme: **arginase,** which is located primarily in the liver and is inhibited by ornithine.

6. **Urea** passes into the blood and is excreted by the kidneys.

   – The urea excreted each day by a healthy adult (about 30 g) accounts for about 90% of the nitrogenous excretory products.

7. **Ornithine** is transported back into the mitochondrion where it can be used for another round of the cycle.

   a. When the cell requires additional **ornithine,** it is synthesized from glucose via glutamate (see Figure 7-9).

   b. **Arginine** is a nonessential amino acid. It is synthesized from glucose via ornithine and the first four reactions of the urea cycle.

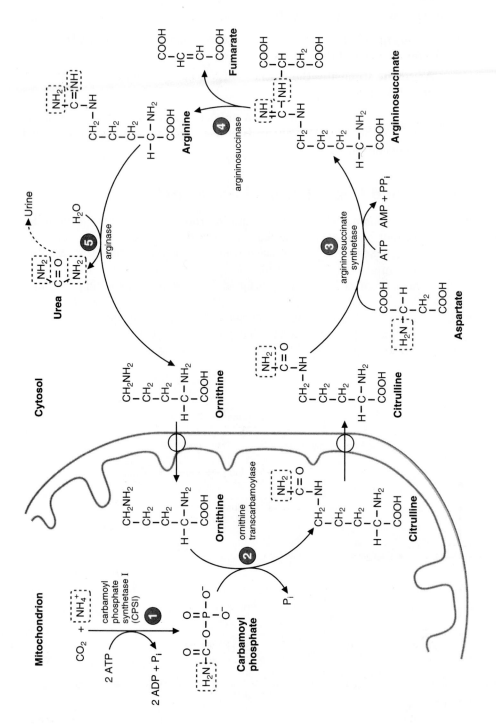

Figure 7-5. The urea cycle. The *dashed boxes* indicate the nitrogen-containing groups from which urea is formed. *Numbers* correspond to the steps described in the text in section III B.

C. Regulation of the urea cycle

1. *N*-**Acetylglutamate** is an activator of carbamoyl phosphate synthetase I, the first enzyme of the urea cycle.

   – **Arginine** stimulates the synthesis of *N*-acetylglutamate from acetyl CoA and glutamate.

2. Although the liver normally has a great capacity for urea synthesis, the enzymes of the urea cycle are **induced** if a high-protein diet is consumed for 4 days or more.

IV. Synthesis and Degradation of Amino Acids

- Of the 20 amino acids commonly found in proteins, 11 are not essential in the adult diet because they can be synthesized in the body.
- Ten of the nonessential amino acids contain carbon skeletons that can be derived from glucose (Figure 7-6).
- Tyrosine is produced by hydroxylation of the essential amino acid phenylalanine.
- The major products obtained by degradation of the carbon skeletons of the amino acids are pyruvate, intermediates of the TCA cycle, acetyl CoA, and acetoacetate (Figure 7-7).

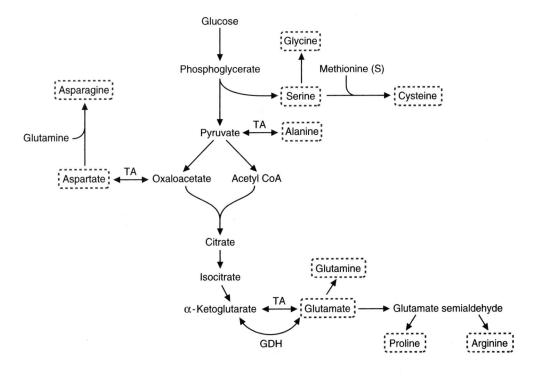

Figure 7-6. Overview of the synthesis of nonessential amino acids. Ten amino acids can be produced from glucose via intermediates of glycolysis or the TCA cycle. The eleventh nonessential amino acid, tyrosine, is synthesized by hydroxylation of the essential amino acid phenylalanine. *GDH* = glutamate dehydrogenase; *TA* = transamination.

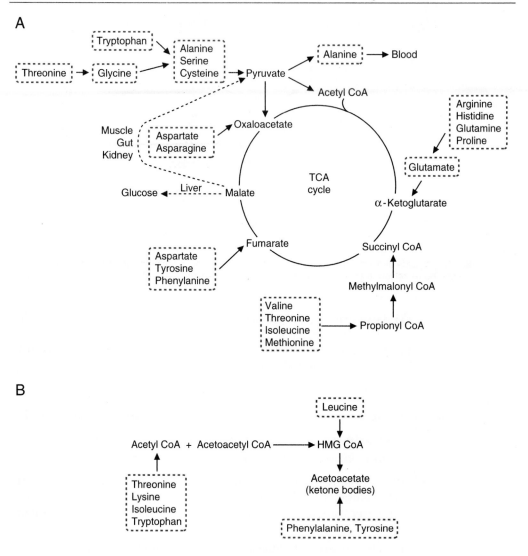

Figure 7-7. Degradation of amino acids. *A*, Amino acids that produce pyruvate or intermediates of the tricarboxylic acid (TCA) cycle. *B*, Amino acids that produce acetyl CoA or ketone bodies. *HMG CoA* = hydroxymethylglutaryl CoA.

A. Synthesis of amino acids

– Messenger RNA contains codons for 20 amino acids. Eleven of these amino acids can be synthesized in the body. The carbon skeletons of 10 of these amino acids can be derived from **glucose.**

1. Amino acids derived from intermediates of glycolysis (Figure 7-8)

– Intermediates of glycolysis serve as precursors for serine, glycine, cysteine, and alanine.

a. Serine can be synthesized from the glycolytic intermediate 3-phosphoglycerate, which is oxidized, transaminated by glutamate, and dephosphorylated.

b. Glycine and **cysteine** can be derived from serine.

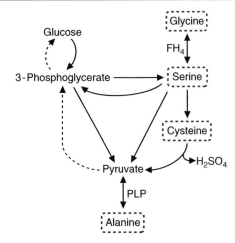

Figure 7-8. Amino acids derived from intermediates of glycolysis. These amino acids can be synthesized from glucose and can be reconverted to glucose in the liver. FH_4 = tetrahydrofolate; PLP = pyridoxal phosphate.

    (1) Glycine can be produced from serine by a reaction in which a methylene group is transferred to tetrahydrofolate.

    (2) Cysteine derives its carbon and nitrogen from serine. The essential amino acid **methionine** supplies the sulfur.

  c. Alanine can be derived by transamination of pyruvate.

2. Amino acids derived from TCA cycle intermediates (see Figure 7-6)

  a. Aspartate can be derived from oxaloacetate by transamination.

    – **Asparagine** is produced from aspartate by amidation.

  b. Glutamate is derived from α-ketoglutarate by the addition of NH_4^+ via the glutamate dehydrogenase reaction or by transamination. **Glutamine, proline, and arginine** can be derived from glutamate (Figure 7-9).

    (1) Glutamine is produced by amidation of glutamate.

    (2) Proline and arginine can be derived from **glutamate semialdehyde,** which is formed by reduction of glutamate.

      – **Proline** can be produced by cyclization of glutamate semialdehyde.

      – **Arginine,** via three reactions of the urea cycle, can be derived from ornithine, which is produced by transamination of glutamate semialdehyde.

3. Tyrosine, the eleventh nonessential amino acid, is synthesized by hydroxylation of the essential amino acid phenylalanine in a reaction that requires tetrahydrobiopterin.

B. Degradation of amino acids

  – When the carbon skeletons of amino acids are degraded, the major products are pyruvate, intermediates of the TCA cycle, acetyl CoA, and acetoacetate (see Figure 7-7).

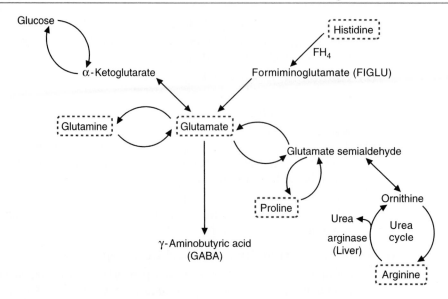

Figure 7-9. Amino acids related through glutamate. These amino acids contain carbons that can be converted to glutamate, which can be converted to glucose in the liver. All of these amino acids except histidine can be synthesized from glucose.

- Amino acids that form pyruvate or intermediates of the TCA cycle in the liver are **glucogenic** (or gluconeogenic); that is, they provide carbon for the synthesis of glucose (see Figure 7-7*A*).
- Amino acids that form acetyl CoA or acetoacetate are **ketogenic;** that is, they form ketone bodies (see Figure 7-7*B*).
- Some amino acids (isoleucine, tryptophan, phenylalanine, and tyrosine) are both glucogenic and ketogenic.

1. **Amino acids that are converted to pyruvate** (see Figure 7-8).

   - The amino acids that are synthesized from intermediates of glycolysis (serine, glycine, cysteine, and alanine) are degraded to form pyruvate.

   a. **Serine** is converted to 2-phosphoglycerate, an intermediate of glycolysis, or directly to pyruvate and NH_4^+ by serine dehydratase, an enzyme that requires pyridoxal phosphate.

   b. **Glycine,** in a reversal of the reaction utilized for its synthesis, reacts with methylene tetrahydrofolate to form serine.

      (1) Glycine also reacts with tetrahydrofolate and NAD^+ to produce CO_2 and NH_4^+.

      (2) Glycine can be converted to glyoxylate, which can be oxidized to CO_2 and H_2O or converted to oxalate.

   c. **Cysteine** forms pyruvate. Its sulfur, which was derived from methionine, is converted to H_2SO_4, which is excreted by the kidneys.

   d. **Alanine** can be transaminated to pyruvate.

2. **Amino acids that are converted to intermediates of the TCA cycle** (see Figure 7-7).

   - Carbons from four groups of amino acids form the TCA cycle intermediates **α-ketoglutarate, succinyl CoA, fumarate,** and **oxaloacetate.**

a. Amino acids that form α-ketoglutarate (see Figure 7-9).

(1) Glutamate can be deaminated by glutamate dehydrogenase or transaminated to form α-ketoglutarate.

(2) Glutamine is converted by glutaminase to glutamate with the release of its amide nitrogen as NH_4^+.

(3) Proline is oxidized so that its ring opens, forming glutamate semi-aldehyde, which is reduced to glutamate.

(4) Arginine is cleaved by arginase in the liver to form urea and ornithine. Ornithine is transaminated to glutamate semialdehyde, which is oxidized to glutamate.

(5) Histidine is converted to formiminoglutamate (FIGLU). The for-mimino group is transferred to tetrahydrofolate (FH_4), and the remaining five carbons form glutamate.

b. Amino acids that form succinyl CoA (Figure 7-10)

– Four amino acids are converted to **propionyl CoA,** which is carboxylated in a biotin-requiring reaction to form methylmalonyl CoA, which is rearranged to form succinyl CoA in a reaction that requires vitamin B_{12}.

(1) Threonine is converted by a dehydratase to NH_4^+ and α-ketobutyrate, which is oxidatively decarboxylated to propionyl CoA.

– In a different set of reactions, threonine is converted to glycine and acetyl CoA.

(2) Methionine provides **methyl groups** for the synthesis of various compounds; its sulfur is incorporated into **cysteine;** and the remaining carbons form **succinyl CoA.**

– Methionine and ATP form *S*-adenosylmethionine (SAM), which donates a methyl group and forms homocysteine.

– **Homocysteine** is reconverted to methionine by accepting a methyl group from the tetrahydrofolate pool via vitamin B_{12}.

– **Homocysteine** can also react with serine to form **cystathionine.** The cleavage of cystathionine produces cysteine, NH_4^+, and α-ketobutyrate, which is converted to propionyl CoA.

(3) Valine and isoleucine, two of the three branched chain amino acids, form succinyl CoA (see Figure 7-10)

– Degradation of all three branched chain amino acids begins with a **transamination** followed by an **oxidative decarboxylation** catalyzed by the branched chain α-keto acid dehydrogenase complex (Figure 7-11). This enzyme, like pyruvate dehydrogenase and α-ketoglutarate dehydrogenase, requires thiamine pyrophosphate, lipoic acid, coenzyme A, FAD, and NAD^+.

– **Valine** is eventually converted to succinyl CoA via propionyl CoA and methylmalonyl CoA.

– **Isoleucine** also forms succinyl CoA after two of its carbons are released as acetyl CoA.

c. Amino acids that form fumarate

– Three amino acids (phenylalanine, tyrosine, and aspartate) are converted to fumarate (see Figure 7-7)

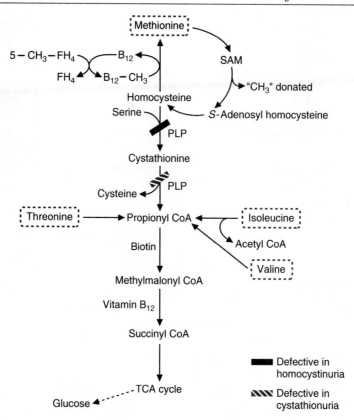

Figure 7-10. Amino acids that can be converted to succinyl CoA. The amino acids methionine, threonine, isoleucine, and valine, which form succinyl CoA via methylmalonyl CoA, are all essential. Because succinyl CoA can form glucose, these amino acids are glucogenic. The carbons of serine are converted to cysteine and do not form succinyl CoA by this pathway. A defect in cystathionine synthase causes homocystinuria. A defect in cystathionase causes cystathionuria. *PLP* = pyridoxal phosphate; *SAM* = S-adenosylmethionine.

(1) Phenylalanine is converted to **tyrosine** by phenylalanine hydroxylase in a reaction requiring tetrahydrobiopterin and O_2 (Figure 7-12).

(2) Tyrosine, obtained from the diet or by hydroxylation of phenylalanine, is converted to homogentisic acid. The aromatic ring is opened and cleaved, forming **fumarate** and **acetoacetate**

(3) Aspartate is converted to fumarate via reactions of the **urea cycle** and the **purine nucleotide cycle.**

– Aspartate reacts with IMP to form AMP and fumarate in the purine nucleotide cycle.

d. Amino acids that form oxaloacetate (see Figure 7-7)

(1) Aspartate is transaminated to form oxaloacetate.

(2) Asparagine loses its amide nitrogen as NH_4^+, forming aspartate in a reaction catalyzed by asparaginase.

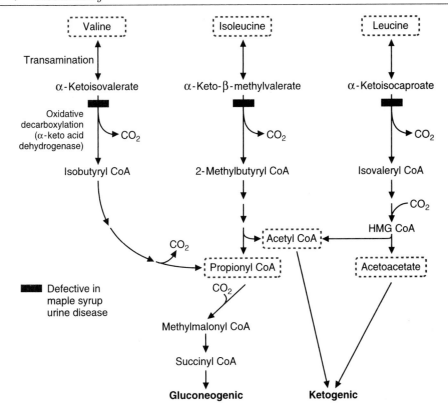

Figure 7-11. Degradation of the branched chain amino acids. Valine forms propionyl CoA. Isoleucine forms propionyl CoA and acetyl CoA. Leucine forms acetoacetate and acetyl CoA.

    3. Amino acids that are converted to acetyl CoA or acetoacetate (see Figure 7-12)

        – Four amino acids (**lysine, threonine, isoleucine,** and **tryptophan**) can form acetyl CoA, and **phenylalanine** and **tyrosine** form acetoacetate. **Leucine** is degraded to form both acetyl CoA and acetoacetate.

V. Interrelationships of Various Tissues in Amino Acid Metabolism

- During fasting, amino acids from muscle protein are released into the blood, predominantly as alanine and glutamine (Figure 7-13).
- The branched chain amino acids are oxidized by muscle to produce energy. Some of the carbons are converted to glutamine and alanine (Figure 7-14). Alanine is also produced by the glucose-alanine cycle.
- The gut takes up glutamine from the blood and converts it to alanine, citrulline, and ammonia, which are released.
- The kidney takes up glutamine from the blood and releases ammonia into the urine and alanine and serine into the blood.
- The liver takes up alanine and other amino acids from the blood and converts the nitrogen to urea and the carbons to glucose and ketone bodies, which are released into the blood and oxidized by tissues for energy.

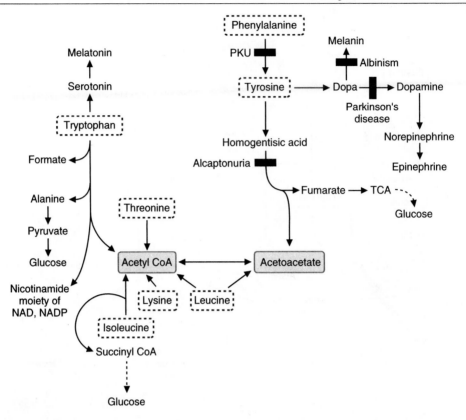

Figure 7-12. Ketogenic amino acids. Some of these amino acids (tryptophan, phenylalanine, and tyrosine) also contain carbons that can form glucose. Leucine and lysine are strictly ketogenic; they do not form glucose. A deficiency in various steps leads to the diseases indicated. *PKU* = phenylketonuria; *TCA* = tricarboxylic acid.

- Thus, amino acids from muscle protein serve as a source of energy for many other tissues.

A. Amino acid metabolism in muscle

- During **fasting,** amino acids are released from muscle protein. Some of the **amino acids** are **partially oxidized** in muscle and their remaining carbons are converted to **alanine** and **glutamine**. Thus, although about 50% of the amino acids released into the blood from muscle are alanine and glutamine, these two amino acids constitute much less than 50% of the total amino acid residues in muscle protein.

1. **Branched chain amino acids** are oxidized in muscle. Some of their carbons are converted to glutamine and alanine before they are released into the blood (see Figure 7-14).

   a. **Valine** and **isoleucine** produce succinyl CoA, which feeds into the TCA cycle and forms malate, generating energy.

   b. **Malate** can be converted by the malic enzyme to pyruvate, which is transaminated to alanine or oxidatively decarboxylated to acetyl CoA.

   c. Malate can also continue around the TCA cycle to α-ketoglutarate, generating additional energy.

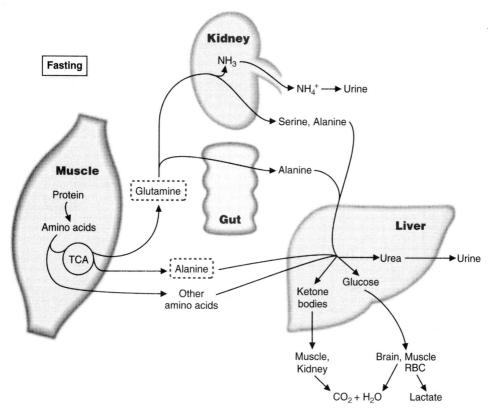

Figure 7-13. Interrelationships of various tissues in amino acid metabolism. During fasting, muscle releases amino acids, particularly alanine and glutamine. Glutamine is converted by the kidney to alanine and serine or by the gut to alanine. Alanine is taken up by the liver. The liver converts the carbons of alanine and other amino acids to glucose or to ketone bodies and the nitrogens to urea. Glucose and ketone bodies are oxidized by other tissues. Muscle can oxidize glucose, forming alanine, which is reconverted to glucose in the liver (the glucose-alanine cycle).

> **d. α-Ketoglutarate** forms glutamate, which produces glutamine.

> **2.** The **alanine** released by muscle is also produced by the **glucose-alanine cycle,** which involves the transport of glucose from the liver to muscle and the return of carbon atoms to the liver as alanine.

> **a.** Glucose is oxidized in muscle to **pyruvate,** producing energy.

> **b.** Pyruvate can be transaminated to **alanine,** which travels to the liver carrying nitrogen for urea synthesis and carbon for gluconeogenesis.

B. Amino acid metabolism in the gut (see Figure 7-13)

> – The gut takes up **glutamine** and releases alanine, citrulline, and ammonia.

> **1.** In the gut, **glutamine** is converted to NH_4^+ and glutamate, which forms α-ketoglutarate.

> **2. α-Ketoglutarate** is converted to malate, generating energy. In the cytosol, malate is decarboxylated by the malic enzyme to form pyruvate, which is transaminated to **alanine.**

> **3. Glutamate** is also converted to ornithine, which forms **citrulline.**

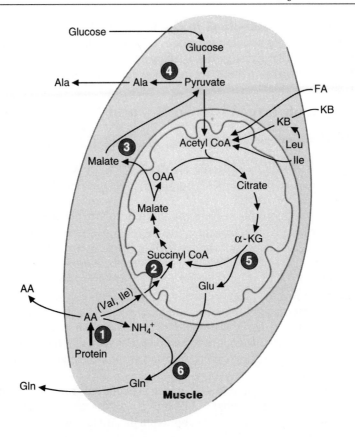

Figure 7-14. Conversion of muscle protein to alanine and glutamine. During fasting, muscle protein is degraded (1). Amino acids *(AA)* are either directly released into the blood or converted to alanine (2, 3, 4) or glutamine (2, 5, 6) and then released into the blood. αKG = α-ketoglutarate; *FA* = fatty acid; *KB* = ketone bodies; *OAA* = oxaloacetate.

C. Amino acid metabolism in the kidney (see Figure 7-13)

– The kidney takes up **glutamine,** which is deaminated by glutaminase, forming ammonia and glutamate, which is converted to alanine and serine.

1. **Ammonia** (NH_3) is released into the **urine,** where it forms NH_4^+, **buffering** the hydrogen ions produced by phosphoric acid, sulfuric acid (produced from cysteine), and various metabolic acids (e.g., lactic acid and the ketone bodies, acetoacetic acid and β-hydroxybutyric acid).

2. **Alanine** and **serine** produced from glutamate are released into the **blood**.

   a. **Glutamate** is deaminated or transaminated to form α-ketoglutarate, which enters the TCA cycle and is converted to malate.

   b. **Malate** enters the cytosol and is oxidized to oxaloacetate, which is converted by phosphoenolpyruvate carboxykinase to phosphoenolpyruvate (PEP).

   c. **Phosphoenolpyruvate** feeds into glycolysis and forms alanine and serine, which are released into the blood.

D. Amino acid metabolism in the liver (see Figure 7-13)
- The liver takes up alanine, serine, and other amino acids from the blood and converts their **nitrogen to urea** and their **carbons to glucose or to ketone bodies**, which are released into the blood and oxidized by other tissues.

VI. Tetrahydrofolate, Vitamin B$_{12}$, and S-Adenosylmethionine

- Groups containing a single carbon atom can be transferred from one compound to another.
- One-carbon groups at lower levels of oxidation than CO_2 are transferred by tetrahydrofolate (FH$_4$), vitamin B$_{12}$, and S-adenosylmethionine. (CO_2 is transferred by biotin.)
- FH$_4$, which is produced from the vitamin folate, obtains one-carbon groups from serine, glycine, histidine, formaldehyde, and formate. The one-carbon groups are oxidized and reduced while they are attached to FH$_4$. The most reduced form, methyl-FH$_4$, however, cannot be oxidized.
- The one-carbon groups carried by FH$_4$ are transferred to dUMP to form dTMP; to glycine to form serine; to purine precursors to form C2 and C8 of the purine ring; and to vitamin B$_{12}$.
- Vitamin B$_{12}$ is involved in two reactions in the body. It is used in the rearrangement of the methyl group of methylmalonyl CoA to form succinyl CoA, and it transfers a methyl group from 5-methyl-FH$_4$ to homocysteine to form methionine.
- S-Adenosylmethionine (SAM), which is produced from methionine and ATP, is involved in the transfer of methyl groups to compounds which form creatine, phosphatidylcholine, epinephrine, melatonin, and methylated polynucleotides.

A. Tetrahydrofolate

1. The nature of tetrahydrofolate (FH$_4$) and its derivatives

    a. **FH$_4$** cannot be synthesized in the body. It is produced from the vitamin folate.
- **NADPH** and **dihydrofolate reductase** convert folate to dihydrofolate (**FH$_2$**), which undergoes a second reduction by the same enzyme to form **FH$_4$** (Figure 7-15A).

    b. The **one-carbon groups** of FH$_4$ can be oxidized and reduced (see Figure 7-15B).
- The most reduced form, N^5-methyl-FH$_4$, cannot be reoxidized under physiologic conditions.

2. Sources of one-carbon groups carried by FH$_4$
- Serine, glycine, formaldehyde, histidine, and formate transfer one-carbon groups to FH$_4$ (Figure 7-16 *top*).

    a. **Serine, glycine,** and **formaldehyde** produce N^5,N^{10}-methylene-FH$_4$.

        (1) **Serine** transfers a one-carbon group to FH$_4$ and is converted to glycine in a reversible reaction. Because serine can be derived from glucose, this one-carbon group can be obtained from dietary carbohydrate.

        (2) When **glycine** transfers a one-carbon unit to FH$_4$, NH$_4^+$ and CO_2 are produced.

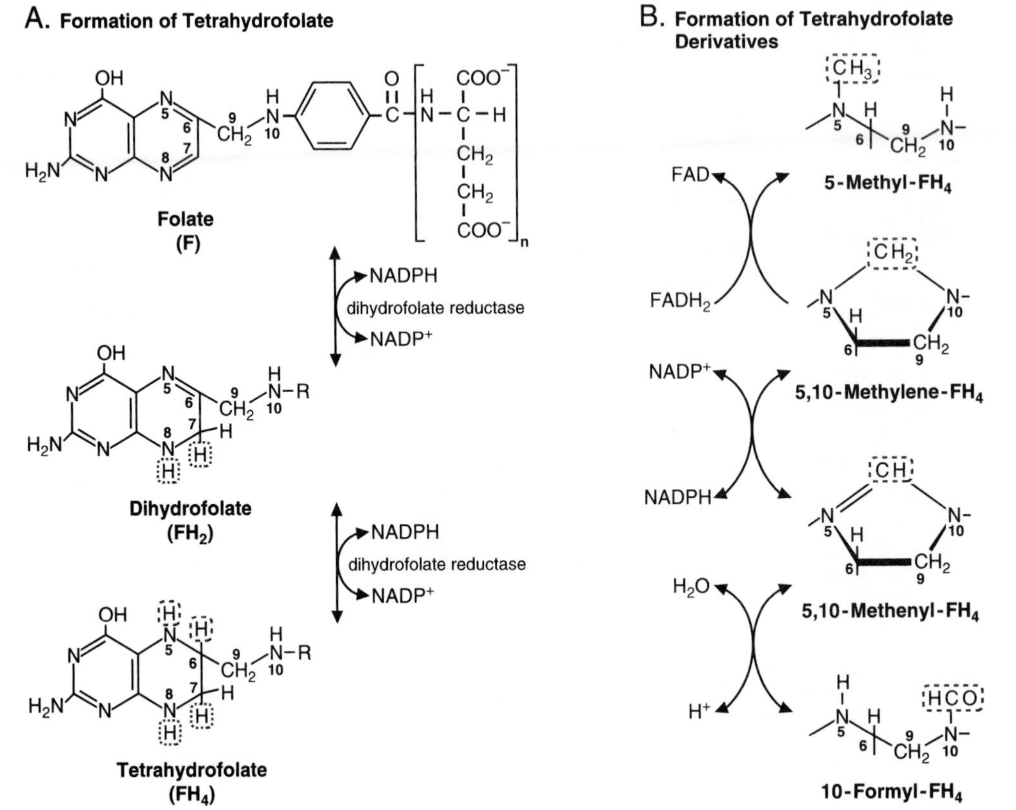

A. Formation of Tetrahydrofolate

B. Formation of Tetrahydrofolate Derivatives

Figure 7-15. Tetrahydrofolate (FH_4). *A*, Reduction of folate by dihydrofolate reductase. *B*, The one-carbon groups carried by FH_4. The one-carbon groups are indicated by *dashed boxes*. Only atoms 5, 6, 9, and 10 of FH_4 are shown. The remainder of the structure is shown in A.

    (3) Formaldehyde, which can be produced from the -N-CH$_3$ of epinephrine, forms N^5,N^{10}-methylene-FH$_4$.

  b. Histidine is degraded to formiminoglutamate (FIGLU). The formimino group reacts with FH$_4$, releasing NH$_4^+$ and producing glutamate and N^5,N^{10}-methenyl-FH$_4$.

  c. Formate, which can be derived from tryptophan, produces N^{10}-formyl-FH$_4$.

3. Recipients of one-carbon groups

  – The one-carbon groups that tetrahydrofolate receives are transferred to various compounds (see Figure 7-16, *bottom*).

  a. Purines precursors obtain carbons 2 and 8 from FH$_4$. Purines are required for DNA and RNA synthesis.

  b. dUMP forms dTMP by accepting a one-carbon group from FH$_4$ (Figure 7-17). This reaction produces the **thymine** required for **DNA synthesis.**

    (1) The methylene group is reduced to a methyl group in this reaction, and tetrahydrofolate is oxidized to dihydrofolate (FH$_2$).

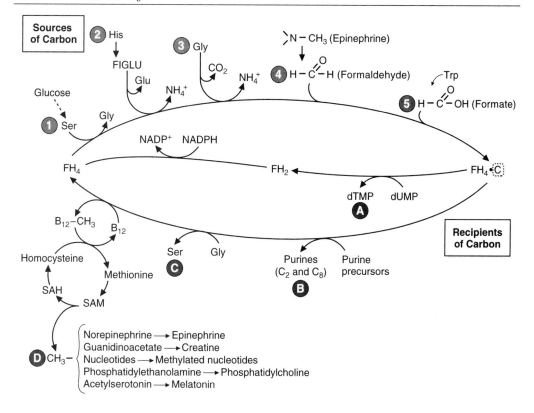

Figure 7-16. The sources of carbon (1–5) for the FH$_4$ pool and the recipients of carbon (A–D) from the pool. *FH$_2$* = dihydrofolate; *FH$_4$ • C* = FH$_4$ carrying a one-carbon unit; *FIGLU* = formiminoglutamate; *SAH* = *S*-adenosylhomocysteine; *SAM* = *S*-adenosylmethionine.

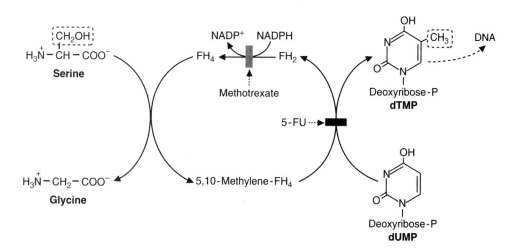

Figure 7-17. The transfer of a one-carbon unit from serine to deoxyuridine monophosphate (dUMP) to form deoxythymidine monophosphate (dTMP). Tetrahydrofolate (FH$_4$) is oxidized to dihydrofolate (FH$_2$) in this reaction. FH$_2$ is reduced to FH$_4$ by dihydrofolate reductase. The carbon group that is transferred is indicated by *dashed boxes*. *Rectangles* indicate the steps at which the antimetabolites methotrexate and 5-fluorouracil (5-FU) act.

(2) FH_2 is reduced to FH_4 in the NADPH-requiring reaction catalyzed **by dihydrofolate reductase**.

c. **Glycine** obtains a one-carbon group from FH_4 to form **serine**.

d. **Vitamin B$_{12}$** obtains a methyl group from 5-methyl-FH_4. The methyl group is transferred from methyl-B$_{12}$ to homocysteine to form **methionine** (see Figure 7-16, *bottom*). This is the only fate of 5-methyl-FH_4.

B. Vitamin B$_{12}$

1. Source of vitamin B$_{12}$

a. Vitamin B$_{12}$ is produced by microorganisms, but not by plants.

b. Animals obtain vitamin B$_{12}$ from their intestinal flora, from bacteria in their food supply, or by consuming the tissues of other animals.

c. **Intrinsic factor,** produced by gastric parietal cells, is required for absorption of vitamin B$_{12}$ by the intestine.

d. Vitamin B$_{12}$ is stored and efficiently recycled in the body.

2. Functions of vitamin B$_{12}$

– Vitamin B$_{12}$ contains **cobalt** in a corrin ring that resembles a porphyrin (Figure 7-18).

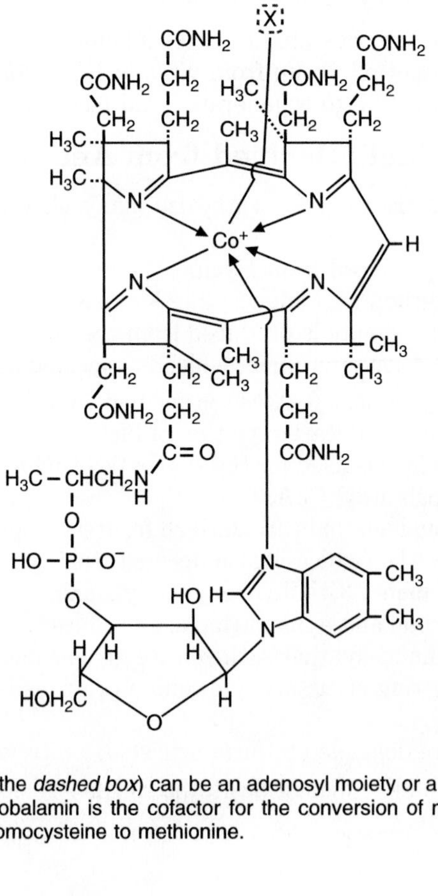

Figure 7-18. Vitamin B$_{12}$. *X* (in the *dashed box*) can be an adenosyl moiety or a methyl group in the coenzyme forms of the vitamin. Adenosylcobalamin is the cofactor for the conversion of methylmalonyl CoA to succinyl CoA and methylcobalamin for homocysteine to methionine.

    a. Vitamin B$_{12}$ is the cofactor for methylmalonyl CoA mutase, which catalyzes the rearrangement of **methylmalonyl CoA to succinyl CoA** (see Figure 7-10).

    – This reaction is involved in the production of succinyl CoA from valine, isoleucine, threonine, methionine, thymine, and the propionyl CoA formed by oxidation of fatty acids with an odd number of carbons.

    b. Vitamin B$_{12}$ is involved in the transfer of methyl groups from FH$_4$ to **homocysteine to form methionine** (see Figure 7-10).

C. *S*-Adenosylmethionine

    1. *S*-Adenosylmethionine (SAM) is synthesized from **methionine** and **ATP**.

    2. Methyl groups are supplied by SAM for the following conversions (see Figure 7-16):

        a. Guanidinoacetate to **creatine**

        b. Phosphatidylethanolamine to **phosphatidylcholine**

        c. Norepinephrine to **epinephrine**

        d. Acetylserotonin to **melatonin**

        e. Polynucleotides to **methylated polynucleotides**

    3. When *S*-adenosylmethionine transfers its methyl group to an acceptor, S-adenosylhomocysteine is produced.

    4. *S*-adenosylhomocysteine releases adenosine to form homocysteine, which obtains a methyl group from vitamin B$_{12}$ to form methionine. Methionine reacts with ATP to regenerate SAM (see Figures 7-10 and 7-16).

VII. Special Products Derived from Amino Acids

- Amino acids are used to synthesize many nitrogen-containing compounds in the body.
- Creatine is produced from glycine, the guanidinium group of arginine, and the methyl group of *S*-adenosylmethionine.
  - Creatine phosphate is produced from creatine and ATP. It spontaneously cyclizes to form creatinine, which is excreted in the urine.
- γ-Aminobutyric acid (GABA) is formed by decarboxylation of glutamate and histamine by decarboxylation of histidine.
- Ceramide, which is used for the synthesis of sphingolipids, is produced from serine and palmitoyl CoA.
- Serotonin and melatonin are derived from tryptophan, as is the nicotinamide portion of NAD$^+$ (which is also derived from the vitamin niacin).
- Thyroid hormone, 3,4-dihydroxyphenylalanine (dopa), melanin, dopamine, norepinephrine, and epinephrine are produced from tyrosine.
- During purine biosynthesis, the entire glycine molecule is incorporated into the growing ring structure; glutamine provides N3 and N9; and aspartate provides N1.
  - Purines are degraded to form uric acid, a nitrogenous excretory product.
- During pyrimidine biosynthesis, the ring is formed by carbamoyl phosphate and aspartate.

- Heme is produced from glycine and succinyl CoA via a series of porphyrins.
  – Heme is degraded to bilirubin, which is excreted in the bile.

A. Creatine (Figure 7-19)

1. **Creatine** is produced from glycine, arginine, and SAM.
   – Glycine combines with arginine to form ornithine and guanidinoacetate, which is methylated by *S*-adenosylmethionine to form creatine.

2. **Creatine** travels from the liver to other tissues where it is converted to **creatine phosphate.**
   – ATP phosphorylates creatine to form creatine phosphate in a reaction catalyzed by **creatine kinase.**

   a. **Muscle** and **brain** contain large amounts of **creatine phosphate.**

   b. **Creatine phosphate** provides a small reservoir of high-energy phosphate that readily regenerates ATP from ADP. It plays a particularly important role during the early stages of exercise in muscle, where the largest quantities of creatine phosphate are found.

   c. Creatine also transports high-energy phosphate from mitochondria to actomyosin fibers.

3. Creatine phosphate spontaneously cyclizes, forming **creatinine,** which is **excreted by the kidney.**

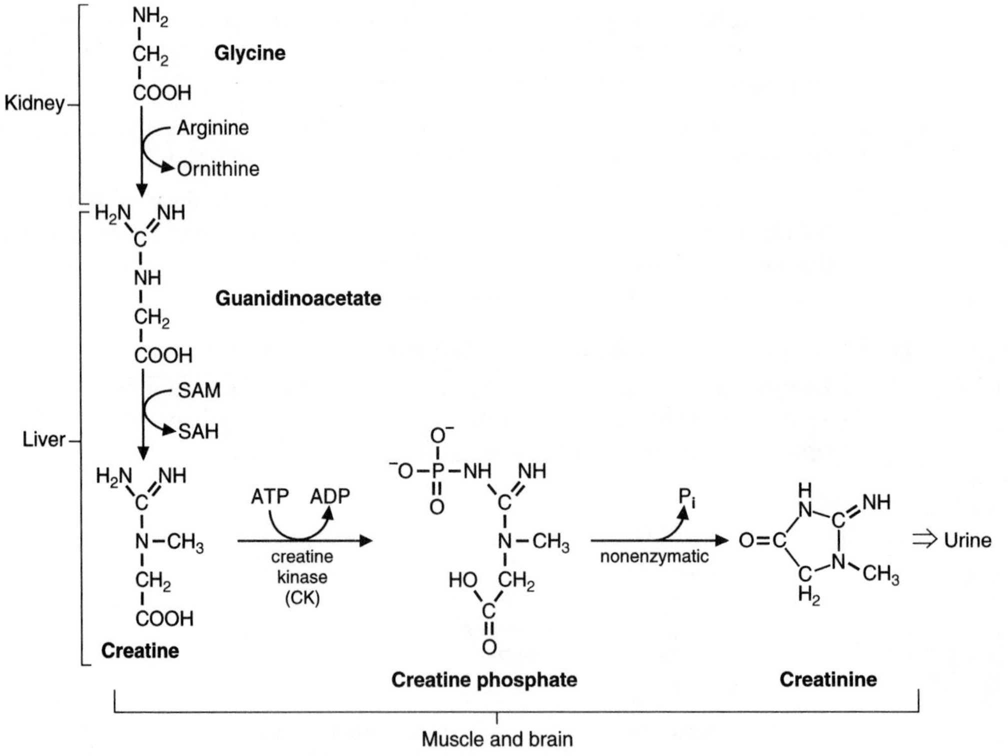

Figure 7-19. The synthesis of creatine phosphate and its spontaneous (nonenzymatic) conversion to creatinine. *SAH* = *S*-adenosylhomocysteine; *SAM* = *S*-adenosylmethionine.

– The amount of **creatinine** excreted per day depends on **body muscle mass** and **kidney function** and is constant at about 15 millimoles for the average person.

B. Products formed by amino acid decarboxylations

– **Amines** are produced by decarboxylation of amino acids in reactions that use **PLP** as a cofactor.

1. γ-Aminobutyric acid (**GABA**), an inhibitory neurotransmitter, is produced by decarboxylation of **glutamate** (Figure 7-20).

2. **Histamine** is produced by decarboxylation of **histidine.**

   – Histamine causes vasodilation and bronchoconstriction. In the stomach, it stimulates the secretion of HCl.

3. The initial step in **ceramide** formation involves the condensation of **palmitoyl CoA** with **serine,** which undergoes a simultaneous decarboxylation.

   – Ceramide forms the sphingolipids (e.g., sphingomyelin, cerebrosides, gangliosides) (see Figure 6-17).

4. The production of **serotonin** from tryptophan and of **dopamine** from tyrosine involves decarboxylations of amino acids.

C. Products derived from tryptophan

– **Serotonin, melatonin,** and the nicotinamide moiety of **NAD** and **NADP** are formed from tryptophan (see Figure 7-12).

1. **Tryptophan** is hydroxylated in a **tetrahydrobiopterin**-requiring reaction similar to the hydroxylation of phenylalanine. The product, 5-hydroxytryptophan, is decarboxylated to form **serotonin.**

2. **Serotonin** undergoes acetylation by acetyl CoA and methylation by *S*-adenosylmethionine to form **melatonin** in the pineal gland.

3. Tryptophan can be converted to the nicotinamide moiety of **NAD** and **NADP** (see Figure 7-12), although the major precursor of nicotinamide is the vitamin niacin (nicotinic acid). Thus, to a limited extent, tryptophan can spare the dietary requirement for niacin.

D. Products derived from phenylalanine and tyrosine

– **Phenylalanine** can be hydroxylated to form **tyrosine** in a reaction that requires **tetrahydrobiopterin**. Tyrosine can be hydroxylated to form **dopa** (3,4-dihydroxyphenylalanine) (see Figure 7-12).

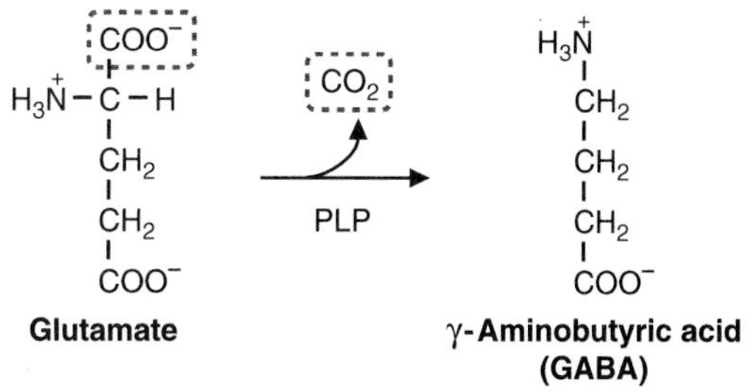

Figure 7-20. The decarboxylation of glutamate to form γ-aminobutyric acid (GABA). *PLP* = pyridoxal phosphate.

1. The **thyroid hormones,** triiodothyronine (**T₃**) and thyroxine (**T₄**), are produced in the thyroid gland from tyrosine residues in **thyroglobulin** (see Chapter 8).

2. **Melanins,** which are pigments in skin and hair, are formed by polymerization of oxidation products (quinones) of **dopa**.

   – In this case, dopa is formed by hydroxylation of tyrosine by an enzyme that uses copper rather than tetrahydrobiopterin.

3. The **catecholamines** (dopamine, norepinephrine, and epinephrine) are derived from tyrosine in a series of reactions (see Figure 7-12).

   a. Synthesis of the catecholamines

   (1) Phenylalanine forms tyrosine, which forms dopa. In this case, both these hydroxylation reactions require **tetrahydrobiopterin.**

   (2) Decarboxylation of dopa forms the neurotransmitter **dopamine.**

   (3) Hydroxylation of dopamine by an enzyme that requires copper and vitamin C yields the neurotransmitter **norepinephrine.**

   (4) Methylation of norepinephrine in the adrenal medulla by *S*-adenosylmethionine forms the hormone **epinephrine.**

   b. Inactivation of the catecholamines

   (1) The catecholamines are inactivated by monoamine oxidase (**MAO**), which produces NH_4^+ and H_2O_2 and converts the catecholamine to an aldehyde, and by catecholamine *O*-methyltransferase (**COMT**), which methylates the 3-hydroxy group.

   (2) The major urinary excretory product of the deaminated, methylated catecholamines is **VMA** (vanillylmandelic acid, or 3-methoxy-4-hydroxymandelic acid).

E. Purine and pyrimidine metabolism

   – De novo purine and pyrimidine biosynthesis occurs in the liver and, to a limited extent, in the brain.

   – The nucleotides that are produced in the liver are converted to nucleosides and bases, which travel in red blood cells to other tissues where they are reconverted to nucleotides and further metabolized.

1. **Purine synthesis** (Figure 7-21, *left*)

   a. The **purine base** is synthesized on the **ribose moiety.**

   (1) 5′-Phosphoribosyl-1′-pyrophosphate (**PRPP**), which provides the ribose moiety, reacts with **glutamine** to form phosphoribosylamine.

   – This first step in purine biosynthesis produces N9 of the purine ring and is inhibited by AMP and GMP.

   (2) The entire **glycine** molecule is added to the growing purine precursor. Then C8 is added by **methenyl tetrahydrofolate**, N3 by **glutamine**, C6 by CO_2, N1 by **aspartate**, and C2 by **formyl tetrahydrofolate** (see Figure 7-21, *bottom*).

   (3) **Inosine monophosphate (IMP),** which contains the base hypoxanthine, is generated.

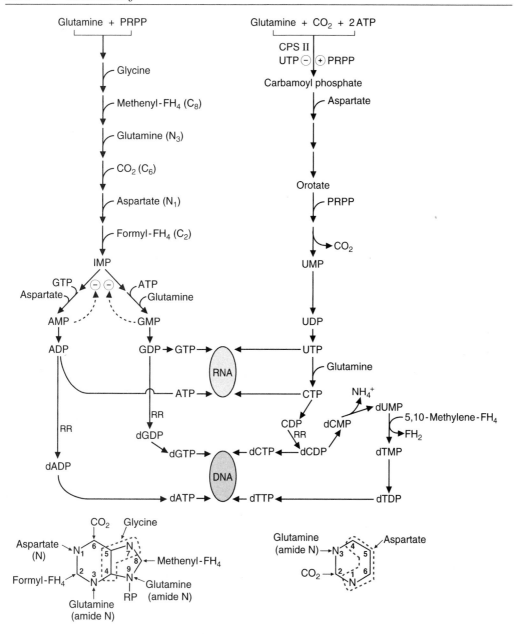

Figure 7-21. De novo synthesis of purines and pyrimidines. Ribonucleotide reductase *(RR)* catalyzes the reduction of the ribose moiety in ADP, GDP, and CDP to deoxyribose. The source of each of the atoms is indicated in the boxes at the bottom of the figure. In hereditary orotic aciduria, the enzymes converting orotate to UMP are defective; *FH₄* = tetrahydrofolate; *PRPP* = 5'-phosphoribosyl-1'-pyrophosphate.

– IMP is cleaved in the liver. Its free base, or nucleoside, travels to various tissues where it is reconverted to the nucleotide.

b. IMP is the precursor of both AMP and GMP.

    (1) Each product, by feedback inhibition, regulates its own synthesis from the IMP branch point as well as inhibits the initial step in the pathway.

(2) AMP and GMP can be phosphorylated to the triphosphate level.

(3) The nucleotide triphosphates (ATP and GTP) can be used for energy-requiring processes or for **RNA synthesis.**

c. **Reduction of the ribose moiety to deoxyribose** occurs at the diphosphate level and is catalyzed by **ribonucleotide reductase,** which requires the protein thioredoxin.

– After the diphosphates are phosphorylated, dATP and dGTP can be used for **DNA synthesis.**

d. **Purine bases** can be salvaged by **reacting with PRPP** to re-form nucleotides (Figure 7-22). The purine-salvage enzymes are hypoxanthine-guanine phosphoribosyl transferase **(HGPRT)** and adenine phosphoribosyl transferase **(APRT).**

2. **Purine degradation** (Figure 7-23*A*)

– In the degradation of the purine nucleotides, **phosphate** and **ribose** are removed first; then the nitrogenous base is oxidized.

a. Degradation of **guanine** produces **xanthine.**

b. Degradation of **adenine** produces **hypoxanthine,** which is oxidized to **xanthine** by xanthine oxidase; this enzyme requires molybdenum.

c. **Xanthine** is oxidized to **uric acid** by xanthine oxidase.

d. **Uric acid,** which is not very water soluble, is **excreted** by the **kidneys.**

3. **Pyrimidine synthesis** (see Figure 7-21, *right*)

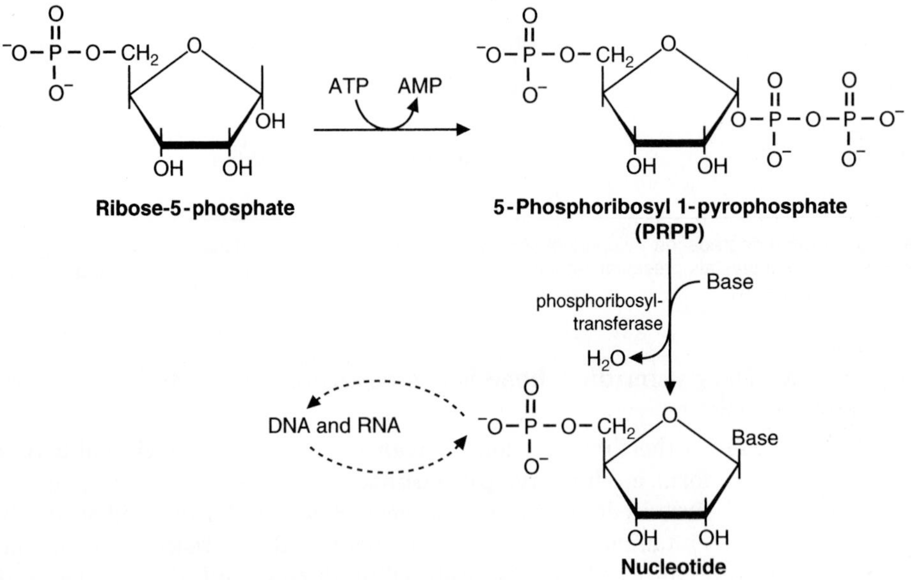

Figure 7-22. Salvage of the purine bases. Salvage of guanine, adenine, and hypoxanthine occurs in reactions catalyzed by phosphoribosyl transferase.

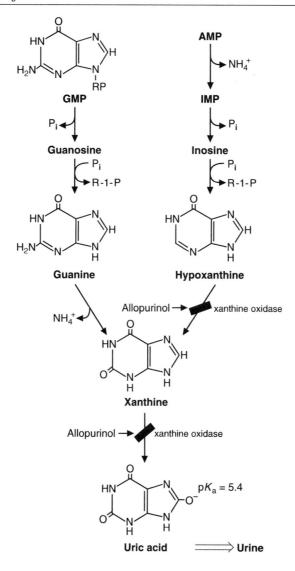

Figure 7-23. Purine degradation. Allopurinol *(AP)*, which inhibits xanthine oxidase, is used to treat gout. Gout occurs when uric acid crystals precipitate in joints because of an increased concentration in the blood. *R-1-P =* ribose 1-phosphate.

a. The **pyrimidine base** is synthesized prior to addition of the ribose moiety.

(1) In the first reaction, **glutamine** reacts with CO_2 and **2 ATP** to form **carbamoyl phosphate**. This reaction is analogous to the first reaction of the urea cycle. However, for pyrimidine synthesis, glutamine provides the nitrogen and the reaction occurs in the cytosol, where it is catalyzed by **carbamoyl phosphate synthetase II,** which is inhibited by UTP.

(2) The entire **aspartate** molecule adds to carbamoyl phosphate. The molecule closes to yield a ring, which is oxidized, forming orotate.

(3) Orotate reacts with PRPP, producing orotidine 5′-phosphate, which is decarboxylated to form uridine monophosphate (UMP).

b. UMP is phosphorylated to UTP, which obtains an amino group from glutamine to form CTP. UTP and CTP are used in the synthesis of **RNA.**

c. The ribose moiety of CDP is reduced to **deoxyribose,** forming dCDP. **Ribonucleotide reductase** is the enzyme.

(1) dCDP is deaminated and dephosphorylated to form **dUMP.**

(2) dUMP is converted to **dTMP** by methylene tetrahydrofolate.

(3) Phosphorylations produce dCTP and dTTP, which are precursors of **DNA.**

4. Pyrimidine degradation

– In pyrimidine degradation, the carbons produce CO_2 and the nitrogens produce urea.

F. Heme metabolism

– Heme, which consists of a **porphyrin ring** coordinated with **iron,** is found mainly in **hemoglobin,** but is also present in **myoglobin** and the **cytochromes.**

1. Heme synthesis (Figure 7-24)

a. In the first step of heme synthesis, **glycine** and **succinyl CoA** condense to form δ-aminolevulinic acid (δ-ALA). **Pyridoxal phosphate** is the cofactor for δ-aminolevulinic acid synthase. Glycine is decarboxylated in this reaction.

b. Two molecules of **δ-aminolevulinic acid** condense to form the pyrrole, porphobilinogen.

c. Four **porphobilinogens** form the first in a series of porphyrins.

d. The **porphyrins** are altered by decarboxylation and oxidation, and protoporphyrin IX is formed.

e. Protoporphyrin IX binds **iron,** forming **heme.**

(1) Iron is obtained from the diet, travels in the blood in the protein **transferrin,** and is stored as **ferritin** in tissues such as liver and spleen (see Figure 7-24).

(2) Vitamin C increases the uptake of iron from the intestinal tract.

(3) Ceruloplasmin, a protein that contains copper, is involved in the oxidation of iron.

(4) Excess iron is stored as **hemosiderin.**

f. Heme regulates its own **production** by repressing the synthesis of δ-aminolevulinic acid synthase in the liver.

g. Erythropoietin induces heme synthesis in bone marrow.

h. Heme stimulates synthesis of the protein **globin** by maintaining the translational initiation complex on the ribosome in its active state.

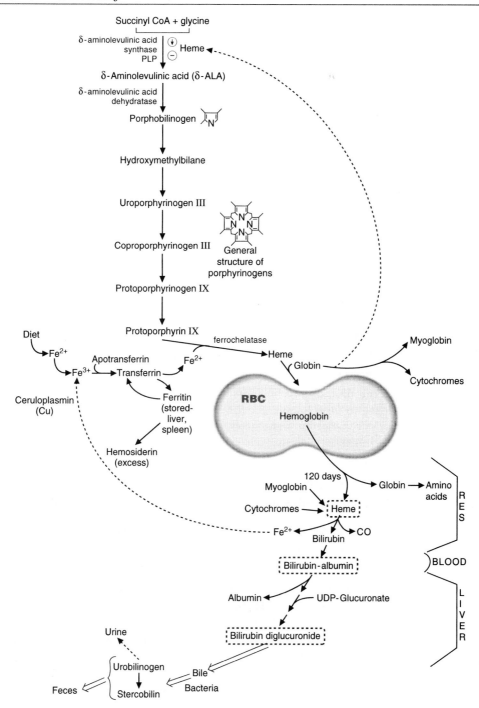

Figure 7-24. Hemoglobin synthesis and degradation. Regulation of heme synthesis occurs by repression of the synthesis of the enzyme δ-ALA synthase, by inhibition of this enzyme by heme in the liver, and by induction of the enzyme by erythropoietin in bone marrow. Bilirubin is converted to urobilinogens and stercobilins by bacterial flora in the intestine. *PLP* = pyridoxal phosphate; *RES* = reticuloendothelial system; ⊕ = repression of enzyme synthesis; ⊖ = inhibition; δ-ALA = δ-aminolevulinic acid.

2. **Heme degradation** (see Figure 7-24)

 – After **red blood cells,** which contain hemoglobin, reach their lifespan of about 120 days, they are **phagocytosed** by cells of the reticuloendothelial system. Globin is released and converted to amino acids. Heme is degraded to **bilirubin,** which is excreted in the bile.

 a. **Heme** is oxidized and cleaved to produce carbon monoxide and biliverdin, a green pigment.

 b. **Iron** is released, oxidized, and returned by transferrin to the iron stores of the body.

 c. **Bilirubin,** produced by reduction of biliverdin, is carried by the protein albumin to the liver.

 d. In the liver, bilirubin reacts with **UDP-glucuronate** to form bilirubin monoglucuronide, which is converted to the diglucuronide.

 e. Formation of the diglucuronide increases the solubility of the pigment, and **bilirubin diglucuronide** is **secreted** into the **bile.**

 f. **Bacteria** in the intestine convert bilirubin to **urobilins** and **stercobilins,** which give feces its brown color.

VIII. Clinical Correlations

A. Liver disease

Many important steps in nitrogen metabolism occur in the liver. If liver disease is severe enough, urea production can be compromised. Blood urea nitrogen **(BUN) levels decrease,** and levels of the toxic compound **ammonia increase.** Because the liver is normally involved in converting bilirubin to the diglucuronide that is excreted in the bile, in liver disease, the levels of **bilirubin increase** in the body and **jaundice** can occur. When liver cells are damaged, enzymes such as aspartate transaminase **(AST)** and alanine transaminase **(ALT)** leak into the blood.

B. Renal failure

Nitrogenous excretory products are removed from the body mainly in the urine. In renal failure, these products are retained. **BUN, creatinine,** and **uric acid levels rise.**

C. Inborn errors of amino acid metabolism

Although the individual diseases caused by defective enzymes in amino acid metabolism are rare, a large number of these diseases occur, and studies of these diseases have helped to elucidate the pathways of amino acid metabolism in the human.

1. **Defective membrane-transport systems** for amino acids result in decreased absorption of amino acids from the intestine and resorption of amino acids by the kidney (and thus increased excretion in the urine). In **cystinuria,** transport of cysteine is defective. Cysteine is synthesized in the body and oxidized to cystine, which can crystallize, forming kidney stones. In **Hartnup's disease,** the transport of neutral amino acids is defective, resulting in **deficiencies of essential amino acids** because they are not absorbed from the diet.

2. In **phenylketonuria (PKU),** the conversion of phenylalanine to tyrosine is defective. Some cases of PKU are due to defects in phenylalanine hydroxylase and some to defects in the synthesis of tetrahydrobiopterin. Phenylalanine accumulates and is converted to compounds such as the **phenylketones**, which give the urine a musty odor. **Mental retardation** occurs. PKU is treated by restriction of phenylalanine in the diet.

3. In **alcaptonuria,** homogentisic acid, a product of phenylalanine and tyrosine metabolism, accumulates because homogentisate oxidase is defective (see Figure 7-12). Homogentisic acid autooxidizes and the products polymerize, forming dark-colored pigments, which accumulate in various tissues and are sometimes associated with a **degenerative arthritis.**

4. In **histidinemia,** histidase, which converts histidine to urocanate, is defective. Early cases were reported to be associated with mental retardation, but more recently, deleterious consequences have not been observed.

5. In **maple syrup urine disease,** the enzyme complex that decarboxylates the transamination products of the branched chain amino acids (the α-keto acid dehydrogenase) is defective (see Figure 7-11). Valine, isoleucine, and leucine accumulate. Urine has the odor of maple syrup. **Mental retardation** occurs.

6. In **homocystinuria,** cystathionine synthase is defective. Therefore, homocysteine does not react with serine to form cysteine (see Figure 7-10). The homocysteine that accumulates is oxidized to homocystine and excreted in the urine. Some cases respond to increased doses of vitamin B_6, which forms PLP, the cofactor for the synthase enzyme. Other causes of elevated levels of homocyst(e)ine (homocysteine or homocystine) in the blood or urine are deficiencies of the enzyme methionine synthetase (that converts homocysteine to methionine) or dietary deficiencies of the vitamin cofactors for this enzyme (folate and B_{12}). Elevated levels of homocyst(e)ine are associated with increased risk of **coronary artery disease.**

D. Disorders of purine and pyrimidine metabolism

1. **Gout** is a group of diseases caused by an increased conversion of purine bases to uric acid or a decreased excretion of **uric acid** by the kidney. (Lead and metabolic acids—lactic acid, acetoacetic acid, and 3-hydroxybutyric acid—interfere with uric acid excretion.) Accumulation of uric acid, which is very insoluble, results in the precipitation of urate crystals in the joints. An **acute inflammatory arthritis** results. Chronic cases are treated with allopurinol, a base that forms a nucleotide that inhibits xanthine oxidase and prevents hypoxanthine and xanthine from being converted to uric acid (see Figure 7-23).

2. **Lesch-Nyhan syndrome** is caused by a defective hypoxanthine-guanine phosphoribosyl transferase **(HGPRT).** Purine bases cannot be salvaged (i.e., reconverted to nucleotides). The purines are converted instead to uric acid, which rises in the blood. **Mental retardation** and **self-mutilation** are characteristics of the disease.

3. In **hereditary orotic aciduria,** orotic acid is excreted in the urine because the enzymes that convert it to uridine monophosphate (orotate phosphoribosyl transferase and orotidine 5′-phosphate decarboxylase) are defec-

tive (see Figure 7-21). Pyrimidines cannot be synthesized, and therefore, **growth retardation** occurs. Oral administration of **uridine** bypasses the metabolic block and provides the body with a source of pyrimidines.

E. Diseases related to heme metabolism

1. **Porphyrias,** a group of rare inherited disorders, are caused by deficiencies of enzymes in the pathway of heme biosynthesis. **Neuropsychiatric symptoms** result from accumulation of intermediates in the pathway that have toxic effects on the nervous system. **Photosensitivity** results from accumulation of porphyrinogens, which react with light to form porphyrins that produce oxygen radicals that damage the skin.

2. **Dietary deficiencies of iron or of vitamin B$_6$** result in the production of small, pale red blood cells. A microcytic, hypochromic anemia results.

3. In **lead poisoning**, δ-amino levulinic acid (δ-ALA) and protoporphyrin IX accumulate because lead inhibits δ-ALA dehydratase and ferrochelatase. Heme production is decreased, and anemia results from a lack of hemoglobin.

4. **Excessive levels of bilirubin or bilirubin diglucuronide** result in a yellowish discoloration of various tissues of the body (**jaundice**), which is particularly evident in the whites of the eyes. Causes of jaundice include overproduction of bilirubin due to **hemolytic anemia**, an inability of the liver to conjugate and excrete bilirubin due to **liver disease**, or an **obstruction of the bile duct** that prevents bilirubin diglucuronide from passing from the liver into the intestine. **Neonatal jaundice** is common and is caused by an **immaturity of the system for conjugating and excreting bilirubin**. As the enzymes in the pathway develop, the condition resolves. Phototherapy, which converts bilirubin to other compounds that can be excreted in the urine, is used to prevent permanent damage to the nervous system (kernicterus).

F. Diseases related to the metabolism of other nitrogen-containing compounds

1. In **Parkinson's disease,** dopamine levels are decreased because of a deficiency in conversion of dopa to dopamine (see Figure 7-12). The common characteristics are **tremors**, difficulty initiating voluntary movement, a **masked face** with a staring expression, and a **shuffling gait**.

2. **Pheochromocytomas** are tumors that produce norepinephrine and epinephrine and cause **hypertension.**

3. In **albinism,** tyrosinase is defective and tyrosine cannot be converted to the skin pigment melanin. Characteristics are very **light-colored skin, hair,** and **eyes.**

G. Vitamin deficiencies that affect amino acid metabolism

1. **Pellagra** is caused by a deficiency of the vitamin **niacin** or of **tryptophan**. Niacin is required for the production of NAD and NADP. These compounds can also be generated from tryptophan. Pellagra results in the four Ds: **dermatitis, diarrhea, dementia, and death.**

2. Vitamin B_6 is required for the formation of pyridoxal phosphate, an important cofactor in nitrogen metabolism. **Deficiencies of vitamin B_6** are caused by a lack of the vitamin in the diet or by the administration of drugs such as isoniazid, which interfere with its metabolism. Synthesis of neurotransmitters, NAD, and heme are decreased, resulting in **neurologic** and **pellagra-like symptoms** and **anemia**.

3. **Folate and vitamin B_{12} deficiencies** result in decreased DNA and RNA synthesis, which causes a **megaloblastic anemia**. Tetrahydrofolate (FH_4) is directly involved in providing carbon for thymine (and thus DNA) synthesis and for synthesis of the purines (see Figure 7-21), which are required for both DNA and RNA synthesis. In a folate deficiency, normal cell proliferation cannot occur, and megaloblasts develop. If vitamin B_{12}, which accepts methyl groups from 5-methyl-FH_4, is deficient, 5-methyl-FH_4 accumulates. Since this compound cannot be reconverted to other FH_4 derivatives, a folate deficiency is secondarily produced (the methyl trap theory). Vitamin B_{12} also is involved in converting methylmalonyl CoA to succinyl CoA (see Figure 7-10). In a **vitamin B_{12} deficiency**, methylmalonic acid is excreted in the urine, and, in addition to a megaloblastic anemia, **neurologic symptoms**, which cannot be alleviated by administration of folate, occur. They are due to demyelination of nerves, and, thus are irreversible. The **absence of intrinsic factor**, which is produced by the stomach and necessary for vitamin B_{12} absorption in the intestine, causes **pernicious anemia.**

H. Chemotherapeutic drugs that affect nitrogen metabolism (see Figure 7-17)

1. **5-Fluorouracil** produces a nucleotide that binds to thymidylate synthetase and prevents the conversion of dUMP to dTMP. This inhibition of the synthesis of thymine **prevents DNA synthesis** and thus affects the proliferation of cells.

2. **Methotrexate** inhibits dihydrofolate reductase, which catalyzes the reduction of FH_2 to FH_4. When dUMP is converted to dTMP, N^5, N^{10}-methylene tetrahydrofolate is converted to FH_2, which must be reduced to FH_4 in order for the production of thymine to continue. If the reductase is inhibited by methotrexate, thymine synthesis is also inhibited, thus **preventing DNA synthesis.** In addition, dietary folate cannot be reduced to FH_4 by dihydrofolate reductase, thus a deficiency of FH_4 results.

Review Test

Directions: Each of the numbered items or incomplete statements in this section is followed by answers or by completions of the statement. Select the **one** lettered answer or completion that is **best** in each case.

1. A deficiency of which of the following proteolytic enzymes has the greatest effect on the digestion of proteins?

(A) Trypsin
(B) Chymotrypsin
(C) Carboxypeptidase A
(D) Pepsin
(E) Aminopeptidase

2. In liver disease, the enzymes aspartate transaminase (AST) and alanine transaminase (ALT) leak into the blood from damaged liver cells. Both of these enzymes

(A) transfer ammonia to α-keto acids to form amino acids
(B) form intermediates of glycolysis from amino acids
(C) require thiamine pyrophosphate as a cofactor
(D) catalyze irreversible reactions
(E) convert α-ketoglutarate to glutamate

3. In the urea cycle,

(A) carbamoyl phosphate is derived directly from glutamine and CO_2
(B) ornithine reacts with aspartate to generate argininosuccinate
(C) the α-amino group of arginine forms one of the nitrogens of urea
(D) ornithine directly reacts with carbamoyl phosphate to form citrulline
(E) N-acetylglutamate is a positive allosteric effector of ornithine transcarbamoylase

4. Via enzymes of the urea cycle, aspartate

(A) provides nitrogen for synthesis of arginine
(B) provides carbon for the synthesis of arginine
(C) is converted to malate
(D) is converted to oxaloacetate

5. An infant who appeared normal at birth began to develop lethargy, hypothermia, and apnea within 24 hours. These problems were traced to a deficiency of argininosuccinate synthetase. This infant would most likely have

(A) high blood levels of urea (blood urea nitrogen)
(B) high blood levels of citrulline
(C) high blood levels of arginine
(D) low blood levels of ammonia

6. Isocitrate dehydrogenase is required for the synthesis from glucose of the amino acid

(A) serine
(B) alanine
(C) aspartate
(D) glutamate
(E) cysteine

7. The pathway for serine biosynthesis begins with the glycolytic intermediate

(A) pyruvate
(B) fructose 1,6-bisphosphate
(C) dihydroxyacetone phosphate
(D) 3-phosphoglycerate
(E) glucose 6-phosphate

8. The carbons of cysteine are derived from

(A) threonine
(B) serine
(C) homocysteine
(D) methionine

9. Which of the following statements about serine is correct?

(A) It is converted to pyruvate and urea by a dehydratase
(B) It may be synthesized from glucose via an intermediate of the TCA cycle
(C) It is converted to glycine by a reaction requiring tetrahydrofolate
(D) It is the only amino acid that contains a hydroxyl group
(E) It is an essential amino acid

273

10. Which of the following statements concerning glutamate is TRUE?

(A) It is produced in a transamination reaction in which aspartate reacts with oxaloacetate
(B) It undergoes a series of reactions in which it cyclizes to produce histidine
(C) It can be converted to arginine by a series of reactions, some of which require urea cycle enzymes
(D) It is produced by the action of glutamate dehydrogenase, an enzyme that requires NH_4^+ and FAD

11. A common intermediate in the synthesis of arginine, serine, and aspartate from glucose is

(A) oxaloacetate
(B) glyceraldehyde 3-phosphate
(C) pyruvate
(D) α-ketoglutarate
(E) ornithine

12. During the metabolism of the branched chain amino acids

(A) valine is deaminated rather than transaminated
(B) none of the carbons of isoleucine is converted to succinyl CoA
(C) lipoic acid is not required
(D) leucine is converted to acetoacetate

13. The plasma and urine of patients with maple syrup urine disease contain

(A) elevated levels of valine
(B) elevated levels of phenylketones
(C) low levels of leucine
(D) low levels of tyrosine
(E) normal levels of isoleucine

14. A deficiency of pyridoxal phosphate would directly affect which of the following reactions?

(A) glutamate + NH_3 + ATP → glutamine + ADP + P_i
(B) glutamate + NAD^+ → α-ketoglutarate + NH_4^+ + NADH + H^+
(C) glutamine + H_2O → glutamate + NH_3
(D) pyruvate + glutamate → alanine + α-ketoglutarate

15. The major amino acid that is released from muscle and converted to glucose in the liver is

(A) alanine
(B) glutamine
(C) valine
(D) aspartate
(E) glutamate

16. Which of the following statements about the kidney is correct?

(A) It uses ammonia released from glutamine to buffer acids in the urine
(B) It excretes creatine phosphate
(C) It produces glutamate from alanine and releases it into the blood
(D) It synthesizes most of the urea that is excreted into the urine

17. For which of the following reactions does S-adenosylmethionine (SAM) serve as a methylating agent?

(A) Conversion of dopamine to norepinephrine
(B) Synthesis of creatinine from creatine phosphate
(C) Synthesis of phosphatidylcholine from phosphatidylethanolamine
(D) Conversion of dUMP to dTMP
(E) Formation of methionine from homocysteine

18. Pregnant women frequently suffer from folate deficiencies. A deficiency of folate would decrease the production of

(A) creatine phosphate from creatine
(B) all of the pyrimidines required for RNA synthesis
(C) the thymine nucleotide required for DNA synthesis
(D) phosphatidylcholine from diacylglycerol and CDP-choline

19. The conversion of propionyl CoA to succinyl CoA requires

(A) biotin
(B) vitamin B_{12}
(C) biotin and vitamin B_{12}
(D) biotin, vitamin B_{12}, and tetrahydrofolate

20. Compared with a healthy person, a person with pernicious anemia

(A) produces less intrinsic factor
(B) excretes less methylmalonic acid in the urine
(C) requires less methionine in the diet
(D) has a higher rate of purine biosynthesis
(E) has lower blood levels of FIGLU

21. A 24-hour urine collection showed that an individual's excretion of creatinine was much lower than normal. Decreased excretion of creatinine could be caused by

(A) decreased dietary intake of creatine
(B) a higher than normal muscle mass resulting from weight lifting
(C) a genetic defect in the enzyme that converts creatine phosphate to creatinine
(D) kidney failure

22. A genetic defect in the ability to synthesize tetrahydrobiopterin would result in increased conversion of

(A) phenylalanine to phenylketones
(B) tyrosine to dopamine
(C) dopa to melanin
(D) serotonin to melatonin

23. Phenylketonuria, alcaptonuria, and albinism are caused by deficiencies in enzymes involved in the metabolism of

(A) tryptophan
(B) tyrosine
(C) histidine
(D) valine
(E) lysine

24. Which of the following statements about nitrogen metabolism is correct?

(A) Cysteine "spares" methionine; that is, ingestion of cysteine reduces the need for methionine in the diet
(B) The enzyme glutamate dehydrogenase catalyzes the transamination of glutamate
(C) Creatine requires glycine, ornithine, and methionine for synthesis of its carbon skeleton
(D) Formiminoglutamate (FIGLU) is an intermediate in glutamine degradation

25. Excessive degradation of AMP and GMP would result in increased urinary excretion of

(A) creatinine
(B) urea
(C) uric acid
(D) thiamine
(E) thymine

26. De novo pyrimidine synthesis requires

(A) phosphoribosyl pyrophosphate (PRPP) for the initial step
(B) tetrahydrofolate for the incorporation of carbons 2 and 8
(C) both carbon and nitrogen of aspartate to form the ring
(D) NH_4^+ as a substrate for carbamoyl phosphate synthetase II
(E) glycine as the source of two nitrogens in the ring

27. 5-Fluorouracil (5-FU) is an effective chemotherapeutic agent because it interferes with DNA synthesis by directly inhibiting the reaction in which

(A) $FH_2 \rightarrow FH_4$
(B) $dUMP \rightarrow dTMP$
(C) glutamine + PRPP $\rightarrow$ phosphoribosylamine
(D) methyl $B_{12} \rightarrow B_{12}$

28. Which of the following statements about heme and iron metabolism is correct?

(A) Iron is stored in the liver as transferrin
(B) Iron (as Fe^{3+}) is inserted into protoporphyrin IX in the last step of heme synthesis
(C) δ-Aminolevulinate (δ-ALA) synthase catalyzes the regulated and rate-limiting step in heme biosynthesis.
(D) The major route for bilirubin excretion is via the urine
(E) The iron produced by heme degradation is excreted in the feces

29. Which of the following statements about bilirubin is TRUE?

(A) It is made more soluble in the liver by attachment of residues of glucose
(B) It is excreted mainly in the urine
(C) It is produced by oxidation of heme, with loss of carbon monoxide (CO)
(D) It contains iron in the Fe^{2+} state

30. In the biosynthetic pathways for the synthesis of heme, creatine, and guanine, which of the following amino acids directly provides carbon atoms that appear in the final product?

(A) serine
(B) aspartate
(C) cysteine
(D) glutamate
(E) glycine

Directions: Each group of items in this section consists of lettered options followed by a set of numbered items. For each item, select the **one** lettered option that is most closely associated with it. Each lettered option may be selected once, more than once, or not at all.

Questions 31–35

(A) Pepsin
(B) Trypsin
(C) Carboxypeptidase A
(D) Enteropeptidase

Match each property below with the appropriate enzyme.

31. Digests dietary proteins in the stomach

32. Is synthesized by intestinal cells

33. Cleaves bonds at the carboxyl end of the arginine and lysine residues within a polypeptide chain

34. Acts as an exopeptidase

35. Is produced by the action of HCl on its precursor

Questions 36–40

(A) Vitamin B_{12}
(B) Tetrahydrofolate (FH_4)
(C) Biotin
(D) Thiamine
(E) Pyridoxal phosphate

Each of the reactions below would be affected by a vitamin deficiency. Match each reaction with the appropriate vitamin.

36. Decarboxylation of the transamination product of valine

37. Synthesis of deoxythymidylate from deoxyuridylate

38. Synthesis of serine from glycine

39. Conversion of methylmalonyl CoA to succinyl CoA

40. Conversion of histidine to histamine

Questions 41–46

(A) Tyrosine
(B) Tryptophan
(C) Threonine
(D) Thymine

Match the descriptions below with the appropriate compound.

41. Can be converted to epinephrine

42. Contains nonring carbons that can be cleaved from the ring structure to form alanine

43. Is synthesized by hydroxylation of an essential amino acid

44. Can be converted to serotonin by reactions requiring tetrahydrobiopterin and molecular oxygen

45. Can be converted to the moiety of NAD^+ that can also be derived from niacin

46. Can be produced from uracil

Questions 47–50

(A) Leucine
(B) Homocysteine
(C) Glutamate
(D) Tryptophan

Match each of the metabolites below with the compound to which it is related.

47. NAD^+

48. HMG CoA

49. Proline

50. Methionine

Questions 51-54

(A) Folate
(B) Vitamin B_{12}
(C) Either folate or vitamin B_{12}
(D) Neither folate nor vitamin B_{12}

Each of the conditions below can result from a vitamin deficiency. For each condition, choose the vitamin or set of vitamins which, if in deficient supply, would produce that condition.

51. Megaloblastic anemia

52. Neurologic symptoms caused by demyelination

53. Homocysteinemia

54. Non-classic phenylketonuria

Questions 55–58

(A) Low blood urea nitrogen (BUN); high blood NH_4^+ and high total bilirubin levels
(B) Dark brown stool; elevated total bilirubin in blood
(C) Low hematocrit; small, pale red blood cells
(D) Light-colored stool; elevated conjugated bilirubin in blood

Match each of the conditions below with the most likely clinical findings.

55. Bile duct obstruction

56. Hemolytic anemia

57. Iron deficiency anemia

58. Hepatitis

Questions 59–62

(A) Bilirubin
(B) Uric acid
(C) Creatine kinase
(D) Blood urea nitrogen (BUN)

Match each condition below with the component that would be elevated to the greatest extent in the blood.

59. Gout

60. Myocardial infarction

61. Hepatitis

62. Kidney disease

Questions 63–67

(A) Parkinson's disease
(B) Cystinuria
(C) Pellagra
(D) Lesch-Nyhan syndrome
(E) Hartnup's disease

Match each description below with the appropriate condition.

63. Can be caused by a dietary tryptophan deficiency

64. Caused by a genetic defect in hypoxanthine guanine phosphoribosyl-transferase (HGPRT)

65. Caused by a defective transporter on intestinal epithelial cells for essential amino acids

66. Caused by a defective transporter on kidney tubule cells for a nonessential amino acid

67. Caused by decreased production of dopamine from dopa

Answers and Explanations

1–A. Trypsin cleaves and, thus, activates the pancreatic zymogens, converting chymotrypsinogen to the active form, chymotrypsin, and the procarboxypeptidases to the active carboxypeptidases. It even autocatalyses its own activation–the conversion of trypsinogen to trypsin (which is also catalyzed by enteropeptidase).

2–E. These transaminases convert amino acids to their corresponding α-keto acids in reactions that are readily reversible. α-Ketoglutarate and glutamate serve as the other α-keto acid/amino acid pair. Pyruvate (the end product of glycolysis) is the α-keto acid corresponding to alanine, and oxaloacetate (an intermediate of the TCA cycle) is the partner of aspartate. Pyridoxal phosphate is the cofactor.

3–D. Carbamoyl phosphate is formed from NH_4^+, CO_2, and ATP. It reacts with ornithine to form citrulline, which reacts with aspartate to form argininosuccinate. Fumarate is released from arginino-succinate, and arginine is formed. Urea is produced from the guanidinium group on the side chain of arginine, not from the amino group. Ornithine is regenerated. N-acetylglutamate is an allosteric activator of carbamoyl phosphate synthetase I.

4–A. When argininosuccinate is cleaved to form arginine, the carbons that were derived from aspartate are released as fumarate and the nitrogen of aspartate is incorporated into arginine.

5–B. With this defect in the urea cycle, urea would not be produced at a normal rate, thus the blood urea nitrogen would be low. Arginine would also be low, but the compound before the block, citrulline, would be elevated, as would ammonia.

6–D. Formation of glutamate from glucose involves the TCA cycle intermediate α-ketoglutarate, which is formed from isocitrate in a reaction catalyzed by isocitrate dehydrogenase. α-Ketoglutarate is converted to glutamate either by glutamate dehydrogenase or a transaminase. Formation of serine, alanine, aspartate, and cysteine from glucose do not require isocitrate dehydrogenase.

7–D. Serine is synthesized from glucose. The pathway branches from glycolysis at 3-phosphoglycerate, which is oxidized, transaminated, and dephosphorylated by phosphoserine phosphatase to form serine.

8–B. Serine reacts with homocysteine to form cystathionine, which is cleaved to form cysteine, NH_4^+, and α-ketobutyrate. Methionine provides the sulfur via homocysteine.

9–C. Both serine and threonine contain a hydroxyl group. Serine dehydratase produces pyruvate and ammonia from serine. Serine can be produced from glucose via the 3-phosphoglyceric acid intermediate of glycolysis; thus, it is nonessential. Tetrahydrofolate (FH_4) reacts with serine to form glycine and N^5, N^{10}-methylene-FH_4.

10–C. Glutamate can be reduced to glutamate semialdehyde and then transaminated to form ornithine, which can be converted to arginine via enzymes of the urea cycle. Glutamate semialdehyde cyclizes to form proline. (Histidine cannot be synthesized in the human.) Aspartate and α-ketoglutarate undergo a transamination reaction that produces oxaloacetate and glutamate. The reaction catalyzed by glutamate dehydrogenase requires NADH or NADPH; it produces glutamate from α-ketoglutarate and NH_4^+.

11–B. In the synthesis of these three amino acids from glucose, serine is produced from the glycolytic intermediate 3- phosphoglycerate. Arginine is produced from the TCA cycle intermediate α-ketoglutarate, and aspartate by transamination of oxaloacetate. Therefore, glyceraldehyde-3-phosphate, the precursor of 3-phosphoglycerate in glycolysis, is the only common intermediate on this list.

12–D. Valine, isoleucine, and leucine (the branched chain amino acids) are transaminated and then oxidized by an α-keto acid dehydrogenase that requires lipoic acid as well as thiamine pyrophosphate, coenzyme A, FAD, and NAD$^+$. Four of the carbons of valine and isoleucine are converted to succinyl CoA. Isoleucine also produces acetyl CoA. Leucine is converted to HMG CoA, which is cleaved to acetoacetate and acetyl CoA.

13–A. In maple syrup urine disease (MSUD), the branched chain amino acids (valine, leucine, and isoleucine) can be transaminated but not oxidatively decarboxylated because the α-keto acid dehydrogenase is defective. Therefore, these amino acids and their transamination products (the corresponding α-keto acids) will be elevated. Phenylketones are elevated in phenylketonuria (PKU) not in MSUD. Tyrosine levels should be normal in MSUD.

14–D. Transamination reactions require pyridoxal phosphate.

15–A. Alanine and glutamine are the major amino acids released from muscle. Glutamine is further metabolized in the gut and the kidney. Alanine is the major amino acid that is converted to glucose in the liver.

16–A. Glutaminase acts on glutamine to release ammonia, which enters the urine and serves as a buffer by forming NH$_4^+$. The kidney excretes creatinine, a compound produced by nonenzymatic cyclization of creatine phosphate. The kidney takes up glutamine and releases serine and alanine into the blood. Most of the urea that is excreted by the kidney is produced in the liver.

17–C. The conversion of dopamine to norepinephrine involves a hydroxylation reaction. (SAM methylates norepinephrine to form epinephrine.) The synthesis of creatine requires SAM, not the conversion of creatine phosphate to creatinine. Tetrahydrofolate is involved in the conversion of dUMP to dTMP. The formation of methionine from homocysteine requires B$_{12}$ and methyl-FH$_4$. 3 SAMs are required to convert phosphatidyl ethanolamine to phosphatidylcholine.

18–C. The only pyrimidine that requires folate for its synthesis is thymine (dUMP → dTMP). Folate is required for incorporation of carbons 2 and 8 into all purine molecules. The synthesis of creatine phosphate and of phosphatidylcholine do not require folate. Folate deficiencies during pregnancy can lead to neural tube defects (e.g., spina bifida) in the fetus.

19–C. The conversion of propionyl CoA to methylmalonyl CoA requires biotin, and the conversion of methylmalonyl CoA to succinyl CoA requires vitamin B$_{12}$. FH$_4$ is not involved.

20–A. Pernicious anemia occurs when the stomach does not produce adequate intrinsic factor for absorption of vitamin B$_{12}$, which is required for the conversion of methylmalonyl CoA to succinyl CoA and of homocysteine to methionine. A vitamin B$_{12}$ deficiency results in the excretion of methylmalonic acid in the urine and an increased dietary requirement for methionine. The methyl group transferred from vitamin B$_{12}$ to homocysteine to form methionine comes from 5′-methyl tetrahydrofolate, which accumulates in a vitamin B$_{12}$ deficiency, causing a decrease in free folate levels and symptoms of folate deficiency, including increased levels of FIGLU and decreased purine biosynthesis.

21–D. Creatine is synthesized from glycine, arginine, and SAM. In muscle, creatine is converted to creatine phosphate, which is nonenzymatically cyclized to form creatinine. The amount of creatinine excreted by the kidneys each day depends on body muscle mass. In kidney failure, the excretion of creatinine into the urine will be low.

22–A. Tetrahydrobiopterin is involved in hydroxylation reactions that occur in the conversion of phenylalanine to tyrosine, tyrosine to dopamine, and tryptophan to serotonin, but not in the conversion of dopa to melanin or of serotonin to melatonin. A deficiency of tetrahydrobiopterin would cause phenylalanine to be converted to phenylketones rather than to tyrosine.

23–B. PKU is caused by a deficiency of phenylalanine hydroxylase, which converts phenylalanine to tyrosine. A defect in tyrosine degradation causes homogentisic acid to accumulate and produce dark pigments (alcaptonuria). A defect in the conversion of tyrosine to the skin pigment melanin causes albinism.

24–A. Because the sulfur of methionine is used for cysteine synthesis, as cysteine increases in the diet, less methionine is required. Glutamate dehydrogenase catalyzes the addition of ammonia to α-ketoglutarate to form glutamate. For creatine synthesis, arginine, not ornithine, is required in addition to glycine and SAM. FIGLU is produced during the degradation of histidine.

25–C. The purine bases, adenine (A) and guanine (G), are oxidized to uric acid, which is excreted in the urine. Excessive production of uric acid can result in the condition known as gout.

26–C. Options A and B are true for purine but not pyrimidine biosynthesis. During pyrimidine synthesis, the entire aspartate molecule is incorporated into the ring. Glutamine is the substrate for carbamoyl phosphate synthetase II, the enzyme involved in pyrimidine biosynthesis. (NH_4^+ is the substrate for synthetase I used in urea synthesis.) Glycine supplies one nitrogen for purine synthesis.

27–B. Methotrexate inhibits reaction A. 5-FU inhibits reaction B. The remaining reactions are not directly affected by 5-FU. Reaction C is the first step in purine biosynthesis, and reaction D provides the methyl group for the biosynthesis of methionine from homocysteine.

28–C. The first and rate-limiting step in heme biosynthesis involves the condensation of glycine and succinyl CoA to form δ-ALA. Iron is stored as ferritin and transported in the blood in transferrin. As Fe^{2+}, it is inserted into protoporphyrin IX to form heme. When heme is degraded to form bilirubin (which is excreted mainly via the intestine), iron is returned to the body's iron stores and is not excreted. Bleeding is the only significant means by which iron is lost from the body.

29–C. Bilirubin is produced by oxidation of heme after its iron is released; CO is produced in this reaction. Bilirubin diglucuronide, which contains two glucuronic acid (not glucose) residues, is excreted into the bile by the liver.

30–E. Glycine reacts with succinyl CoA in the first step of heme synthesis and with arginine in the first step of creatine synthesis. The entire glycine molecule is incorporated into the growing purine ring.

31–A. Pepsin acts in the stomach.

32–D. Enteropeptidase, which is produced by intestinal cells, cleaves trypsinogen to trypsin.

33–B. Trypsin is an endopeptidase that cleaves polypeptide chains at arginine and lysine residues.

34–C. Carboxypeptidases A and B are pancreatic exopeptidases, which cleave one amino acid at a time from the C-terminal end of a polypeptide chain.

35–A. Pepsin is produced as pepsinogen (a zymogen), which autocatalyzes its own cleavage to pepsin when exposed to HCl.

36–D. The branched chain amino acids (valine, isoleucine, and leucine) are transaminated and then oxidatively decarboxylated by an enzyme that requires thiamine, lipoic acid, coenzyme A, FAD, and NAD.

37–B. N^5,N^{10}-methylene tetrahydrofolate reacts with dUMP to form dTMP. Dihydrofolate is produced and then reduced to FH_4 by dihydrofolate reductase.

38–B. N^5,N^{10}-methylene-FH_4 is involved in the conversion of glycine to serine.

39–A. Vitamin B_{12} is required for the conversion of methylmalonyl CoA to succinyl CoA.

40–E. Decarboxylations of amino acids require pyridoxal phosphate.

41–A. Tyrosine can be converted to dopa, dopamine, norepinephrine, and then to epinephrine.

42–B. The nonring carbons of tryptophan are cleaved from the ring to form alanine.

43–A. Tyrosine is synthesized by hydroxylation of the essential amino acid phenylalanine.

44–B. Tryptophan is hydroxylated by a mixed-function oxidase that requires tetrahydrobiopterin and O_2. The product, 5-hydroxytryptophan, is decarboxylated to form serotonin.

45–B. The ring portion of tryptophan can be converted to the nicotinamide moiety of NAD, which can also be derived from the vitamin niacin.

46–D. Uracil as dUMP is converted to thymine (dTMP).

47–D. The nicotinamide moiety of NAD can be derived from tryptophan.

48–A. Leucine forms HMG CoA, which is cleaved to form acetyl CoA and acetoacetate.

49–C. Proline is derived from glutamate and can be converted to glutamate.

50–B. Methionine reacts with ATP to form S-adenosylmethionine (SAM), which donates a methyl group and forms S-adenosylhomocysteine. After release of adenosine, homocysteine is produced. Homocysteine is converted to methionine when it receives a methyl group from vitamin B_{12} (which obtains it from methyl-FH_4).

51–C. A dietary deficiency of folate or a folate deficiency secondary to a B_{12} deficiency can cause a megaloblastic anemia. (In a B_{12} deficiency, folate is "trapped" as methyl-FH_4.)Without adequate folate, thymine and purine bases are not produced. Red blood cell precursors attempt to divide, but become megaloblasts because they lack the precursors to fully replicate their DNA.

52–B. A B_{12} deficiency can result in a megaloblastic anemia as described in question 51. In addition, because B_{12} is also required for the conversion of methylmalonyl CoA to succinyl CoA, a B_{12} deficiency causes neurologic symptoms that result from demyelination.

53–C. In a dietary folate deficiency or one secondary to a B_{12} deficiency (see question 51), there is decreased conversion of homocysteine to methionine. Elevated blood homocysteine levels result and are associated with coronary heart disease.

54–D. Non-classic phenylketonuria is caused by a decreased ability to produce tetrahydrobiopterin, not by a folate or a B_{12} deficiency. (Classic PKU is caused by a genetic defect in the enzyme phenylalanine hydroxylase that converts phenylalanine to tyrosine.)

55–D. If the bile duct is obstructed, conjugated bilirubin from the liver does not enter the gut but instead backs up into the blood. The dark brown color of stool is caused by stercobilin, a pigment produced by bacterial oxidation of bilirubin in the gut. When less bilirubin than normal enters the gut, the stool will be light in color.

56–B. Increased hemolysis of red blood cells causes bilirubin to be elevated in the blood. The liver conjugates the bilirubin and excretes it into the gut where it is converted to stercobilin, the compound that gives feces its brown color.

57–C. A lower than normal amount of heme is produced from protoporphyrin IX in an iron-deficiency anemia. Red blood cells are pale and small.

58–A. In hepatitis, the liver's ability to produce urea from NH_4^+ and to conjugate and excrete bilirubin is decreased.

59–B. In gout, uric acid crystals precipitate in joints, causing severe pain.

60–C. When heart muscle is damaged, cellular enzymes leak into the blood. Creatine kinase (CK) is found mainly in muscle cells and to a lesser extent in the brain. The presence of the MB fraction of CK in blood is indicative of a heart attack.

61–A. Bilirubin is conjugated and excreted by the liver. If the liver is sick, bilirubin will accumulate in the blood and in tissues, producing jaundice.

62–D. The kidney excretes urea. If the kidney is diseased, urea will accumulate in the blood. Uric acid would also accumulate, but to a much lesser extent.

63–C. Pellagra (and the 4 Ds: diarrhea, dermatitis, dementia, death) can be caused by a deficiency of niacin or tryptophan.

64–D. A defect in the purine salvage enzyme HGPRT causes Lesch-Nyhan syndrome.

65–E. An inability to absorb certain essential amino acids from the gut causes Hartnup's disease.

66–B. In cystinuria, a defect in resorption results in the formation of cystine stones in the urine.

67–A. The loss of brain cells that produce dopamine results in Parkinson's disease.

8

Molecular Endocrinology

Overview

- Communication between cells is essential for human survival and is provided mainly by the nervous and endocrine systems.
- Endocrine glands produce hormones that travel through the blood to other tissues where they elicit a response (Table 8-1).
- The action of hormones at the molecular level involves receptors.
  - Polypeptide hormones and epinephrine react with receptors in the cell membrane, triggering an alteration in the structure or concentration of intracellular com-

Table 8-1. Abbreviations for Hormones and Related Compounds

ACTH	Adrenocorticotropic hormone
ABP	Androgen binding protein
ADH	Antidiuretic hormone (also known as VP)
ANP	Atrionatriuretic peptide (or atriopeptin)
CRH	Corticotropin releasing hormone
1,25-DHC	1,25-Dihydroxycholecalciferol
DHEA	Dehydroepiandrosterone
DHT	Dihydrotestosterone
E_2	Estradiol
FSH	Follicle stimulating hormone
GH	Growth hormone
GRH	Growth hormone releasing hormone (GHRH)
GnRH	Gonadotropin releasing hormone
hCG	Human chorionic gonadotropin
IGF	Insulin-like growth factor
LH	Luteinizing hormone
LPH	Lipotropin
MSH	Melanocyte stimulating hormone
POMC	Pro-opiomelanocortin
PRH	Prolactin releasing hormone
PRIH	Prolactin release inhibiting hormone (PIH)
PRL	Prolactin
PTH	Parathyroid hormone
T_3	Triiodothyronine
T_4	Thyroxine (tetraiodothyronine)
TRH	Thyrotropin releasing hormone
TSH	Thyroid stimulating hormone
VP	Vasopressin (also known as ADH)

pounds (usually second messengers) that allow the external signal from the hormone to produce its intracellular effects.

– Steroid hormones (as well as thyroid hormone, 1,25-dihydroxycholecalciferol, and retinoic acid) cross the cell membrane and bind to intracellular receptors. Ultimately, the hormone-receptor complex binds to DNA and activates or inactivates genes that produce proteins that have physiologic effects.

- Hormones often act as a chain of chemical messengers. For example, a hormone produced by the hypothalamus may stimulate the anterior pituitary to produce another hormone that subsequently causes an endocrine gland to produce yet another hormone that ultimately acts on its target cells.

I. Synthesis of Hormones

- An amino acid can be converted to a compound that serves as a hormone (e.g., epinephrine, thyroid hormone), or a series of amino acids may be joined by peptide bonds to produce a polypeptide hormone (e.g., insulin, prolactin).
- The steroid nucleus can be biochemically modified to produce a number of hormones (e.g., progesterone, cortisol).

A. Epinephrine

1. **Tyrosine**, produced by hydroxylation of the essential amino acid phenylalanine, is further hydroxylated to form **dihydroxyphenylalanine** (dopa), which is subsequently decarboxylated to form **dopamine.**

2. An additional hydroxylation reaction produces **norepinephrine,** which is methylated (mainly in the adrenal medulla) to produce **epinephrine.**

B. Thyroid Hormones (Figure 8-1)

1. The follicular cells of the thyroid gland produce the protein **thyroglobulin,** which is secreted into the colloid.

2. **Iodine,** concentrated in the follicular cells by a pump in the cell membrane, is oxidized by a peroxidase. Iodination of **tyrosine residues** in thyroglobulin produces monoiodotyrosine (MIT) and diiodotyrosine (DIT), which undergo **coupling reactions** to produce 3,5,3'-triiodothyronine (T_3) and 3,5,3',5'-tetraiodothyronine (T_4), which is also known as thyroxine.

3. Thyroid stimulating hormone (**TSH**) stimulates **pinocytosis** of thyroglobulin, and **lysosomal proteases** cleave peptide bonds, releasing free **T_3** and **T_4** from thyroglobulin. These hormones enter the blood.

C. Polypeptide hormones

1. Polypeptide hormones are **gene products.**

3,5,3',5'-Tetraiodothyronine (T_4)   **3,5,3'-Triiodothyronine (T_3)**

Figure 8-1. The thyroid hormones. T_4 = thyroxine.

2. mRNA is transcribed from the gene and translated on ribosomes attached to the rough endoplasmic reticulum (RER). A polypeptide **precursor** (or preprohormone) larger than the active hormone is usually formed.

3. Removal of the **signal peptide** in the RER produces the **prohormone**.

4. Modification of the prohormone occurs in the Golgi complex, and the **mature hormone** is secreted from the cell by the process of **exocytosis**.

D. **Steroid hormones**

– Steroid hormones are derived from **cholesterol** (Figure 8-2), which forms **pregnenolone** by cleavage of its side chain.

1. **Progesterone** is produced by oxidation of the A ring of **pregnenolone**.

2. **Testosterone** is produced from **progesterone** by removal of the side chain of the D ring. Testosterone is also produced from **pregnenolone** via dehydroepiandrosterone (DHEA).

3. **17β-Estradiol** (E$_2$) is produced from **testosterone** by aromatization of the A ring.

4. **Cortisol** and **aldosterone,** the adrenal steroids, are produced from **progesterone.**

5. **1,25-Dihydroxycholecalciferol** (1,25-DHC or calcitriol), the active form of vitamin D$_3$ (see Figure 4-10), can be produced by two hydroxylations of **dietary vitamin D$_3$** (cholecalciferol). The first hydroxylation occurs at position 25 (in the liver), and the second occurs at position 1 (in the kidney). In addition, 7-dehydrocholesterol, a precursor of cholesterol produced from acetyl CoA, can be converted by **ultraviolet light** in the **skin** to cholecalciferol and then hydroxylated to form 1,25-DHC.

II. General Mechanisms of Hormone Action

- Hormones interact with receptors that are located either inside the cell or within the cell membrane.
- Cells are exposed to many hormones. Whether a given hormone will elicit a response in a particular cell depends on the complement of receptors that the cell contains.
- Insulin, a polypeptide hormone, binds to the insulin receptor on the cell membrane, causing the receptor to phosphorylate itself on tyrosine residues and then to phosphorylate intracellular proteins, initiating a series of events that result in cellular responses.
- In general, other polypeptide hormones and epinephrine act through second messengers. The hormone (the first messenger) reacts with receptors in the cell membrane, altering the intracellular concentration of compounds known as second messengers (e.g., cyclic AMP [cAMP], cyclic GMP [cGMP], inositol trisphosphate [IP$_3$], diacylglycerol [DAG], and Ca^{2+}). These second messengers permit an external signal from the hormone to produce intracellular effects.
- The steroid and thyroid hormones, 1,25-DHC, and retinoic acid cross the cell membrane and bind to intracellular receptors, forming complexes that activate or inactivate genes.

A. **Hormones that bind to cell membrane receptors**

1. **Hormones that activate tyrosine kinases** (Figure 8-3)

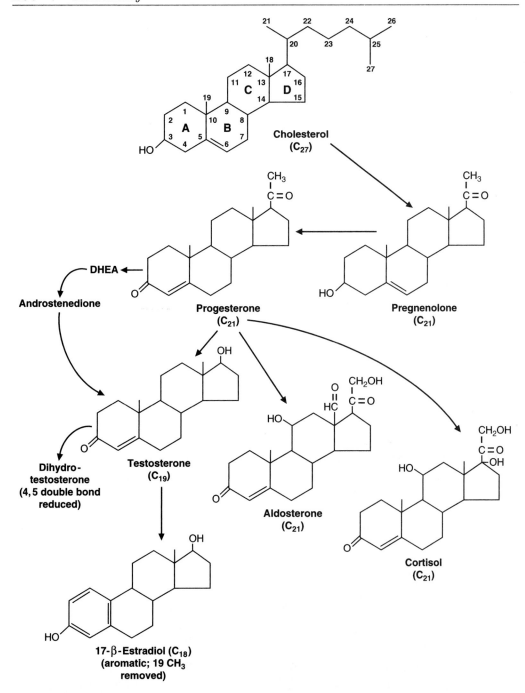

Figure 8-2. Synthesis of the steroid hormones. The rings of the precursor, cholesterol, are *lettered.* Dihydrotestosterone is produced from testosterone by reduction of the C-C double bond in ring A. *DHEA* = dehydroepiandrosterone.

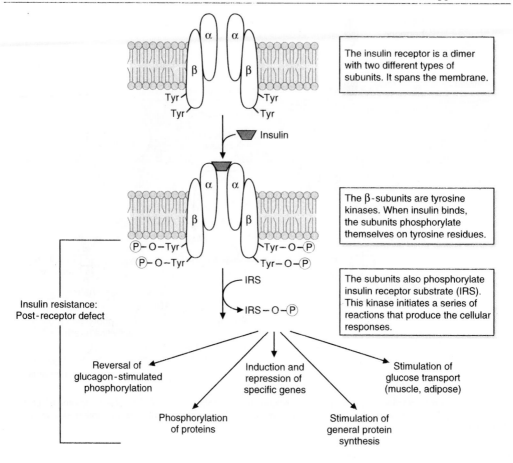

The insulin receptor is a dimer with two different types of subunits. It spans the membrane.

The β-subunits are tyrosine kinases. When insulin binds, the subunits phosphorylate themselves on tyrosine residues.

The subunits also phosphorylate insulin receptor substrate (IRS). This kinase initiates a series of reactions that produce the cellular responses.

Insulin resistance: Post-receptor defect

Reversal of glucagon-stimulated phosphorylation

Induction and repression of specific genes

Stimulation of glucose transport (muscle, adipose)

Phosphorylation of proteins

Stimulation of general protein synthesis

Figure 8-3. The actions of insulin. Insulin resistance or Type 2 diabetes mellitus is caused by a postreceptor defect. Ⓟ = phosphate.

a. Insulin binds to a receptor on the cell surface, causing the β subunits of the receptor (that extend through the membrane) to **phosphorylate** themselves on **tyrosine residue**s located on the inner surface.

b. The phosphorylated receptor acts as a **kinase**, phosphorylating an intracellular protein known as **insulin receptor substrate** (IRS).

c. Phosphorylated IRS then activates other signal transduction proteins, **initiating a sequence of events** that ultimately produce the intracellular effects of insulin.

2. **Hormones that act through cyclic nucleotides** (Figure 8-4)

a. Epinephrine and certain polypeptide hormones, such as glucagon, bind to **receptors on the external surface** of the cell membrane. These hormone-receptor complexes interact with **G proteins** (so-called because they bind guanine nucleotides) (Figure 8-5), and activate **adenylate cyclase,** which **converts ATP to cAMP.** cAMP activates **protein kinase A**, which subsequently **phosphorylates** certain intracellular proteins, altering their activity.

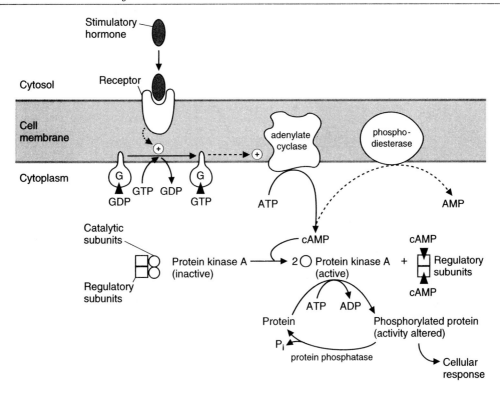

Figure 8-4. The production and action of cyclic adenosine monophosphate (cAMP). G = G proteins (G proteins function when GTP is bound); 0 = free catalytic subunits; □ = regulatory subunits of protein kinase A; ⊕ = stimulates.

– The activity of these proteins can be returned to their previous state by **phosphatases** that **dephosphorylate** these proteins. The activity of the phosphatases is controlled by hormones such as insulin, which opposes the action of glucagon (see Chapter 5 IV F).

b. Some of these hormone-receptor complexes **lower cAMP** levels, either by inhibiting adenylate cyclase or by activating the **phosphodiesterase** that cleaves cAMP to AMP.

c. At least one hormone, **atrionatriuretic peptide (ANP),** activates guanylate cyclase, which produces cGMP.

– **cGMP** activates **protein kinase G.**
– ANP is released from atrial cells of the heart and produces effects that include increased urine volume, excretion of sodium ions, and vasodilation.

3. Hormones that act through calcium and the phosphatidylinositol bisphosphate (PIP$_2$) system (Figure 8-6)

– Some hormones (e.g., thyrotropin releasing hormone [TRH] and oxytocin) interact with G proteins to alter the amount and distribution of calcium ions within the cell and activate **protein kinase C.**

a. Hormone-G protein complexes **open calcium channels** within the cell membrane, allowing extracellular calcium to move into the cell.

A. Before hormone binds

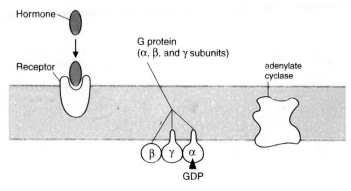

B. After hormone binds

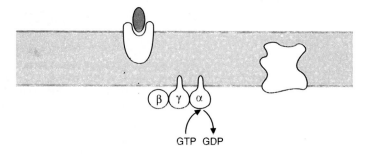

C. G proteins dissociate

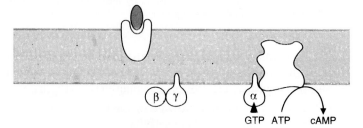

D. GTPase cleaves GTP to GDP and P$_i$

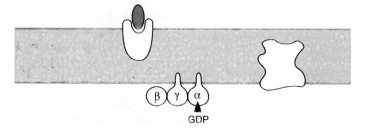

Figure 8-5. The G proteins. *A,* Before the hormone binds. *B,* After the hormone binds. GDP on the α-subunit of the G proteins is exchanged for GTP. *C,* G protein subunits dissociate. The α-subunit with GTP activates adenylate cyclase, which converts ATP to cAMP. *D,* GTPase cleaves GTP to GDP and P$_i$. α, β, and γ subunits of the G proteins reassociate. Adenylate cyclase is no longer active.

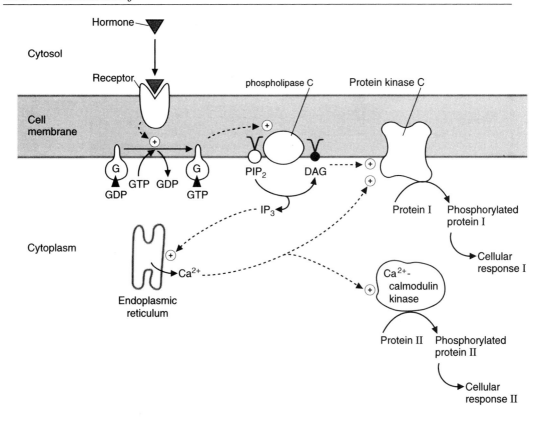

Figure 8-6. Signal transduction involving Ca^{2+} and the phosphatidylinositol bisphosphate (PIP_2) system. *DAG =* diacylglycerol; IP_3 = inositol 1,4,5-trisphosphate; *G* = G proteins; ⊕ = stimulates.

    b. Some complexes **activate phospholipase C,** which cleaves PIP_2 in the cell membrane to produce two messengers, diacylglycerol (DAG) and phosphatidyl inositol bisphosphate (IP_3) (Figure 8-7).

        (1) DAG activates protein kinase C, which phosphorylates certain proteins, altering their activity.

        (2) IP_3 causes Ca^{2+} to be released from intracellular stores, such as those in the endoplasmic reticulum.

          – Ca^{2+}, either directly or complexed with calmodulin, interacts with proteins, altering their activity.

B. Hormones that bind to intracellular receptors and activate genes (Figure 8-8)

    1. Steroid and **thyroid** hormones, **1,25-DHC,** and **retinoic acid** cross the cell membrane and bind to **intracellular receptors.**

    2. These **receptors** contain domains that bind the hormone and domains that bind to **regulatory elements** [i.e., hormone response elements (HRE)] **on DNA** that stimulate or inhibit the synthesis of mRNA (see Figure 8-8). Translation of this mRNA produces **proteins** that are responsible for the physiologic effects of the hormone.

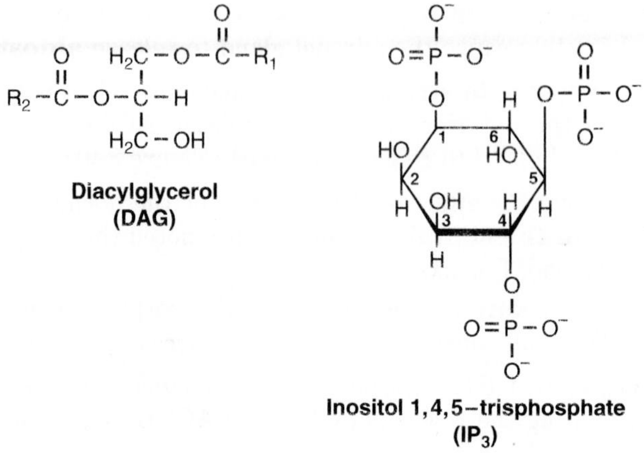

Diacylglycerol (DAG)

Inositol 1,4,5–trisphosphate (IP₃)

Figure 8-7. Structures of diacylglycerol and inositol trisphosphate.

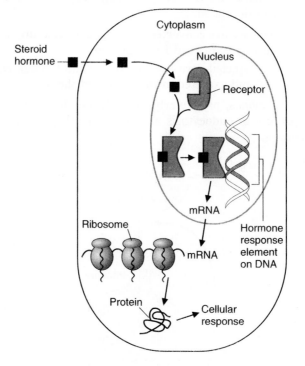

Figure 8-8. The mechanism of action of hormones of the steroid-thyroid family. 1,25-DHC (the active form of vitamin D₃) and retinoic acid (produced from vitamin A) are members of this family of hormones.

III. Regulation of Hormone Levels

- In order to maintain homeostasis or to repeat physiologic processes such as the menstrual cycle, hormone levels must be regulated.

A. Regulation of hormone synthesis and secretion

1. The **release of hormones** is stimulated either by changes in the environment or physiologic state or by a stimulatory hormone from another tissue that acts on the cells that release the hormone. For example:

    a. A **decrease** in **blood pressure** initiates a sequence of events that ultimately cause the adrenal gland to release **aldosterone.**

    b. In response to **stress**, the hypothalamus releases **CRH**, which stimulates the anterior pituitary to release **ACTH**. ACTH stimulates the adrenal gland to release **cortisol** (Figure 8-9).

  2. The physiologic effect of the hormone or the hormone itself causes a **decrease in the signal** that initially promoted the synthesis and release of the hormone. For example:

    a. Aldosterone causes an increased resorption from the kidney tubule of Na^+, and consequently of water, increasing blood pressure.

    b. Cortisol feeds back on the hypothalamus and the anterior pituitary, inhibiting the release of CRH and ACTH (see Figure 8-9).

B. Hormone inactivation

  1. After hormones exert their physiologic effects, they are inactivated and excreted or degraded.

  2. Some hormones are converted to compounds that are no longer active and may be readily **excreted** from the body.

    – Cortisol, a steroid hormone, is reduced and conjugated with glucuronide or sulfate and excreted in the urine and the feces.

  3. Some hormones, particularly the polypeptides, are taken up by cells by the process of endocytosis and subsequently **degraded by lysosomal enzymes.**

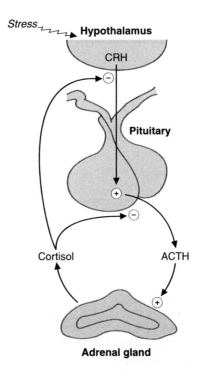

Figure 8-9. Hormone feedback regulation. *ACTH* = adrenocorticotropic hormone; *CRH* = corticotropin releasing hormone; ⊕ = activates; ⊖ = inhibits.

– The **receptor,** which is internalized along with the hormone, can either be **degraded** by lysosomal proteases, or it can be **recycled** to the cell membrane.

IV. Actions of Specific Hormones

- Tissues that produce hormones include the hypothalamus, anterior and posterior pituitary, adrenal cortex and medulla, gonads, thyroid and para- thyroid glands, heart, brain, cells of the gastrointestinal tract, and the pan- creas.

A. Hypothalamic hormones (Figure 8-10)

– The hypothalamus produces **vasopressin (VP)** and **oxytocin (OT),** and it produces **other hormones** (mainly peptides and polypeptides) that regulate the synthesis and release of hormones from the anterior pituitary.

B. Hormones of the posterior pituitary (see Figure 8-10)

– **VP** (also called antidiuretic hormone [ADH]) and **oxytocin** are synthesized in the hypothalamus and travel through nerve axons to the posterior pitu- itary where they are stored, each complexed with a neurophysin. They are released into the blood in response to the appropriate stimulation.

1. **VP,** in response to decreased blood volume or increased Na^+ concentration, **stimulates** the **resorption of water** by kidney tubules.

2. **Oxytocin promotes** the **ejection of milk** from the mammary gland in response to suckling and the **contraction of the uterus** during childbirth.

C. Hormones of the anterior pituitary (see Figure 8-10)

1. **Prolactin (PRL),** released in response to PRH from the hypothalamus caused by suckling of an infant, stimulates the **synthesis of milk proteins** during lactation. Dopamine from the hypothalamus inhibits PRL release.

2. **Growth hormone (GH)** stimulates the **release of insulin-like growth factors** (IGFs) and **antagonizes** the **effects of insulin on carbohy- drate and fat metabolism.** The release of GH is stimulated by GHRH and inhibited by somatostatin from the hypothalamus.

3. **TSH,** produced in response to TRH from the hypothalamus, **stimulates** the release of T_3 and T_4 from the thyroid gland.

4. Luteinizing hormone (**LH**) and follicle stimulating hormone (**FSH**) **stimu- late** the **gonads** to release hormones that are involved in reproduction. The release of LH and FSH is stimulated by GnRH and inhibited by GnRIH from the hypothalamus.

5. The protein product of the **proopiomelanocortin (POMC)** gene, pro- duced in response to CRH from the hypothalamus, is cleaved to generate a number of polypeptides.

   a. **Adrenocorticotropic hormone (ACTH)** stimulates the production of cortisol and has a permissive effect on the production of aldosterone by the adrenal cortex.

   b. **Lipotropin (LPH)** may be cleaved to form melanocyte stimulating hormone and endorphins.

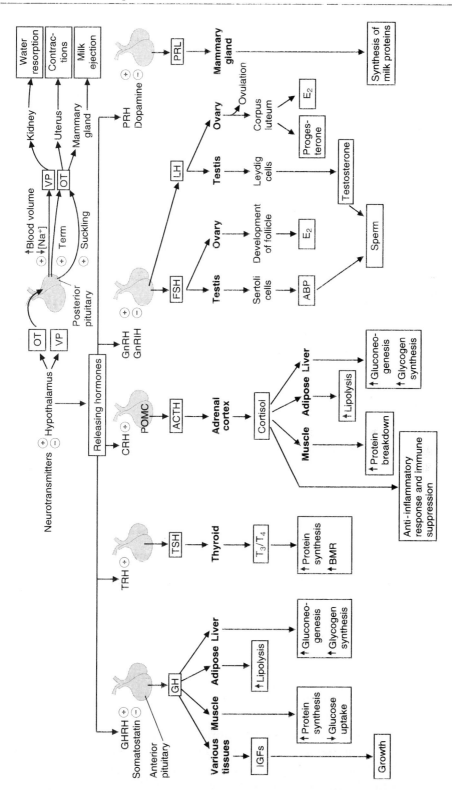

Figure 8-10. The actions of hypothalamic and pituitary hormones on their target cells. See Table 8-1 for abbreviations.

    c. Melanocyte stimulating hormone (MSH), which is part of ACTH and LPH, stimulates the production of the pigment melanin by the melanocytes in the skin.

    d. Endorphins produce analgesic effects.

D. Thyroid hormone

    1. T_3 is much more active metabolically than T_4.

        a. Although the thyroid secretes some T_3, the majority is produced by **deiodination of T_4,** a process that occurs in nonthyroidal tissue.

        b. During starvation, T_4 is converted to reverse T_3 (rT_3), which is not active.

    2. Thyroid hormone binds to nuclear receptors and **regulates the expression of many genes.**

    3. Thyroid hormone is necessary for **growth, development,** and **maintenance** of almost all tissues of the body. It **stimulates** oxidative metabolism and causes the **basal metabolic rate** (BMR) to increase.

E. Hormones that stimulate growth

    – **Insulin** and **GH** stimulate growth and promote protein synthesis.

    – However, **GH antagonizes** many of the metabolic actions of **insulin,** stimulating gluconeogenesis and promoting lipolysis. The result is that alternative fuels are made available so that muscle protein (i.e., growth) can be preserved.

F. Hormones that mediate the response to stress

    – **Glucocorticoids** (particularly cortisol) and **epinephrine** act in concert to supply fuels to the blood so that energy can be produced to combat stressful situations.

    1. Glucocorticoids (Figure 8-11)

        – In response to ACTH, the adrenal cortex produces glucocorticoids. **Cortisol** is the major glucocorticoid in humans.

        a. Glucocorticoids have **anti-inflammatory effects.**

            – They induce the synthesis of **lipocortin,** a protein that inhibits phospholipase A_2, the rate-limiting enzyme in prostaglandin, thromboxane, and leukotriene synthesis (see Figure 6-18).

        b. Glucocorticoids **suppress the immune response** by causing the lysis of lymphocytes.

        c. Glucocorticoids **influence metabolism** by causing the movement of fuels from peripheral tissues to the liver, where gluconeogenesis and glycogen synthesis are stimulated (see Figures 8-10 and 8-11).

            (1) Amino acids are released from muscle protein.

            (2) Lipolysis occurs in adipose tissue.

            (3) In addition to providing amino acids and glycerol as carbon sources, **glucocorticoids promote gluconeogenesis** by **inducing** synthesis of the enzyme phosphoenolpyruvate carboxykinase (**PEPCK**).

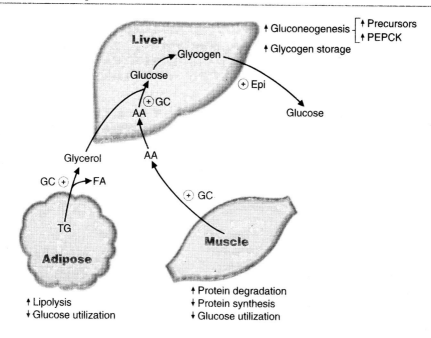

Figure 8-11. The effects of glucocorticoids (GC) on fuel metabolism. Chronic stress causes GC to stimulate the breakdown of fuels in peripheral tissues, and gluconeogenic precursors are converted to glycogen in the liver. Acute stress causes the release of epinephrine (Epi), which stimulates the breakdown of liver glycogen to produce blood glucose as fuel for "fight or flight." Epinephrine also stimulates glycogen breakdown in muscle to produce ATP for muscle contraction, and it stimulates lipolysis in adipose tissue and gluconeogenesis in the liver. PEPCK = phosphoenolpyruvate carboxykinase.

(4) **Glucose,** produced by gluconeogenesis promoted by glucocorticoids, is **stored as glycogen** in the liver.

(5) Glucocorticoids prepare the body during stressful conditions so that fuel stores are ready for the "alarm" reaction mediated by epinephrine.

2. **Epinephrine**

– Epinephrine increases blood glucose by **stimulating liver glycogenolysis** (see Figure 8-11). It also **stimulates lipolysis** in adipose tissue and **glycogen degradation in muscle.** Overall, it makes fuels available for "fight or flight."

G. **Hormones that regulate salt and water balance**

– In addition to **VP** (see IV B) and **ANP** (see II A 2 c), **aldosterone** is involved in regulating salt and water balance.

1. **Synthesis of aldosterone**

a. **Renin** (produced by the juxtaglomerular cells of the kidney in response to decreased blood pressure, blood volume, or sodium ion concentration) **cleaves angiotensinogen to angiotensin I.**

b. **Angiotensin I** is **cleaved** to **angiotensin II** by angiotensin converting enzyme (**ACE**), which is made in the lung.

– Further cleavage to angiotensin III occurs.

    c. Angiotensin II acts directly on vascular smooth muscle cells, causing **vasoconstriction,** which increases blood pressure.

    d. Angiotensin II and III (and also decreased serum [Na^+] and increased serum [K^+]) **stimulate** the glomerulosa cells of the adrenal cortex to produce and secrete **aldosterone.**

        – ACTH has a permissive effect (i.e., it maintains cells so that they can respond to angiotensin II).

2. Action of aldosterone

    a. Aldosterone causes the production of proteins in cells of the distal tubule and the collecting ducts of the kidney.

        (1) A **permease** is **produced** that allows Na^+ to enter cells from the lumen.

        (2) Citrate synthase is **induced,** which increases the capacity of the tricarboxylic acid (TCA) cycle for the generation of ATP.

        (3) Energy is thus provided to drive the **Na^+ -K^+ ATPase,** which may also be induced.

    b. Overall, K^+ and H^+ are lost; Na^+ is retained; water is resorbed; and blood volume and pressure are increased.

H. Hormones that control reproduction (see Figure 8-10)

    – The hypothalamus produces gonadotropin releasing hormone (**GnRH**), which causes the anterior pituitary to release **FSH** and **LH,** which act on both the **ovary** and the **testis.**

1. The action of FSH and LH on the ovary

    a. The menstrual cycle

        (1) Initially, **FSH acts on** the **follicles** to promote maturation of the ovum and to stimulate estradiol (E_2) production and secretion.

        (2) Estradiol acts on the uterine **endometrium,** causing it to thicken and vascularize in preparation for implantation of a fertilized egg.

        (3) A **surge of LH** at the midpoint of the menstrual cycle **stimulates** the ripe **follicle to ovulate,** leaving the residual follicle, which forms the **corpus luteum** and **secretes** both **progesterone and estradiol.**

        (4) Progesterone causes the endometrium to continue to thicken and vascularize and increase its secretory capacity.

    b. Events in the absence of fertilization

        (1) The **corpus luteum regresses** due to declining LH levels. It produces diminishing amounts of progesterone and estradiol.

        (2) Because of the low steroid hormone levels, the cells die and the degenerating **endometrium is sloughed** into the uterine cavity and excreted (**menstruation**).

        (3) The low levels of estradiol and progesterone cause feedback inhibition to be relieved, and the hypothalamus releases GnRH, initiating a new menstrual cycle.

c. **Events following fertilization**

(1) The **corpus luteum** is **maintained** initially by **human chorionic gonadotropin (hCG)** produced by the cells of the developing embryo (trophoblast).

(2) Subsequently, the **placenta produces hCG and progesterone.**

(3) After the corpus luteum dies, the **placenta** continues to produce large amounts of **progesterone.**

(4) Near **term,** hCG and, subsequently, **progesterone levels fall.**
– Fetal cortisol may cause the decline in progesterone.

(5) **Prostaglandin $F_{2\alpha}$ ($PGF_{2\alpha}$)** and **oxytocin** (released from both maternal and fetal pituitaries) stimulate uterine contractions, and the infant is delivered.

2. **The action of FSH and LH on the testis**

a. **LH stimulates Leydig cells** to produce and secrete testosterone.

b. **FSH** acts on **Sertoli cells** of the seminiferous tubule to promote the synthesis of androgen binding protein **(ABP).**

c. **ABP binds testosterone** and transports it to the site of spermatogenesis, where **testosterone is reduced** to the more potent androgen, dihydrotestosterone **(DHT).**

d. **Testosterone** plays a role in **spermatogenesis** in the adult male.

(1) Testosterone is responsible for **masculinization** during early development.

(2) At puberty, testosterone promotes **sexual maturation** of the male.

I. **Hormones that promote lactation** (see Figure 8-10)
– Many hormones are necessary for development of the mammary glands during adolescence.

1. **Preparation of the mammary gland for lactation**

a. During pregnancy, **prolactin, glucocorticoids, and insulin** are the major hormones responsible for differentiation of mammary alveolar cells into secretory cells capable of producing milk.

b. **PRL stimulates** the **synthesis of the milk proteins,** particularly casein and α-lactalbumin.

(1) **α-Lactalbumin,** the major protein in human milk, serves as a **nutrient.**

(2) α-Lactalbumin binds to galactosyl transferase, decreasing its K_m for glucose and, thus, **stimulating synthesis** of the milk sugar **lactose** (see Chapter 5 VII B 2 b).

c. **Progesterone inhibits milk protein production** and secretion during pregnancy.

d. At term, when progesterone levels fall, the inhibition of milk protein synthesis is relieved.

2. **Regulation of milk secretion during lactation**

   a. **PRL causes milk proteins to be produced** and secreted into the alveolar lumen.

   b. **Oxytocin causes contraction** of the myoepithelial cells surrounding the alveolar cells and the lumen, and **milk is ejected** through the nipple.

   c. The **secretion** of both PRL and oxytocin by the pituitary is stimulated by **suckling** of the infant and by other factors.

J. **Hormones involved in growth and differentiation**

   1. **Retinoids are produced** in the body from dietary **vitamin A** (see Figure 4-10). The major dietary source, β-carotene, is cleaved to 2 molecules of retinal.

   2. **Retinal** (an aldehyde) and **retinol** (an alcohol) are interconverted by oxidation and reduction reactions. **Retinoic acid** is produced by oxidation of retinal and cannot be reduced.

   3. **Retinol**, the **transport** form, is stored as retinyl esters.

   4. **Retinal** is a functional component of the reactions of the **visual cycle.**

   5. **Retinoic acid** is involved in **growth** and also in **differentiation** and **maintenance** of **epithelial tissue**. The functions of **retinoic acid** result from its ability to **activate genes** (i.e., it acts like a steroid hormone).

K. **Hormones that regulate Ca^{2+} metabolism**

   – **Calcium** has many important functions. It is involved in blood coagulation, activation of muscle phosphorylase, and secretory processes. It combines with phosphate to form the hydroxyapatite of bone. Parathyroid hormone **(PTH)**, **1,25-DHC**, and **calcitonin** are the major regulators of Ca^{2+} metabolism.

   1. **Parathyroid hormone (PTH),** produced in response to low calcium levels, acts to **increase Ca^{2+}** levels in the extracellular fluid.

      a. PTH promotes Ca^{2+} and phosphate mobilization from **bone**.

      b. PTH acts on **renal tubules** to resorb Ca^{2+} and excrete phosphate.

      c. PTH stimulates the **hydroxylation of 25-hydroxycholecalciferol** to form 1,25-DHC, the active hormone.

   2. **1,25-Dihydroxycholecalciferol** stimulates the synthesis of a protein involved in **Ca^{2+} absorption** by **intestinal** epithelial cells. 1,25-DHC acts synergistically with PTH in **bone resorption** and promotes resorption of Ca^{2+} by **renal tubular cells**.

   3. **Calcitonin lowers Ca^{2+}** levels by inhibiting its release from bone and stimulating its excretion in the urine.

L. **Hormones that regulate the utilization of nutrients**

   1. **Gut hormones**

      a. **Gastrin** from the gastric antrum and the duodenum stimulates gastric acid and pepsin secretion.

    b. Cholecystokinin (CCK) from the duodenum and jejunum stimulates contraction of the gallbladder and the secretion of pancreatic enzymes.

    c. Secretin from the duodenum and jejunum stimulates the secretion of bicarbonate by the pancreas.

    d. Gastric inhibitory polypeptide (GIP) from the small bowel enhances insulin release and inhibits secretion of gastric acid.

    e. Vasoactive intestinal polypeptide (VIP) from the pancreas relaxes smooth muscles and stimulates bicarbonate secretion by the pancreas

2. Insulin and glucagon

    – The two major hormones that **regulate fuel metabolism,** insulin and glucagon, are produced by the pancreas. Their actions (discussed extensively in Chapters 5, 6, and 7) are summarized in Table 8-2.

V. Clinical Correlations

A. Hypothyroidism

In patients with hypothyroidism, the stimulatory effect of thyroid hormone on the oxidation of fuels is diminished. As a consequence, the generation of ATP is reduced, causing a sense of **weakness, fatigue,** and **hypokinesis.** The **reduced basal metabolic rate (BMR)** is associated with diminished heat production, causing **cold intolerance** and **decreased sweating.** With less demand for the delivery of fuels and oxygen to peripheral tissues, the circulation is slowed, causing a reduction in heart rate and, when far advanced, a reduction in blood pressure. In hypothyroidism, **TSH levels are elevated** and an enlarged thyroid (**goiter**) can occur.

B. Hyperthyroidism

When the thyroid gland secretes excessive quantities of thyroid hormone, the rate of oxidation of fuels by muscle and other tissues is increased (i.e., the **BMR** is **increased**). With enhanced oxidative metabolism, heat production is increased, leading to a sense of **heat intolerance** and the need to dissipate heat through **increased sweating.** Thyroid hormone excess raises the tone of the sympathetic (adrenergic) nervous system, **raising** the **heart rate** and **systolic blood pressure.** In addition, **tremulousness,** a sense of **restless-**

Table 8-2 Actions of Insulin and Glucagon

Insulin	Glucagon
Elevated in the fed state	Elevated during fasting
Promotes the storage of fuels: glycogen and triacylglycerol	Increases the availability of fuels (glucose and fatty acids) in the blood
Stimulates:	*Stimulates:*
Glycogen synthesis in liver and muscle	Glycogen degradation in liver, but *not* in muscle
Triacylglycerol synthesis in liver and conversion to very low density lipoprotein (VLDL)	Gluconeogenesis
Triacylglycerol storage in adipose tissue	Lipolysis (breakdown of triacylglycerols) in adipose tissue
Glucose transport into muscle and adipose cells	
Protein synthesis and growth	

ness, and **insomnia** often occur. Since stored fuels in muscle and fat tissue are being utilized at an excessive rate, **weight loss** occurs despite increased caloric intake. In hyperthyroidism, **TSH levels are low** and an enlarged thyroid (**goiter**) can occur.

C. Growth hormone excess

Excessive secretion of growth hormone (GH) occurs as a result of a **benign tumor** of the **anterior pituitary gland.** If the hypersecretion begins prior to closure of the growth centers in the long bones, excessive height (**gigantism**) occurs. If hypersecretion begins after the growth centers have closed, the bones grow in bulk and width, leading to a condition called **acromegaly.** Soft tissue overgrowth occurs as well, leading to **organomegaly, thickness of the skin,** and **coarseness of the facial features.**

Chronic GH excess may lead to **glucose intolerance** and **diabetes mellitus** because GH stimulates gluconeogenesis and slows glucose uptake by muscle. If the pituitary tumor grows beyond the confines of the sella turcica, the tumor may encroach on the optic nerves, causing **visual difficulties,** or may lead to other cranial nerve dysfunction, progressive headaches, and eventually, symptoms of increased intracranial pressure.

D. Prolactin excess

The most common secretory neoplasm of the anterior pituitary gland is a **prolactin-secreting adenoma** (prolactinoma). An early symptom of prolactin excess is a **milky discharge from the breasts** (galactorrhea). Because hyperprolactinemia suppresses the secretion of gonadotropic hormones (e.g., LH, FSH), **menstrual irregularity, amenorrhea,** and **infertility** can occur in women. In men, gonadotropic hormone dysfunction can lead to reduced libido, sexual impotence, and infertility.

E. Hypoglycemia

Whenever **insulin levels** in the blood are chronically **elevated,** which occurs, for example, in patients with insulin-secreting pancreatic tumors or in patients inadvertently given excessive quantities of exogenous insulin, the transport of glucose from the blood into tissues such as skeletal muscle and fat cells is enhanced, leading to hypoglycemia. The clinical manifestations of a **reduction in blood glucose levels** are those related to stimulation of the sympathetic nervous system by **hypoglycemia** (e.g., **sweating, palpitations** of the heart, **tremulousness**) and those due to inadequate delivery of glucose to the brain, also known as **neuroglycopenic sequelae** (e.g., irritability, slurring of speech, confusion, drowsiness, and eventually, coma).

F. Hyperparathyroidism

When the secretion of parathyroid hormone is excessive, the physiologic effects of this peptide on the gut, the skeleton, and the kidney tubules are enhanced. The percentage of dietary calcium absorbed into the circulation is increased; calcium ions are released from bone and enter the blood more rapidly; and the renal tubules reabsorb more calcium than usual from the luminal urine, all leading to **hypercalcemia.** Chronic hypercalcemia is associated with vague generalized musculoskeletal pain, fatigue, and eventually, slowed mentation.

The osteolytic effect of excessive parathyroid hormone action may lead to demineralization of the skeleton (**osteoporosis**) and fracture. Chronic renal

filtration of blood rich in calcium leads to saturation of the tubular fluid with calcium salts; as a consequence, **renal calculi** (kidney stones) can occur.

G. Menopause

Clinically, menopause is defined as the **last physiologic menstrual cycle** in which pituitary gonadotropins (e.g., LH, FSH) have stimulated the maturation of a primordial follicle and caused ovulation. The transition from full reproductive potential to final ovarian failure is known as the **climacteric,** a period that begins about age 40. As estradiol levels in the blood gradually fall below normal, the early symptoms of the climacteric occur, including anxiety, mood swings, irritability, and in some instances, depression. Vasomotor instability with early morning paresthesias in the extremities and ascending bouts of sweating and flushing (**"hot flashes"**) also occur.

Late symptoms of the climacteric are those related to chronic exposure of the urogenital tract to less than normal physiologic levels of estradiol. These include vaginal dryness and laxity of the supportive tissues of the urogenital tract, causing a predisposition to **urinary tract infections** and **painful intercourse.**

H. Glucocorticoid excess

Hypercortisolemia has an adverse effect on virtually every tissue of the body. Central nervous system effects range from **hyperirritability** to **depression.** The catabolic effect on protein-containing tissues leads to a reduction in the ground substance of bone and eventually to **osteoporosis,** loss of muscle protein causing **weakness**, and thinning and tearing of dermal and epidermal structures, which is manifest as reddish stripes, or **striae**, over the lower abdomen, the lateral thorax, and other areas where skin tension is increased. Similar catabolic effects on the elastin of vessel walls leads to vascular fragility with **easy bruising** and hemorrhaging of the skin. A suppressive effect on immunocompetence may increase the likelihood of infection.

The diabetogenic actions of cortisol may lead to **glucose intolerance** or overt **diabetes mellitus.** A peculiar tendency for the disposition of fat in the face (**moon facies**), posterior neck (**buffalo hump**), thorax, and abdomen, while sparing the distal extremities, causes a distinct "**central obesity.**"

This constellation of clinical signs and symptoms resulting from chronic hypercortisolemia is referred to as **Cushing's syndrome** if the condition is caused by excessive production of **cortisol** by an **adrenal tumor** or by intake of **exogenous glucocorticoids. Cushing's disease** refers to hypercortisolemia caused by excessive secretion of **ACTH** by a **pituitary tumor**.

I. Mineralocorticoid deficiency

A deficiency of adrenocortical secretion of aldosterone is usually accompanied by a reduction in the secretion of other adrenal steroid hormones as well. The loss of adrenocortical steroids is known as **Addison's disease.**

The mineralocorticoid deficiency leads to a net loss of sodium ions and water into the urine with a reciprocal retention of potassium ions (**hyperkalemia**) and hydrogen ions (**mild metabolic acidosis**). The subsequent contraction of the effective plasma volume may lead to a **reduction in blood pressure**. If volume loss is profound, perfusion of vital tissues such as the brain could lead to lightheadedness and possible loss of consciousness.

Review Test

Directions: Each of the numbered items or incomplete statements in this section is followed by answers or by completions of the statement. Select the **one** lettered answer or completion that is **best** in each case.

1. A key intermediate for the synthesis of both estradiol and cortisol from cholesterol is

(A) 7-hydroxycholesterol
(B) pregnenolone
(C) aldosterone
(D) retinoic acid

2. Which of the following is true of epinephrine?

(A) It acts only through the phosphatidylinositol bisphosphate system
(B) It is synthesized from tyrosine
(C) It causes the level of cAMP in liver cells to decrease
(D) It functions like a steroid hormone

3. Which of the following is true of testosterone?

(A) It is converted to a more active androgen in its target cells
(B) It acts by binding to receptors on the cell surface
(C) It is produced from estradiol (E_2)
(D) It stimulates the synthesis of gonadotropin releasing hormone (GnRH) by the hypothalamus

4. In the synthesis of 1,25-DHC from 7-dehydrocholesterol

(A) the steroid ring structure remains intact
(B) cholesterol is an intermediate
(C) ultraviolet light is required
(D) three hydroxylations occur

5. Which of the following acts to increase the release of Ca^{2+} from the endoplasmic reticulum?

(A) Diacylglycerol (DAG)
(B) Inositol triphosphate (IP_3)
(C) Parathyroid hormone(PTH)
(D) 1,25-Dihydroxycholecalciferol (1,25-DHC)

6. A dietary deficiency of iodine would

(A) directly affect the synthesis of thyroglobulin on ribosomes
(B) result in increased secretion of thyroid stimulating hormone (TSH)
(C) result in decreased production of thyrotropin releasing hormone (TRH)
(D) result in increased heat production

7. A patient with central obesity, thin limbs, and purple striae on the abdomen complained of muscle weakness, depression, and blurred vision. The patient's blood glucose was 280 mg/dL (reference range = 80–100 mg/dL). No ketone bodies were present in the urine. Plasma cortisol levels were 56 μg/mL (reference range = 3–31 μg/mL), and plasma ACTH levels were 106 pg/mL (reference range = 0–100 pg/mL). A low dose (1 mg) of dexamethasone (a synthetic glucocorticoid) was administered in the evening. This dose failed to suppress the plasma cortisol level by the next morning. After a high-dose (8 mg) dexamethasone suppression test, the plasma cortisol level was 21 μg/mL. Based on this information, if the patient's problem is due to a single cause, the most likely diagnosis is

(A) Type 2 diabetes mellitus
(B) Type 1 diabetes mellitus
(C) a secretory tumor of the anterior pituitary
(D) a secretory tumor of the posterior pituitary
(E) a secretory tumor of the adrenal cortex

8. GnRH stimulates the release of

(A) GH
(B) T_3 and T_4
(C) PRL
(D) IGF
(E) LH and FSH

Questions 9–11

A patient complains of nervousness, palpitations, sweating, and weight loss without loss of appetite and has a goiter. Suspecting a defect in thyroid function, the physician orders a total serum T_4. The test is performed by radioimmunoassay. The standard curve for the assay, which measures T_4 in 0.1 mL of serum, is shown below. Normal levels of T_4 = 4 - 10 μg/dL. In an assay of 0.1 mL of the patient's serum, 15% of the radioactive T_4 was bound to the antibody.

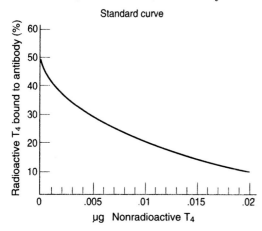

9. According to the radioimmunoassay, the approximate blood levels of T_4 are

(A) 0.015 μg/dL
(B) 0.15 μg/dL
(C) 15 μg/dL
(D) 20 μg/dL
(E) 30 μg/dL

10. The patient is

(A) hypothyroid
(B) normal
(C) hyperthyroid

11. TSH levels in the patient's blood were also measured by radioimmunoassay. If pituitary function is normal, the patient's TSH levels will most likely be

(A) higher than normal
(B) normal
(C) lower than normal

12. A 24-year-old accountant complains of a white discharge from his breasts. He most likely has

(A) a tumor of the posterior pituitary that could be surgically removed.
(B) excessive production of oxytocin in the hypothalamus.
(C) deficient testosterone receptors in the mammary glands.
(D) a prolactinoma that would decrease its secretory activity in response to bromocriptine (an analog of dopamine).

13. A female patient with thinning scalp hair, excessive facial hair, and high ACTH and low cortisol levels in the blood would most likely have

(A) a tumor of the anterior pituitary that produces abnormally large amounts of proopiomelanocortin (POMC).
(B) a tumor of the adrenal medulla that secretes abnormally large amounts of its normal hormone product.
(C) a genetic deficiency of an enzyme in the pathway for cortisol synthesis.
(D) a mutation in the gene for corticotropin releasing hormone that decreases production of this polypeptide.

14. Following an automobile accident, a 14-year-old girl developed diabetes insipidus (excessive loss of water in the urine), amenorrhea (lack of menses), and cold intolerance, and her growth rate slowed markedly. Her symptoms

(A) are all related to damage to her kidneys and ovaries caused by the accident.
(B) are all related to damage to her pituitary gland
(C) could be relieved by treatment with oral doses of anterior and posterior pituitary hormones.
(D) would require long-term treatment with estrogen, thyroxine, and glucocorticoid tablets and also restriction of water intake.

Directions: Each group of items in this section consists of lettered options followed by a set of numbered items. For each item, select the **one** lettered option that is most closely associated with it. Each lettered option may be selected once, more than once, or not at all.

Questions 15–20

(A) Luteinizing hormone (LH)
(B) Prolactin (PRL)
(C) Thyroid stimulating hormone (TSH)
(D) Growth hormone (GH)
(E) Follicle stimulating hormone (FSH)

Match each characteristic below with the appropriate hormone.

15. Has its release inhibited by thyroxine

16. Binds to receptors on Leydig cells

17. Stimulates production of insulin-like growth factor (IGF)

18. Stimulates the synthesis of milk proteins

19. Stimulates the production of progesterone by the corpus luteum

20. Stimulates the production of estradiol by the immature ovarian follicle

Questions 21–25

(A) Cortisol
(B) Aldosterone
(C) Both cortisol and aldosterone
(D) Neither cortisol nor aldosterone

Match each characteristic below with the appropriate steroid hormone.

21. Action mediated by a second messenger

22. Synthesized from cholesterol by cells of the adrenal cortex

23. Receptors have a DNA binding domain

24. Associated with induction of phosphoenolpyruvate carboxykinase (PEPCK)

25. Secreted in response to angiotensin II

Questions 26–29

(A) Oxytocin
(B) Vasopressin
(C) Both oxytocin and vasopressin
(D) Neither oxytocin nor vasopressin

Match each characteristic below with the appropriate hormone.

26. Produced by the anterior pituitary

27. Found associated with neurophysin in secretory granules

28. Associated with diuresis

29. Produced from the proopiomelanocortin (POMC) gene

Questions 30–33

(A) Elevated blood levels of aldosterone and renin resulting from an atherosclerotic plaque in a renal artery.
(B) Hyperprolactinemia due to a pituitary tumor
(C) Acromegaly due to a growth hormone (GH)-producing tumor that developed in adulthood.
(D) Cushing's syndrome due to an adrenal tumor

For each description of a patient given below, choose the most likely cause from the list above.

30. A large, protruding jaw, large hands and feet, normal height, and an elevated blood glucose level.

31. Thin limbs, central obesity, fat cheeks, a ruddy complexion, and an elevated blood glucose level

32. Hypertension and heart disease

33. Galactorrhea, amenorrhea, and blurred vision

Answers and Explanations

1–B. Both pregnenolone and progesterone are intermediates in the synthesis of steroid hormones from cholesterol. 7-Hydroxycholesterol is an intermediate in the conversion of cholesterol to bile salts, and aldosterone is a mineralocorticoid produced well beyond the branch point for the synthesis of the adrenal and gonadal steroids. Retinoic acid acts like a steroid hormone, but it is derived from vitamin A.

2–B. Epinephrine is synthesized from tyrosine. It functions like a polypeptide hormone, binding to receptors on the cell membrane. cAMP levels rise in response to epinephrine.

3–A. Testosterone is reduced to dihydrotestosterone (DHT), the more active hormone. Testosterone is a steroid hormone, thus it activates genes. It is a precursor of E_2. Testosterone inhibits the synthesis of GnRH.

4–C. 1,25-DHC is formed from an intermediate in cholesterol synthesis, 7-dehydrocholesterol. The B ring of this compound is cleaved by a reaction requiring ultraviolet light and, subsequently, hydroxyl groups are added at position 25 in the liver and at position 1 in the kidney.

5–B. Phosphatidylinositol bisphosphate is cleaved to IP_3 and DAG. IP_3 causes the release of Ca^{2+} from the endoplasmic reticulum, while DAG activates protein kinase C. PTH stimulates the release of Ca^{2+} from bone, and 1,25-DHC stimulates the absorption of Ca^{2+} from the intestine.

6–B. When iodine is deficient in the diet, the thyroid does not make normal amounts of thyroid hormone. Consequently, there is less feedback inhibition of TRH and TSH production and release. Low levels of thyroid hormone result in decreased heat production.

7–C. Because ACTH and cortisol were initially elevated, the most likely cause is a tumor of the anterior pituitary that is overproducing ACTH, causing cortisol to be overproduced by the adrenal gland. This conclusion is supported by the fact that the administration of a very high dose of a glucocorticoid (dexamethasone) caused the plasma cortisol level to decrease. (Glucorticoids inhibit the release of ACTH.) The patient's hyperglycemia was caused by the elevated cortisol.

8–E. GnRH stimulates the release of two pituitary hormones, LH and FSH. GRH stimulates the release of growth hormone; TSH, the release of T_3 and T_4; and PRH, the release of prolactin. IGF stimulates growth.

9–C. If 15% of the radioactive T_4 is bound to antibody, the amount of T_4 in 0.1 mL of the patient's serum is 0.015 µg/0.1 mL or 15 µg/dL. (1 dL = 100 mL).

10–C. The patient's T_4 level is above the normal range–the patient is hyperthyroid.

11–C. Thyroid hormone suppresses TSH secretion by the anterior pituitary. If thyroid hormone levels are elevated, TSH levels will be lower than normal. This patient probably has Graves' disease, in which thyroid stimulating antibodies promote T_3 and T_4 production by the thyroid gland. These thyroid hormones inhibit release of TSH from the anterior pituitary.

12–D. The accountant has galactorrhea (inappropriate production of milk) caused by a prolactinoma (a tumor of the anterior pituitary that secretes prolactin). Dopamine, the major regulator of prolactin secretion, inhibits prolactin production and release by the anterior pituitary. Bromocriptine is a drug that acts like dopamine to inhibit prolactin release. While oxytocin stimulates ejection of milk from the mammary gland, prolactin is necessary for milk to be produced in the gland.

13–C. Excess production of ACTH by the anterior pituitary is caused by a lack of suppression by cortisol, because cortisol levels are low. A tumor that produces POMC (the precursor of ACTH) would result in high ACTH and high cortisol levels. CRH levels are probably high (because of lack of suppression by cortisol), resulting in the high ACTH levels. The problem must be in the adrenal cortex (not the medulla), which is failing to produce adequate amounts of cortisol in response to ACTH. Because of a deficient enzyme in the cortisol pathway, cortisol precursors are being used to produce excess androgens, which are causing the patient's secondary male sexual characteristics.

14–B. Damage to her pituitary gland that resulted in decreased hormone production could explain all her symptoms. A low vasopressin (ADH) level results in diabetes insipidus. Decreased levels of LH and FSH cause amenorrhea. Decreased TSH leads to low thyroid hormone levels, which result in a decreased basal metabolic rate (and reduced production of body heat). Lack of growth hormone slows growth. Anterior and posterior pituitary hormones are small peptides that would be digested by proteolytic enzymes in the gut if taken orally. Thyroxine and glucocorticoids would alleviate some of her problems, but estrogen alone would not restore menses, and water intake would have to be increased, not restricted.

15–C. Thyroxine inhibits the release of TSH by the anterior pituitary.

16–A. Luteinizing hormone binds to receptors on Leydig cells and stimulates the release of testosterone.

17–D. GH stimulates the release of IGF by the liver and other tissues.

18–B. Prolactin stimulates the synthesis of milk proteins.

19–A. LH stimulates the corpus luteum to produce progesterone.

20–E. FSH stimulates maturation of the ovarian follicle, which produces estradiol.

21–D. Steroid hormones do not act through second messengers. They enter the cell and activate genes.

22–C. Steroid hormones are synthesized from cholesterol. Cortisol and aldosterone are made in the adrenal cortex.

23–C. Steroid hormones bind to receptors and the complexes subsequently bind to DNA, activating genes. 1,25-DHC, thyroid hormone, and retinoic acid (from vitamin A) act in the same fashion.

24–A. Glucocorticoids, such as cortisol, activate the gene for PEPCK.

25–B. Angiotensin II stimulates the synthesis and secretion of aldosterone.

26–D. Oxytocin and vasopressin are produced by the hypothalamus and stored in and secreted from the posterior pituitary.

27–C. Both oxytocin and vasopressin are bound to neurophysins.

28–D. Vasopressin has an antidiuretic action. Neither acts as a diuretic.

29–D. POMC is produced by the anterior pituitary.

30–C. In acromegaly, height is normal, but the jaw, hands, feet, and soft tissues grow. Diabetes mellitus frequently occurs because of the stimulation of gluconeogenesis by GH and the inability of glucose to suppress the release of GH by the tumor.

31–D. Excess production of cortisol causes muscle breakdown (hence thin limbs), fat deposition in the face and abdomen, thin skin (due to protein breakdown), and an increase in red blood cells resulting in a red complexion. Blood glucose is elevated because cortisol stimulates gluconeogenesis.

32–A. The plaque in the renal artery causes the release of renin, which elevates aldosterone, thus raising blood pressure. Atherosclerotic plaques are probably also the cause of the heart disease.

33–B. A tumor of the anterior pituitary that produces prolactin could cause milk production (galactorrhea) and inhibit LH and FSH production, causing amenorrhea. If the tumor grew over the optic nerves, blurred vision would result.

9

The Biochemical Functions of Tissues and Their Clinical Implications

Overview

- The various tissues of the body have different biochemical functions.
- These functions change with the physiologic state (e.g., fed, fasting, starving, exercise) and under different pathologic conditions.
- Biochemical measurements can be made to determine if the body is in a normal or an abnormal state.

I. Use of Biochemical Measurements to Diagnose Pathologic Conditions

- Measurements can be made on body fluids and tissues and used to draw conclusions about clinical problems.

A. Measurements can be made on:

1. **Compounds** that **enter** the body (e.g., carbohydrates, fats, proteins)

2. **Samples of blood, urine, feces**, and various **secretions**

3. **Cells** obtained from **blood, scrapings,** or **biopsies** of tissues

B. Examples of types of measurements

1. The **amounts** of various **chemical compounds** can be measured (e.g., blood glucose, blood urea nitrogen, urinary creatinine).

2. **Enzyme assays** can be performed (e.g., creatine kinase, aspartate or alanine transaminase, alkaline phosphatase).

3. **DNA, RNA,** or **proteins** can be identified (e.g., by hybridization with DNA probes or by reaction with antibodies), or they can be sequenced.

4. **Substances** can be given to a patient to determine whether the body **processes** them normally (e.g., a glucose tolerance test, radioactive iodine uptake by the thyroid gland).

C. Conclusions from measurements

1. From the results of biochemical measurements, conclusions can be drawn about the patient's condition, and, in conjunction with a medical history and physical examination, the information can be used to formulate a **diagnosis** or to determine what **additional tests** need to be done.

309

2. In order to draw useful conclusions, a physician must understand the **biochemical relationships among tissues** and how they are altered by changes in the physiologic state (e.g., fed, fasting, starving, exercise) and the effects of pathologic changes.

   – The intertissue relationships are summarized in Chapter 1 and presented in more detail throughout the book.
   – Some of the effects of pathologic changes are described in the clinical correlations that appear at the end of each chapter.

II. Biochemical Functions of Tissues

- To review the functions and sort them by tissue, we will take a tour of the body, starting in the mouth and ending in the kidney.
- We will consider the major biochemical functions of various tissues and organs and the consequences of abnormalities in these functions caused, for example, by physical or chemical damage, infection, dietary deficiencies or excesses, and mutations in genes.

A. Mouth

– **Salivary glands** produce α-amylase, which cleaves α-1,4 bonds between glucose residues in dietary starch. (Pancreatic α-amylase catalyzes the same reaction.)

B. Stomach

1. Chief cells produce the proteolytic enzyme **pepsin**, as its inactive precursor pepsinogen. Pepsin digests proteins.

2. Parietal cells produce hydrochloric acid **(HCl)** and **intrinsic factor.**

   a. **HCl** causes pepsinogen (the precursor of pepsin) to cleave itself (autocatalysis), producing **pepsin.**

   b. **Intrinsic factor** binds dietary **vitamin B_{12}** and aids in its absorption.
      – **Vitamin B_{12}** is the cofactor for conversion of **homocysteine to methionine** and **methylmalonyl CoA to succinyl CoA.**
      – A **deficiency of intrinsic factor** causes a condition known as **pernicious anemia**, which results in a deficiency of vitamin B_{12} in the body because of inadequate absorption.
      – A **deficiency of vitamin B_{12}** is characterized by a **megaloblastic anemia**, which is caused by a secondary folate deficiency (see II H) and by **neurologic problems** caused by demyelination of nerves.

C. Gallbladder

1. **Bile salts**, synthesized in the liver from cholesterol, pass through the gallbladder into the intestine, where they aid in lipid digestion.

   – A decrease in bile salt availability can be caused by **problems with bile salt production** in the liver or **blockage of secretion** from the gallbladder. The result is an increase of fat in the stool (**steatorrhea**) because of decreased fat digestion and absorption (which can lead to **caloric deficits** and **fat-soluble vitamin** and **essential fatty acid deficiencies**).

2. **Bilirubin diglucuronide**, produced in the liver from bilirubin (the excretory product of heme degradation), passes through the gallbladder into the intestine.

   – **Obstruction of the flow of bile** into the small intestine is one cause of **jaundice** (the accumulation of bilirubin in tissues, producing a yellow color, which is especially obvious in the whites of the eyes).

D. Pancreas

1. The pancreas **produces bicarbonate (HCO$_3^-$),** which neutralizes stomach acid as it enters the intestinal lumen. The subsequent increase in pH in the lumen allows more extensive **ionization of bile salts** (so they serve as better detergents) and increases the **activity of digestive enzymes.**

   – **Pancreatic disorders** that cause a decrease in bicarbonate release lead to decreased activity of digestive enzymes and increased excretion of bile salts in the feces (because they are less ionized, they are more readily excreted). Therefore, **steatorrhea** occurs (increased excretion of dietary fat in the feces).

2. The pancreas produces **digestive enzymes** (e.g., trypsin, chymotrypsin, the carboxypeptidases, elastase, α-amylase, lipase).

   – **Obstruction of the flow of pancreatic secretions** into the intestinal lumen (caused, for example, by a cancer of the head of the pancreas or by cystic fibrosis) leads to **decreased digestion** of nutrients (and, therefore, to deficiencies of calories, vitamins, and other essential nutrients in the body).

3. The B (or β) cells of the endocrine pancreas produce **insulin** (the hormone that stimulates the storage of fuels in the fed state), and the A (or α) cells produce **glucagon** (the hormone that stimulates the release of stored fuels during fasting).

   – **Decreased production of insulin**, which is usually caused by autoimmune destruction of pancreatic B cells, results in **Type 1** (formerly called insulin-dependent) diabetes mellitus. Type 1 diabetes is characterized by **hyperglycemia**, the result of decreased uptake of glucose by cells and increased output of glucose by the liver (due to low insulin and high glucagon levels in the blood).

   – **Decreased release of insulin** from the pancreas or **decreased sensitivity** of tissues to insulin (insulin resistance) results in **Type 2** (formerly called non-insulin dependent) **diabetes mellitus.** This condition also is characterized by **hyperglycemia.**

   – **Excessive** levels of **insulin**, caused by an insulin-secreting tumor of the pancreas (an insulinoma) or by injection of too much insulin, results in **hypoglycemia.**

E. Intestine

1. **Enzymes** from the **exocrine pancreas digest food** in the intestinal lumen

   – Excessive **proliferation of bacteria** within the lumen causes increased **deconjugation** and **dehydroxylation** of **bile salts** leading to increased bile salt excretion and steatorrhea.

2. **Digestive enzymes** are bound to the brush borders of **intestinal epithelial cells** (aminopeptidases, di- and tripeptidases, lactase, sucrase, maltases, and isomaltases).

   – **Lactase deficiency** is very common. In lactase deficiency, ingestion of milk products results in **diarrhea** (caused by the osmotic effect of excess lactose in the lumen of the gut) and bloating (caused by excessive **gas** production that results from the metabolism of lactose by intestinal bacteria).

3. **Absorption** of digestive products occurs through intestinal epithelial cells.

   – Decreased absorption of **neutral amino acids** (due to a deficient transport protein) leads to **Hartnup's disease.**

   – **Celiac disease** (in children) and **nontropical sprue** in adults are caused by absorption of protein fragments that cause **allergic reactions.**

   – **Cholera** is caused by production of an enterotoxin that ADP-ribosylates G proteins. Adenylate cyclase remains active. Increased cAMP causes increased phosphorylation of transport proteins and, thus, inhibits active transport of Na^+ into the intestinal cells. As a result, water accumulates in the gut, causing **severe diarrhea.**

4. Intestinal epithelial cells produce **chylomicrons** from the digestive products of dietary fat (fatty acids and 2-monoacylglycerols) and secrete the chylomicrons into the lymph.

5. Most **bile salts** are **resorbed** in the ileum and **recycled** by the liver. Only **5% are excreted** in the feces. This excretion of bile salts, along with cholesterol secreted by the liver into the gut via the gallbladder, is the major means by which the body disposes of the cholesterol ring system (sterol nucleus).

F. Liver

1. **Functions** of the liver include:

   a. Storage of **glycogen** produced from dietary carbohydrate

   b. Synthesis of very low density lipoprotein (**VLDL**), mainly from dietary carbohydrate

   c. Production of high-density lipoprotein (**HDL**), which transfers C_{II} and E apoproteins to chylomicrons and VLDL, converts cholesterol to cholesterol esters (via the lecithin-cholesterol acyl transferase or LCAT reaction), and reduces blood cholesterol levels by participating in the process by which cholesterol and cholesterol esters are transported from tissues to the liver

   d. **Maintenance of blood glucose** during fasting via glycogenolysis and gluconeogenesis

   e. Production of **urea** from nitrogen derived, in part, from amino acids as they are being converted to glucose (via gluconeogenesis) during fasting

   f. Production of **ketone bodies** from fatty acids derived from lipolysis of adipose triacylglycerols during fasting

g. Synthesis of **cholesterol** (which is also made in other tissues)

h. Conversion of cholesterol to **bile salts**

i. Production of many **blood proteins** (e.g., albumin, blood clotting proteins)

j. Production of purines and **pyrimidines**, which are transported to other tissues via red blood cells

k. Degradation of purines (to uric acid) and **pyrimidines** (to CO_2, H_2O, and urea)

l. Oxidation of drugs and other **toxic compounds** via the cytochrome P_{450} system

m. Conjugation of bilirubin and excretion of bilirubin diglucuronide into the bile

n. Oxidation of alcohol via alcohol and acetaldehyde dehydrogenases and the microsomal ethanol oxidizing system (MEOS)

o. Synthesis of **creatine** (from guanidinoacetate), which is used to produce creatine phosphate, mainly in muscle and brain

p. Conversion of **dietary fructose** to glycolytic intermediates

2. **If liver cell function is compromised** (e.g., in viral hepatitis or alcoholic cirrhosis):

a. NH_4^+, which is **toxic** (particularly to the central nervous system), **increases** in the blood.

b. The blood urea nitrogen (**BUN**) level **decreases** because the liver has a decreased capacity to produce urea.

c. Blood glucose decreases because of decreased glycogenolysis and gluconeogenesis.

d. Blood **cholesterol** levels **decrease**.

e. Production of **bile salts decreases**.

f. Bilirubin levels **increase** in the body (causing jaundice).

g. Lysis of damaged liver cells allows **enzymes** to **leak** into the blood.
 – Lactic dehydrogenase (**LDH**) increases.
 – Alanine transaminase (**ALT**), formerly called serum glutamate pyruvate transaminase (SGPT) increases.
 – Aspartate transaminase (**AST**), formerly called serum glutamate oxaloacetate transaminase (SGOT) increases.
 – **Alkaline phosphatase** increases.

h. Chronic liver problems result in **decreased protein synthesis**.
 – **Serum proteins** (e.g., albumin) decrease.
 – **VLDL** production decreases because of decreased apoprotein B-100, and triacylglycerols accumulate in the liver. A fatty liver results.

3. **Specific diseases** that affect the liver

a. Glycogen storage diseases

- **Von Gierke's:** glucose 6-phosphatase deficiency. Blood glucose cannot be produced by glycogenolysis or gluconeogenesis, resulting in severe hypoglycemia during fasting.
- **Hers':** liver phosphorylase deficiency. Glycogen cannot be converted to blood glucose. Blood glucose is maintained only by gluconeogenesis.
- **Pompe's:** lysosomal α-glucosidase deficiency. Glycogen accumulates in membrane-enclosed vesicles (residual bodies) and interferes with liver function.

b. Alcoholism

(1) Oxidation of ethanol **produces NADH** by reactions that occur in the liver.

$$\underset{\text{Ethanol}}{CH_3\text{-}CH_2OH} \xrightarrow[\text{NAD}^+\quad\text{NADH}]{} \underset{\text{Acetaldehyde}}{CH_3\text{-}\overset{O}{\overset{\|}{C}}\text{-}H} \xrightarrow[\text{NAD}^+\quad\text{NADH}]{} \underset{\text{Acetate}}{CH_3\text{-}\overset{O}{\overset{\|}{C}}\text{-}O^-}$$

(2) Ingestion of ethanol without food intake results in high [NADH]/[NAD$^+$], which can cause:
- Increased conversion of pyruvate to lactate, producing a **lactic acidosis**
- Inhibition of gluconeogenesis, leading to **hypoglycemia**
- Increased levels of glycerol 3-phosphate, which combines with fatty acids from adipose triacylglycerols to form VLDL. Increased VLDL levels in the blood produce a **hyperlipidemia**.

(3) In **chronic alcoholism**,
- **Protein synthesis decreases** in the liver. Thus, VLDL secretion decreases, leading to a **fatty liver** (the accumulation of triacylglycerol).

c. Diabetes mellitus (DM)
- Low insulin levels (Type 1) or insensitivity to insulin (Type 2) results in increased glycogenolysis and gluconeogenesis, which contribute to the **elevated blood glucose levels**.
- Increased ketone body production can lead to **diabetic ketoacidosis** (DKA) particularly in Type 1 DM. Ketone body synthesis increases because of increased release of fatty acids from adipose triacylglycerols.

d. Fructose intolerance
- A **deficiency of aldolase B** results in elevated fructose 1-phosphate and low inorganic phosphate (P_i) levels after fructose ingestion. (Glycolysis is not affected even though the same aldolase is involved.) Glycogenolysis and gluconeogenesis are inhibited, and **hypoglycemia** results.

G. Brain

1. **Glucose** is the major fuel for the brain.

2. The brain can use **ketone bodies**, but only **after 3 to 5 days of fasting when blood ketone body levels are elevated.**

3. The brain needs energy to **think** (i.e., memory involves RNA synthesis), conduct **nerve impulses**, synthesize **neurotransmitters**, etc.
   – Abrupt decreases in blood glucose can result in **coma** from **lack of ATP**.
   – Very elevated blood glucose levels can cause a **hyperosmolar coma**.
   – Synthesis of some neurotransmitters (e.g., GABA, serotonin, dopamine) involves decarboxylation of amino acids and requires pyridoxal phosphate (from vitamin B_6). **Deficiencies of vitamin B_6** can lead to **convulsions**.

H. Red blood cells

1. Red blood cells **lack mitochondria**, so they have no TCA cycle, β-oxidation of fatty acids, electron transport chain, and other pathways that occur in mitochondria.

2. **Glucose** is the **major fuel** for red blood cells.
   – Glucose is converted to pyruvate and lactate.

3. Red blood cells **carry bases** and **nucleosides** from the liver to other tissues.

4. The major function of red blood cells is to **carry O_2** from the lungs to the tissues and to aid in the **return** of CO_2 from the tissues to the lungs.

5. **Problems involving red blood cells**

   a. **Hemoglobinopathies**
      – **Sickle cell anemia** occurs because valine replaces glutamate at position 6 in the β-globin chain. This hydrophobic amino acid permits interactions to occur between globin chains of different hemoglobin molecules. Cells become misshapen ("sickled") and can block blood flow through capillaries. Painful vasoocclusive crises can occur. The misshapen cells are phagocytosed by the spleen, and anemia results.
      – **Thalassemias** are caused by deficiencies of α or β globin chains, which result from many different types of mutations in genes. Decreased hemoglobin levels result in anemia.

   b. **Iron deficiency anemia**
      – Red blood cell precursors cannot produce normal amounts of heme. Cells are small (microcytic) and pale (hypochromic).

   c. **Vitamin B_6 deficiency**
      – Vitamin B_6 is required for the first reaction (glycine + succinyl CoA $\rightarrow$ δ-ALA) in heme biosynthesis in red blood cell precursors. Decreased heme production leads to decreased hemoglobin levels in mature red blood cells and a microcytic, hypochromic anemia.

   d. **Megaloblastic anemia** (caused by folate or B_{12} deficiencies)
      – **Folate** is required for the production of thymine (by the conversion of dUMP to dTMP) and for the production of the purine bases (carbon 2 and carbon 8 come from the tetrahydrofolate one-carbon pool).
      (1) In a **folate deficiency**, the precursors of red blood cells cannot divide because of a lack of thymine and of purines for DNA synthesis. Megaloblasts form, and a **megaloblastic anemia** results.

(2) In a **vitamin B$_{12}$ deficiency**, folate accumulates as methyltetrahydrofolate because the methyl group cannot be transferred to B$_{12}$ (the methyl trap theory). Thus, there is decreased thymine for DNA synthesis and decreased purines for DNA and RNA synthesis. Decreased cell growth and division occur, and red blood cell precursors form **megaloblasts**

(3) In a **B$_{12}$ deficiency** (but **not in a folate deficiency**), decreased conversion of methylmalonyl CoA to succinyl CoA occurs, resulting in **neurologic problems**.

(4) A **deficiency of folate or vitamin B$_{12}$** results in **decreased** conversion of **homocysteine to methionine**.

– Unless dietary methionine is increased, low levels of methionine result in **decreased** synthesis of *S*-adenosylmethionine (**SAM**), and, thus, decreased conversion of norepinephrine to epinephrine, phosphatidyl ethanolamine to phosphatidylcholine, guanidinoacetate to creatine, etc.

e. Pyruvate kinase deficiency

– Deficiency of pyruvate kinase, a key glycolytic enzyme, leads to decreased ATP production from glycolysis. Red blood cells (which depend on glycolysis for energy) cannot maintain their membranes. They crenate (shrink) and are phagocytosed, and an anemia results.

f. Glucose 6-phosphate dehydrogenase deficiency

– Glucose 6-phosphate dehydrogenase, the first enzyme of the pentose phosphate pathway, produces **NADPH**.

– In **glucose 6-phosphate dehydrogenase deficiency**, NADPH production is decreased. Therefore, **glutathionine** is not reduced at a normal rate. Problems arise when demand for NADPH is high (e.g., when drugs that require NADPH for their metabolism are used, such as primaquine for malaria). As hemoglobin (Fe^{2+}) is slowly oxidized to methemoglobin (Fe^{3+}), superoxide (O$_2^-$) is produced. Superoxide dismutase converts superoxide to hydrogen peroxide (H$_2$O$_2$) and O$_2$. Glutathionine peroxidase converts H$_2$O$_2$ to H$_2$O, producing oxidized glutathionine (GS-SG), which must be converted by NADPH to reduced glutathione (GSH). If reduction does not occur rapidly enough, oxidative damage causes red blood cells to lyse and a **hemolytic anemia** results.

g. Hemolytic anemias cause **bilirubin** and **lactate dehydrogenase** to be released into the blood. If bilirubin is produced faster than the liver can conjugate and excrete it, **jaundice** can occur. **Stercobilin**, a pigment produced from bilirubin by intestinal bacteria, increases in the feces, causing the stool to turn dark brown.

I. Adipose tissue

1. The **major fuel** of adipose tissue is **glucose**.

2. Insulin stimulates the **transport of glucose** into adipose cells.

– In diabetes mellitus, the uptake of glucose by adipose tissue is low because of decreased insulin (Type 1) or insulin resistance (Type 2). The decreased uptake of glucose contributes to the elevated blood glucose levels.

3. The function of adipose tissue is to **store triacylglycerol** in the fed state and release it (via **lipolysis**) during fasting.

   a. **In the fed state**, insulin stimulates the synthesis and secretion of lipoprotein lipase (LPL) which degrades the triacylglycerols of chylomicrons and VLDL in the capillaries. Fatty acids from these lipoproteins enter adipose cells and are converted to triacylglycerols and stored. Glucose provides the glycerol moiety. (Glycerol is not used, because adipose cells lack glycerol kinase.)

   b. **During fasting**, hormone-sensitive lipase (phosphorylated and activated via a cAMP-mediated mechanism) initiates lipolysis in adipose cells.

   c. **In diabetes mellitus,** low insulin levels (Type 1) or insulin resistance (Type 2) result in decreased degradation of the triacylglycerols of chylomicrons and VLDL (because of decreased LPL).

      – **Hypertriglyceridemia** results. In addition, lipolysis occurs, causing excessive amounts of fatty acids and glycerol to reach the liver, where they produce VLDL, thus adding to the hypertriglyceridemia.

J. Muscle

1. Muscle uses **all fuels** that are available (glycogen stores, and fatty acids, glucose, ketone bodies, lactate, and amino acids from the blood) to obtain energy for contraction.

2. During fasting, muscle protein is degraded to provide **amino acids** (particularly alanine) for **gluconeogenesis**.

3. **Creatine phosphate** transports high-energy phosphate from the mitochondria to actinomyosin fibers and provides ATP for muscle contraction.

   – **Muscle damage** results in the release into the blood of **creatine kinase** (CK), the enzyme that catalyzes the reversible reaction—creatine + ATP $\leftrightarrow$ creatine phosphate.

4. **Creatinine** is produced nonenzymatically from creatine phosphate, and a **constant amount** (dependent on body muscle mass) is released into the blood each day and excreted by the kidneys.

5. **Muscle glycogen phosphorylase** differs from liver phosphorylase but catalyzes the same reaction (glycogen + P_i $\leftrightarrow$ glucose 1-phosphate).

   – **McArdle's disease** is a glycogen storage disease in which muscle phosphorylase is deficient. Muscle glycogen cannot be degraded at a normal rate. Glycogen stores increase, and lactate is not produced during exercise. Vigorous exercise quickly produces fatigue; however, mild exercise, using fatty acids and glucose from the blood, can be tolerated.

6. **Insulin** stimulates the **transport of glucose** into muscle cells.

   – In Type 1 and Type 2 diabetes mellitus, the uptake of glucose by muscle is low and is one of the factors that contributes to hyperglycemia.

K. Heart

1. The heart is a specialized muscle that uses **all fuels** from the blood.

2. The muscle-brain **(MB) isozyme** of creatine kinase (CK) is found in heart muscle. Its release can be used to monitor a heart attack.

3. **Heart disease**

   a. **Atherosclerotic plaques** can occlude blood vessels, blocking the flow of nutrients and O_2. Muscle tissue beyond the block suffers from a lack of energy and can die. When the amount of functional cardiac muscle tissue that remains is insufficient to pump blood through the body at a normal rate, **heart failure** occurs. The damaged cells release the **MB isozyme** of CK into the blood.

   b. **High blood cholesterol** levels are associated with increased risk of a heart attack (or a stroke, which is caused by a similar process in the brain). Cholesterol is carried in the blood lipoproteins and is elevated in a group of conditions known as the **hyperlipidemias**.
      – **Type I:** chylomicrons are elevated; thus, triacylglycerols are high.
      – **Type II:** LDL receptors are defective; cholesterol is high.
      – **Type III:** a spectrum of partial degradation products of VLDL appear in the blood (a broad β band).
      – **Type IV:** VLDL is elevated; thus, triacylglycerols are elevated. Type IV is often associated with diabetes mellitus.
      – **Type V:** chylomicrons and VLDL are elevated.

   c. **Treatments include:**

      (1) **A diet low in fat** (particularly saturated fat)

      (2) **Decreased dietary carbohydrate** (to lower VLDL)

      (3) **HMG CoA reductase inhibitors** (statins) to decrease blood cholesterol levels (by decreasing cholesterol synthesis). Decreased cellular levels of cholesterol increase synthesis of LDL receptors. Thus, more LDL (composed of almost 50% cholesterol and cholesterol esters) is taken up from the blood.

      (4) **Bile salt sequestrants** to increase excretion of bile salts, a major means by which the cholesterol ring structure is removed from the body.

      (5) **Niacin** to decrease lipolysis in adipose tissue and VLDL synthesis in the liver.

L. Kidney

1. The kidney **excretes substances** from the body via the urine, including **urea** (produced by the urea cycle in the liver), **uric acid** (from purine degradation), **creatinine** (from creatine phosphate), NH_4^+ (from glutamine via glutaminase), H_2SO_4 (produced from the sulfur of cysteine and methionine), and **phosphoric acid**.

2. Daily **creatinine** excretion is **constant** and depends on body muscle mass. It is used as a measure of kidney function (the creatinine clearance rate).

3. **Glutaminase** action increases during **acidosis** and produces NH_3, which enters the urine and reacts with H^+ to form NH_4^+. NH_4^+ buffers the urine and removes acid (H^+) from the body.

4. **Uric acid** excretion is inhibited by lead (Pb) and metabolic acids (ketone bodies and lactic acid). High blood uric acid can result in **gout**. Gout can be caused either by increased production or by decreased excretion of uric acid. Deficiency of the base salvage enzyme hypoxanthine guanine phosphoribosyltransferase (HGPRT) in **Lesch-Nyhan syndrome** results in increased production of uric acid.

5. **Kidney dysfunction** can lead to increased BUN, creatinine, and uric acid in the blood, and decreased levels of these compounds in the urine.

6. During ketoacidosis, **ketone bodies** are excreted by the kidney, and during lactic acidosis, **lactic acid** is excreted.

7. Elevated blood glucose (over 180 mg/dL) in diabetes mellitus results in **excretion of glucose** in the urine.

8. **Enzyme deficiency diseases** that affect various tissues of the body often result in the **excretion** of substances in the **urine**. Examples of these types of diseases include:

    a. **Phenylketonuria (PKU):** phenylalanine hydroxylase deficiency. Decreased conversion of phenylalanine to tyrosine results in the appearance of phenylalanine and its degradation products (e.g., phenylketones) in the urine.

    b. **Maple syrup urine disease (MSUD):** α-keto acid dehydrogenase deficiency. The branched chain amino acids (valine, isoleucine, and leucine) are excreted.

    c. **Alcaptonuria:** homogentisic acid oxidase deficiency. Oxidized products of homogentisic acid give urine a dark color. The condition may be benign but is sometimes associated with arthritis.

    d. **Cystinuria:** deficiency of the intestinal and kidney transport protein for cystine. Cystine is not resorbed and accumulates in the urine, forming kidney stones.

    e. **Homocystinuria:** deficiency of methionine synthase (homocysteine to methionine), cystathionine synthase (homocysteine + serine → cystathionine), or of the cofactors for these enzymes (folate and vitamin B_{12} for methionine synthase, and vitamin B_6 for cystathionine synthase). Homocysteine accumulates, is oxidized to homocystine, and excreted. Homocystinemia (high levels of homocysteine in the blood) is associated with atherosclerotic vascular disease.

    f. **Cystathionuria:** deficiency of cystathionase. Cystathionine is excreted. High doses of vitamin B_6, the precursor of the cofactor (pyridoxal phosphate) for the enzyme, are sometimes beneficial.

    g. **Benign fructosuria:** deficiency of fructokinase. Fructose is not phosphorylated, thus it accumulates and is excreted. There are no deleterious consequences.

    h. **Galactosemia:** deficiency of galactokinase or galactose 1-phosphate uridyl transferase. In a galactokinase deficiency, galactose accumulates, causes cataracts, and spills into the urine. In the uridyl transferase deficiency (classic galactosemia), hypoglycemia, jaundice, and other

problems result, in addition to cataracts and the appearance of galactose in the urine.

i. **MCAD deficiency:** deficiency of the medium-chain fatty acyl CoA dehydrogenase. Fatty acids cannot be completely oxidized. Consequently, more glucose must be oxidized for energy, resulting in hypoglycemia. Increased ω-oxidation of fatty acids produces dicarboxylic acids that are excreted in the urine.

Comprehensive Examination

Directions: Each of the numbered items or incomplete statements in this section is followed by answers or by completions of the statement. Select the **one** lettered answer or completion that is **best** in each case.

1. A patient who needed to lose weight began eating at fast-food restaurants. He did not change his exercise level. However, the composition of his diet was altered in that his carbohydrate intake decreased by 50 g/day and his fat intake increased by 50 g/day. Otherwise, his diet remained the same. On this diet

(A) he gained weight
(B) he lost weight
(C) his weight remained the same

2. A patient who is obese and has hypertension requires a weight reduction diet. She weighs 176 lb and has a sedentary lifestyle. What is the approximate number of calories the patient burns each day at this weight?

(A) 1920
(B) 2500
(C) 4220
(D) 5490

3. Which of the following compounds can be synthesized in humans?

(A) Riboflavin
(B) Linoleic acid
(C) Leucine
(D) Thiamine
(E) Niacin

4. Which of the following metabolites provides carbon for maintenance of blood glucose levels?

(A) Lysine from muscle protein
(B) Glycogen from muscle stores
(C) Glycerol from adipose triacylglycerols
(D) Even-chain fatty acids from adipose triacylglycerols

5. A person who accidentally ingested a compound that completely inhibited fructose 1,6-bis-phosphatase could still form substantial amounts of blood glucose from

(A) muscle glycogen stores
(B) lactate produced by red blood cells
(C) ingested fructose
(D) ingested galactose
(E) ingested fructose or galactose

6. A person who accidentally ingested a compound that completely inhibited phosphoenol-pyruvate carboxykinase could still form substantial amounts of blood glucose from

(A) muscle glycogen stores
(B) lactate produced by red blood cells
(C) ingested fructose
(D) ingested galactose
(E) ingested fructose or galactose

7. A solution contains 2×10^{-3} moles per liter of a weak acid (pK = 3.5) and 2×10^{-3} moles per liter of its conjugate base. Its pH is

(A) 4.1
(B) 3.9
(C) 3.5
(D) 3.1
(E) 2.7

8. Hydroxymethylglutaryl CoA

(A) is formed by catabolism of valine
(B) gives rise to ketone bodies by cleavage to acetate and acetoacetyl CoA
(C) serves as a precursor of cholesterol
(D) is formed from glutamic acid by the direct action of HMG CoA synthetase

9. The cytochrome P_{450} system of liver in normal individuals has a capacity (V_m) to oxidize approximately 10 nmol of drug X per minute per gram of liver. When the concentration of drug X in the liver is 2 μM, oxidation products are formed at the rate of 4 nmol/min/g of liver. What is the K_m of cytochrome P_{450} for this drug?

(A) 4 nM
(B) 5 nM
(C) 10 nM
(D) 2 μM
(E) 3 μM

10. Enzyme Y was purified from a tissue sample obtained from a patient. The kinetic properties of this enzyme and those of the same enzyme isolated from a normal individual are shown in the graph below. Which of the following statements is TRUE?

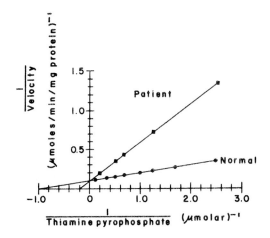

(A) The enzymes do not have the same V_m
(B) A lower concentration of thiamine pyrophosphate (TPP) is required to saturate the patient's enzyme
(C) The patient's enzyme has a K_m for thiamine pyrophosphate that is less than that for the normal enzyme
(D) Administration of thiamine to the patient should result in a greater proportion of the enzyme in the active enzyme-TPP complex

11. A deficiency of pantothenic acid would most directly affect the reaction catalyzed by

(A) citrate synthase
(B) isocitrate dehydrogenase
(C) succinate dehydrogenase
(D) fumarase
(E) malate dehydrogenase

12. In which of the following tissues is glucose the major fuel in prolonged fasting?

(A) muscle
(B) brain
(C) liver
(D) red blood cells
(E) kidney

13. Which of the following statements about adult hemoglobin (HbA) is TRUE?

(A) HbA is composed of two β and two γ subunits
(B) Two subunits combine to form HbA
(C) Each subunit of HbA contains one heme
(D) One mole of HbA binds 1 mole of O_2
(E) The β chain of HbA is more hydrophobic than the β chain of sickle cell hemoglobin (HbS)

14. In scurvy, defective collagen is produced because hydroxylation of procollagen does not occur at the normal rate. Hydroxylation of lysine residues on procollagen

(A) is not required for polymerization of collagen
(B) requires vitamin C, as does hydroxylation of proline residues
(C) occurs before incorporation of lysine into the polypeptide chain
(D) occurs after the mature collagen molecule is secreted from the cell

15. After an overnight fast

(A) fatty acids are the primary fuel for the brain
(B) glucose is synthesized from even-chain fatty acids
(C) ketone bodies are formed in the liver
(D) ketone bodies are a major fuel for red blood cells

16. Protein synthesis in eukaryotes

(A) is initiated by formyl-methionine
(B) begins with the binding of mRNA to the 30S ribosomal subunit
(C) can occur on 80S ribosomes attached to the rough endoplasmic reticulum (RER)
(D) does not require peptidyl transferase for synthesis of peptide bonds
(E) occurs on mRNA that is in the process of being synthesized

17. Which of the following statements concerning genes and transcription in eukaryotes is TRUE?

(A) The conversion of a UAG codon to UAA in mRNA would result in the incorporation of an incorrect amino acid into the polypeptide chain
(B) Genes always occur in one or a small number of copies in the genome
(C) The order of gene sequences in chromosomes is always the same in highly differentiated cells as in germ cells
(D) The primary product of transcription (hnRNA) often contains nucleotide sequences that do not code for the amino acid sequence of the protein encoded by a gene

18. The sequence for a portion of a gene responsible for a lysosomal storage disease (Tay-Sachs) has been determined. The normal gene sequence and the mutant gene sequence are given below. (There is a dot above every fifth base and a number above every tenth base.)

```
         •    10    •    20    •
Normal CGTATATCCTATGGCCCTGACCCAG
Mutant CGTATATCTATCCTATGGCCCTGAC
```

The amino acid sequence in this region of the normal protein is Arg–Ile–Ser–Tyr–Gly–Pro–Asp. Which of the following statements about this portion of the gene sequence is TRUE?

(A) The messenger RNA produced from this region of the mutant gene codes for the amino acid sequence given above
(B) The codon used for arginine in this sequence is AGA
(C) The mutant protein will be shorter than the normal protein
(D) The mutant gene contains a deletion that causes a frameshift mutation
(E) The mutant gene has a point mutation

19. During synthesis of eukaryotic mRNA

(A) RNA polymerase II binds to proteins associated with the TATA box
(B) exons are transcribed from DNA and then cleaved from hnRNA
(C) a cap site serves as the signal for cleavage and addition of the poly(A) tail
(D) the template strand of DNA is covalently bound to histones

20. Bacterial cells growing in a medium containing glucose and all 20 amino acids are transferred to a medium in which the only sugar is lactose and NH_4^+ is the only source of nitrogen. In cells growing in the second medium, compared with those growing in the first medium

(A) cAMP levels will be lower
(B) CAP protein (cAMP-binding protein) will be bound to the *lac* promoter
(C) the *lac* repressor will be bound to the *lac* operator
(D) RNA polymerase will not bind to the *trp* promoter
(E) attenuation of transcription of the *trp* operon will increase

21. The first enzyme to act during base excision repair of DNA is

(A) Ligase
(B) DNA polymerase
(C) Reverse transcriptase
(D) An endonuclease
(E) A glycosylase

22. Use the figures below to answer question 22.

Normal

G   C   A   T

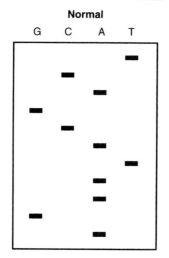

Mutant

G   C   A   T

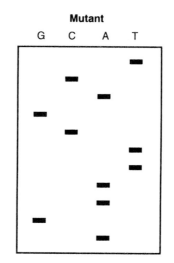

The gene responsible for a recessive genetic disorder was isolated and sequenced by the dideoxynucleotide method. The sequencing gel patterns obtained for a segment of the normal and mutant genes are shown above. A screening test was developed to identify individuals likely to have this disorder. This test used two restriction enzymes: *KpnI*, which cleaves the sequence 5'-GGTACC-3', and *EcoRI*, which cleaves 5'-GAATTC-3'. One of these enzymes produced a DNA fragment from the normal and mutant genes that contained the sequences shown above. The other enzyme cleaved within one of these sequences but not the other. Which of the following statements about the sequences shown on the gels is TRUE?

(A) The normal sequence is cleaved by *KpnI*
(B) The mutant sequence is cleaved by *KpnI*
(C) The normal sequence is cleaved by *EcoRI*
(D) The mutant sequence is cleaved by *EcoRI*

23. Which of the following statements concerning Okazaki fragments is TRUE?

(A) They are produced by the action of an endonuclease on DNA
(B) They are produced from the parental DNA strand that is oriented 3' to 5' in the direction that the replication fork is moving
(C) They are joined by a phosphorylase
(D) They contain a very short sequence of RNA joined by a phosphodiester bond to a short sequence of DNA
(E) They require only DNA polymerase for their synthesis

24. Use the following figure to answer question 24.

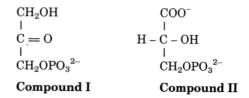

During glycolysis, compound I is converted to compound II shown above. In this conversion

(A) inorganic phosphate is produced
(B) NADH is consumed
(C) ATP is produced
(D) only one enzyme is required

25. After 2 days of fasting, the major process by which blood glucose is produced is

(A) glycolysis
(B) gluconeogenesis
(C) glycogenolysis
(D) the pentose phosphate pathway

26. An individual accidentally ingests a compound that inhibits glucose 6-phosphatase. After an overnight fast, this individual, compared with a healthy person, would have a higher

(A) rate of gluconeogenesis
(B) rate of glycogenolysis
(C) level of liver glycogen
(D) level of blood glucose

27. To determine the genetic father of a child (C), a laboratory test was performed that depended on a restriction fragment length polymorphism (RFLP) in a region upstream from a known gene. This region contains a variable number of tandem repeats (VNTR). Consequently, *HpaI* produces restriction fragments that differ in size. The restriction fragment map is shown below.

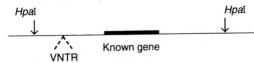

DNA, extracted from a child (C), the child's mother (M), and three men (F1, F2, and F3) was digested with *HpaI* and subjected to electrophoresis. A probe that hybridized to the known gene was used, so that only bands containing this gene were visualized. The gel is shown below. Numbers on the left refer to the size in kilobase (kb) pairs of the *HpaI* restriction fragments that bound the probe.

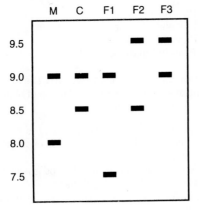

The child's father is most likely to be

(A) F1
(B) F2
(C) F3
(D) none of these men

28. β-Oxidation of even-chain fatty acids

(A) is used to produce energy in all cells of the body
(B) involves a C3-C4 enoyl intermediate
(C) always begins with palmitoyl CoA
(D) can result in ketone body formation
(E) provides carbon for glucose synthesis

29. Which of the following statements concerning digestion of dietary lipids is TRUE?

(A) A deficiency of pancreatic lipase would eventually lead to a prostaglandin deficiency
(B) 2-Monoacylglycerols and free fatty acids are produced by lipoprotein lipase
(C) Phospholipids act as detergents for micelle formation
(D) Bicarbonate ions (HCO_3^-) lower the pH of the small intestine so that lipase and bile salts are more active

30. A muscle-building nutritional supplement that contains succinate was advertised with the statement, "Succinate will provide your muscles with energy even when oxygen is depleted." In the absence of oxygen, the oxidation of 1 mole of succinate in muscle would yield how many moles of ATP?

(A) 0
(B) 1
(C) 2
(D) 3
(E) 5

Questions 31 and 32

Malate + NAD$^+$ → oxaloacetate + NADH + H$^+$
$\Delta G^{\circ\prime} = +7.1$ kcal/mol

Oxaloacetate + acetyl CoA → citrate + CoASH
$\Delta G^{\circ\prime} = -7.7$ kcal/mol

Citrate → isocitrate
$\Delta G^{\circ\prime} = +1.5$ kcal/mol

31. The standard free energy ($\Delta G^{\circ\prime}$) for each of the reactions in the conversion of malate to isocitrate is shown above. What is the $\Delta G^{\circ\prime}$ (in kcal/mol) for the net conversion of malate to isocitrate?

(A) −13.3
(B) −2.1
(C) −0.9
(D) +0.9
(E) +1.5

32. The equilibrium constant for the net conversion of malate to isocitrate is

(A) 0
(B) greater than 1
(C) less than 1

33. The direct conversion of A to B (shown below)

```
      COO⁻          COO⁻
       |             |
      C = O         C = O
       |             |
      CH₃           CH₂
                     |
                    COO⁻

       A             B
```

(A) occurs in the brain, red blood cells, and liver
(B) occurs during gluconeogenesis and lipogenesis
(C) is catalyzed by an enzyme that is allosterically inhibited by acetyl CoA
(D) requires tetrahydrofolate
(E) decreases the level of TCA cycle intermediates

34. In skeletal muscle, increased hydrolysis of ATP during muscular contraction

(A) decreases the rate of palmitate oxidation to acetyl CoA
(B) decreases the rate of NADH oxidation by the electron transport chain
(C) results in activation of phosphofructokinase-1
(D) results in an increased proton gradient across the inner mitochondrial membrane

35. If a person consumed a chemical that irreversibly inhibited all cytochromes in the electron transport chain

(A) the amount of heat generated from NADH oxidation would increase
(B) the rate of succinate oxidation would not change
(C) ATP could still be generated from the oxidation of NADH by transfer of electrons to O$_2$
(D) death would result from a lack of ATP
(E) an electrochemical potential could still be generated

36. In red blood cells, a pyruvate kinase deficiency would be expected to increase

(A) the lifespan of the cells
(B) the rate of fatty acid oxidation
(C) ATP production
(D) the NADH/NAD$^+$ ratio
(E) the activity of hexokinase

37. A person with a deficiency of muscle phosphorylase would

(A) produce a higher than normal amount of lactate during a brief period of intense exercise (push-ups)
(B) be incapable of performing mild exercise of long duration (a 10-mile walk)
(C) have lower than normal amounts of glycogen in muscle tissue
(D) be less dependent than normal on blood glucose to supply energy for exercise
(E) produce normal amounts of blood glucose in response to increased glucagon

38. In the presence of a drug that inhibits cAMP phosphodiesterase, which of the following enzymes would be phosphorylated and inactive in liver?

(A) Phosphorylase kinase
(B) Pyruvate kinase
(C) Phosphorylase
(D) Protein kinase A

39. In a fasting individual, which of the following conditions stimulates the production of blood glucose by gluconeogenesis?

(A) A decreased supply of substrates
(B) Decreased levels of phosphoenolpyruvate carboxykinase
(C) An increase of the portal blood glucose level above the K$_m$ of glucokinase
(D) A cAMP-mediated inactivation of pyruvate kinase

40. A woman with a lactase deficiency who eats no dairy products

(A) cannot produce mucopolysaccharides that contain galactose
(B) cannot produce lactose during lactation
(C) is likely to suffer from a calcium deficiency
(D) is likely to have high cellular levels of galactose 1-phosphate

41. Which of the following liver enzymes becomes less active when a diabetic person in ketoacidosis is treated with insulin?

(A) Fructose 1,6-bisphosphatase
(B) Pyruvate kinase
(C) Pyruvate dehydrogenase
(D) Phosphofructokinase 1 (PFK1)

42. Which of the following statements about proteoglycans is TRUE?

(A) The polysaccharide chain is not covalently linked to the protein
(B) Short chains of repeating disaccharide units are usually present
(C) Sulfation occurs before the monosaccharides are incorporated into the glucosaminoglycan chain
(D) Deficiencies of lysosomal enzymes cause accumulation of partially degraded products

43. Which of the following statements about the carbohydrate structures of glycoproteins is correct?

(A) They do not contain N-acetylneuraminic acid (NANA)
(B) They are degraded in vivo by mitochondrial enzymes
(C) They require nucleoside triphosphate sugars for their synthesis
(D) They are synthesized in the endoplasmic reticulum (ER) and the Golgi complex
(E) They are found on the inner surface of the cell membrane

44. In cystic fibrosis, the pancreatic ducts become obstructed by viscous mucus. Consequently, digestion of which of the following substances would be most impaired?

(A) Starch
(B) Fat
(C) Lactose
(D) Sucrose

45. A gallstone that blocked the upper part of the bile duct would cause an increase in

(A) the formation of chylomicrons
(B) the recycling of bile salts
(C) the excretion of bile salts
(D) the excretion of fat in the feces

46. A 20-year-old woman with diabetes mellitus was admitted to the hospital in a semiconscious state with fever, nausea, and vomiting. Her breath smelled of acetone. A urine sample was strongly positive for ketone bodies. Which of the following statements about this woman is TRUE?

(A) A blood glucose test would probably show that her blood glucose level was well below 80 mg/dL
(B) An insulin injection would decrease her ketone body production
(C) She should be given a glucose infusion to regain consciousness
(D) Glucagon should be administered to stimulate glycogenolysis and gluconeogenesis in the liver
(E) The acetone was produced by decarboxylation of the ketone body β-hydroxybutyrate

47. De novo fatty acid biosynthesis from cytosolic citrate

(A) requires NADH to provide reducing equivalents
(B) is at a maximum when the blood glucagon:insulin ratio is high
(C) is regulated by an enzyme that contains biotin
(D) yields stearic acid as its major product

48. Which of the following statements about the conversion of glucose to triacylglycerol in the liver is correct?

(A) Malate serves to transport acetyl units across the mitochondrial membrane
(B) Reducing equivalents are provided by the reactions of glycolysis
(C) Reducing equivalents are provided by the malic enzyme (a decarboxylating malate dehydrogenase)
(D) The glycerol moiety can be derived from dihydroxyacetone phosphate (DHAP) but not from blood glycerol
(E) 2-Monoacylglycerol is an intermediate

49. Which of the following statements concerning the liver and adipose cells is correct?

(A) Adipose cells contain glycerol kinase
(B) Liver cells contain a hormone-sensitive lipase
(C) Adipose cells have a transport system for glucose that is not regulated by insulin
(D) Liver cells secrete lipoproteins when blood insulin levels are low
(E) Adipose cells secrete lipoprotein lipase when blood insulin levels are high

50. A woman was told by her physician to go on a low-fat diet. She decided to continue to consume the same number of calories by increasing her carbohydrate intake, while decreasing her fat intake. Which of the following blood lipoprotein levels would be decreased as a consequence of this diet?

(A) VLDL
(B) IDL
(C) LDL
(D) Chylomicrons

51. Hormone-sensitive lipase is activated by elevated levels of

(A) cAMP
(B) ADP
(C) insulin
(D) apoprotein CII

52. A person with Type 1 (insulin-dependent) diabetes mellitus failed to take insulin regularly and was found to have high VLDL levels. As a consequence, which of the following compounds in the blood would be elevated?

(A) Triacylglycerols
(B) Cholesterol
(C) Both triacylglycerols and cholesterol
(D) Lipoprotein lipase

53. Which of the following statements about phosphatidylcholine (PC) is correct?

(A) It can transfer a fatty acyl group to cholesterol
(B) It can be synthesized by methylation of phosphatidylserine
(C) It is not produced in the lung
(D) It requires dietary choline for its synthesis

54. Which of the following statements concerning metabolism of arachidonic acid is TRUE?

(A) It is converted to prostaglandins by a process that is stimulated by aspirin
(B) It is converted to prostaglandins by a process that is stimulated by glucocorticoids
(C) It is produced from thromboxanes and leukotrienes
(D) It is derived from palmitate
(E) It is cleaved from membrane phospholipids by a phospholipase

55. A person with a familial hyperlipidemia caused by a deficiency of LDL receptors was treated with an HMG CoA reductase inhibitor. This drug causes

(A) cellular levels of squalene to increase
(B) cellular levels of HMG CoA to decrease
(C) blood cholesterol levels to decrease
(D) blood triacylglycerol levels to increase
(E) cellular acyl cholesterol acyl transferase (ACAT) activity to increase

56. Which of the following statements concerning bile salts is TRUE?

(A) They are derived from cholesterol in all tissues of the body
(B) They contain ionic groups with a positive charge
(C) They can contain glycine or serine residues
(D) They are secreted in the bile and resorbed in the intestine
(E) They are most effective as detergents below pH 3

57. Which of the following statements about reactions of the urea cycle is TRUE?

(A) Aspartate reacts with ornithine to form citrulline
(B) A total of six high-energy phosphate bonds are cleaved during production of one molecule of urea
(C) *N*-acetylglutamate is a positive allosteric effector of carbamoyl phosphate synthetase I
(D) The enzyme arginase releases fumarate from argininosuccinate
(E) Glutamine is the substrate that directly provides the nitrogen for carbamoyl phosphate synthesis

58. A genetic deficiency of which one of the following enzymes could cause an increase in urinary excretion of citrulline?

(A) Argininosuccinate synthetase
(B) Carbamoyl phosphate synthetase I (CPSI)
(C) Formiminotransferase (FIGLU + FH_4 → glutamate + formimino-FH_4)
(D) Ornithine transcarbamolyase (OTC)

59. After an overnight fast, alanine is converted to glucose in the liver. As a result of this conversion

(A) some alanine nitrogen appears in aspartate
(B) none of the alanine nitrogen appears in NH_4^+
(C) one alanine carbon is lost as CO_2
(D) blood urea nitrogen (BUN) levels decrease

60. De novo creatine synthesis requires

(A) alanine
(B) arginine
(C) AMP
(D) NAD^+
(E) urea

61. The cofactor required for the reaction that produces ornithine from glutamate semialdehyde is

(A) tetrahydrofolate
(B) pyridoxal phosphate
(C) thiamine pyrophosphate
(D) NAD^+
(E) vitamin B_{12}

62. A deficiency of which of the following substances could cause blood levels of homocysteine to decrease?

(A) cystathionine synthetase
(B) *S*-adenosylhomocysteine (SAH) cleaving enzyme (SAH → adenosine + homocysteine)
(C) vitamin B_{12}
(D) folate

63. In a person with phenylketonuria (a deficiency of phenylalanine hydroxylase)

(A) phenylalanine can be replaced by tyrosine in the diet
(B) tyrosine is an essential amino acid, but phenylalanine is not
(C) phenylalanine is an essential amino acid, but tyrosine is not
(D) phenylalanine and tyrosine are both essential amino acids

64. A person consuming a diet deficient in methionine would have decreased levels of *S*-adenosylmethionine and, therefore, decreased synthesis of

(A) creatine from glycine
(B) dTMP from dUMP
(C) alanine from glucose
(D) methylmalonyl CoA from propionyl CoA
(E) hydroxymethylglutaryl CoA from acetoacetyl CoA

65. Which of the following cofactors is required for the synthesis of γ-aminobutyric acid, serotonin, epinephrine, dopamine, and histamine from their respective amino acid precursors?

(A) Tetrahydrobiopterin
(B) Tetrahydrofolate
(C) Pyridoxal phosphate
(D) Thiamine pyrophosphate
(E) Vitamin B_{12}

66. Which of the following statements is TRUE of de novo pyrimidine synthesis but not of de novo purine synthesis?

(A) The base is synthesized while attached to ribose-5-phosphate
(B) One-carbon fragments are donated by folic acid derivatives
(C) Carbamoyl phosphate donates a carbamoyl group
(D) The entire glycine molecule is incorporated into a precursor of the base
(E) Glutamine donates nitrogen that becomes one of the atoms in the ring

67. Allopurinol is a drug that is used to prevent the conversion of

(A) IMP to GMP
(B) adenosine to inosine
(C) xanthine to uric acid
(D) dUMP to dTMP
(E) cytosine to uracil

68. Which of the following changes occurs in hemolytic anemia?

(A) A decrease in the rate of formation of bilirubin diglucuronides in the liver
(B) A decrease in the rate of secretion of bilirubin diglucuronides into the gallbladder
(C) An increase in the amount of bile pigments converted to stercobilin in the intestine
(D) An increase in the amount of hemoglobin in the blood

69. When excessive amounts of iron are present in the diet, the excess iron is stored as

(A) hemoglobin
(B) transferrin
(C) hemosiderin
(D) ferritin

70. The symptoms of a dietary deficiency of niacin (which results in pellagra) will be less severe if the diet has a high content of

(A) tyrosine
(B) tryptophan
(C) thiamine
(D) thymine

71. Which of the following statements about nitrogen metabolism is correct?

(A) Glutamate is produced from α-ketoglutarate by release of ammonia or by transamination
(B) In the degradation of histidine, the intermediate formiminoglutamate (FIGLU) is formed
(C) Alanine can be produced from pyruvate by the action of a dehydratase followed by the action of a transaminase
(D) Vitamin B_{12} can transfer a methyl group to propionyl CoA to form methylmalonyl CoA

72. A 52-year-old patient with a round face, acne, and a large hump on the back of his neck complains that he is too weak to mow his lawn. His fasting blood glucose level is 170 mg/dL (reference range = 80–100 mg/dL); plasma cortisol level, 62 μg/mL (reference range = 3–31 μg/mL); and plasma ACTH level, 0 pg/mL (reference range = 0–100 pg/mL). If the patient's condition is due to a single cause, the most likely diagnosis is

(A) Type 2 (non-insulin dependent) diabetes mellitus
(B) Type 1 (insulin-dependent) diabetes mellitus
(C) a secretory tumor of the anterior pituitary
(D) a secretory tumor of the posterior pituitary
(E) a secretory tumor of the adrenal cortex

73. Women who take oral contraceptives (estrogen for 25 days, accompanied by progesterone for the last 10 days)

(A) produce a normal corpus luteum
(B) ovulate on the 14th day of the cycle
(C) have a peak of estradiol on the 13th day of the cycle
(D) have low levels of follicle stimulating hormone (FSH) and luteinizing hormone (LH)

74. As part of the treatment for hypopituitarism caused by damage to the pituitary during surgery

(A) TSH and ACTH should be given orally
(B) water intake should be restricted to compensate for low vasopressin levels
(C) thyroxine tablets should be prescribed and taken regularly by the patient
(D) cortisol should be administered daily except during periods of increased stress
(E) estrogen and progesterone are the only hormones needed by women who wish to remain fertile

75. A woman whose thyroid gland was surgically removed was treated daily with 0.10 mg of thyroxine (tablet form). After 3 months of treatment, her serum TSH levels were constant at 6 MIU/mL (reference range of 0.3–5 MIU/mL). She complained of fatigue, weight gain, and hoarseness. Her dose of thyroid hormone should

(A) be increased
(B) be decreased
(C) remain the same

76. In heart cells deprived of oxygen during a myocardial infarction

(A) the mitochondrial proton pump slows down, preventing ATP synthesis by oxidative phosphorylation
(B) the citric acid cycle will accelerate to provide more electrons for ATP synthesis
(C) the electron transport chain will accelerate to provide more protons for ATP synthesis
(D) anaerobic glycolysis will decrease, and the conversion of glucose to CO_2 will increase
(E) product inhibition by NADH and ADP will slow many of the reactions in the citric acid cycle

Directions: Each group of items in this section consists of lettered options followed by a set of numbered items. For each item, select the **one** lettered option that is most closely associated with it. Each lettered option may be selected once, more than once, or not at all.

Questions 77–80

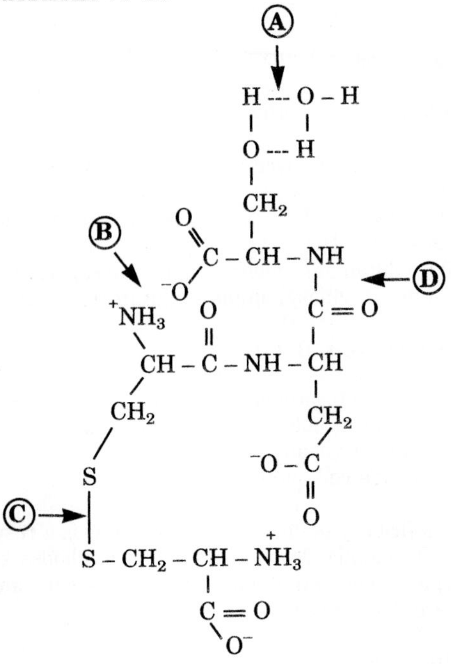

Match the circled letters in the structure shown above with the appropriate type of bond or interaction.

77. Hydrogen bond
78. Electrostatic interaction
79. Disulfide bond
80. Peptide bond

Questions 81–84

(A) Higher
(B) Lower
(C) The same

Indicate whether the blood levels of the compounds below would be higher, lower, or the same in a person with Type 1 (insulin-dependent) diabetes mellitus (DM) who fails to take insulin for 2 days compared with a normal person who has just finished dinner.

81. Glucose
82. Glucagon
83. Urea
84. Ketone bodies

Questions 85–90

(A) rRNA
(B) tRNA
(C) mRNA
(D) hnRNA
(E) DNA

Match each property below with the appropriate type of nucleic acid.

85. Contains a CCA sequence to which an amino acid is attached
86. Is replicated only during the S phase of the cell cycle
87. Is synthesized mainly in the nucleolus of the cell
88. Interacts with histones to form nucleosomes
89. Is found only in the nucleus
90. Contains A-T base pairs

Questions 91–93

(A) UTP
(B) dTTP
(C) ATP
(D) GTP
(E) dUTP

Match each description with the appropriate nucleotide.

91. A precursor that adds nucleotides to growing DNA chains
92. Substrate from which the tail at the 3′ end of mRNA is produced
93. Substrate for the cap structure of hnRNA

Questions 94–96

(A) eIF-2
(B) EF-2
(C) EF-1
(D) Peptidyl transferase

Match each description below with the appropriate component of the translation process in eukaryotes.

94. Required for translocation during protein synthesis
95. Required during the initiation of protein synthesis
96. Required for binding of methionyl-tRNA to codon 36 of an mRNA

Questions 97–99

(A) Initiation
(B) Binding of aminoacyl-tRNA to the "A" site on the ribosome
(C) Peptide bond formation
(D) Translocation

Match each antibiotic below with the appropriate step in translation that it inhibits in prokaryotes.

97. Tetracycline
98. Streptomycin
99. Erythromycin

Questions 100–103

(A) Glucose
(B) Galactose
(C) Fructose
(D) Glucose and galactose
(E) Glucose, galactose, and fructose

The blood levels of glucose, galactose, and fructose were measured in normal persons and in persons with various enzyme deficiencies soon after they drank a milkshake made with milk and sugar. Match each comparison below with the appropriate sugar(s).

100. Lower in the blood of a person with a lactase deficiency than in a normal person
101. Higher in the blood of a person with a galactose 1-phosphate uridyl transferase deficiency than in a normal person
102. Higher in the blood of a person with a fructokinase deficiency than in a normal person
103. Higher in the blood of a person with an aldolase B deficiency than in a normal person

Questions 104–106

(A) Thiamine pyrophosphate
(B) NAD^+
(C) $NADP^+$
(D) Biotin

Match each enzyme below with its required cofactor.

104. Malate dehydrogenase
105. Transketolase
106. Glucose 6-phosphate dehydrogenase

Questions 107–109

(A) Heme
(B) Purines
(C) Pyrimidines
(D) Urea

Each reaction below is the first step in a biosynthetic pathway. In each case, select the final end product of the pathway.

107. Glycine + succinyl CoA $\rightarrow$ δ-aminolevulinic acid + CoASH + CO_2
108. CO_2 + NH_4^+ + 2 ATP $\rightarrow$ carbamoyl phosphate + 2 ADP + P_i
109. Glutamine + phosphoribosyl pyrophosphate $\rightarrow$ phosphoribosyl amine + glutamate + PP_i

Questions 110–115

(A) Megaloblastic anemia
(B) Hypochromic, microcytic anemia
(C) Hemolytic anemia
(D) Sickle cell anemia

A deficiency of each substance below can result in an anemia. For each substance, choose the type of anemia that would occur if the substance were deficient.

110. Iron
111. Intrinsic factor
112. Pyridoxine
113. B_{12}
114. Folate
115. NADPH

Questions 116–120

(A) Increased MB fraction of serum creatine kinase (CK)
(B) Increased blood ketone bodies
(C) Decreased creatinine in the urine
(D) Decreased blood lactate
(E) Decreased blood urea nitrogen (BUN)

For each untreated condition below, select the blood or urine value that best distinguishes that condition from the others. All values are measured after an overnight fast and are compared with those of a normal individual.

116. Type 1 (insulin-dependent) diabetes mellitus (DM)
117. Myocardial infarction
118. Hepatitis
119. Renal failure
120. Alcoholism

Questions 121–123

(A) LH
(B) FSH
(C) GH
(D) ACTH

Match each description below with the most appropriate hormone.

121. Is encoded by the proopiomelanocortin (POMC) gene
122. Stimulates testosterone production
123. Causes acromegaly when secreted in excessive amounts in adults

Questions 124–126

(A) Oxytocin
(B) Aldosterone
(C) Vasopressin
(D) Prolactin

Match each biologic activity below with the appropriate hormone.

124. Increases sodium and water resorption by renal tubule cells
125. Causes synthesis of α-lactalbumin
126. Causes uterine contractions

Questions 127–130

(A) High prolactin (PRL)
(B) High thyroid stimulating hormone (TSH)
(C) High cortisol
(D) Low growth hormone (GH)
(E) Low aldosterone

Each pathologic condition below can be associated with one of the blood hormone levels listed above. For each condition, choose the most appropriate hormone.

127. Hypothyroidism caused by a viral infection of the thyroid gland
128. Elevated levels of somatostatin
129. Low levels of dopamine produced by the hypothalamus
130. Hypotension

Questions 131–135

(A) Ketone bodies
(B) Blood glucose
(C) Fatty acids
(D) Glycogen
(E) Alanine

For each condition below, choose the major fuel that is being used.

131. By the brain after 1 day of fasting.
132. By red blood cells following an overnight fast.
133. By the liver after 2 days of fasting.
134. By the brain after 1 week of fasting.
135. By the chest muscles used during weight lifting.

Questions 136–138

(A) Higher
(B) Lower
(C) The same

Indicate whether the blood levels of the compounds below (following an overnight fast) would be higher, lower, or the same in a person with a carnitine deficiency compared with a normal person.

136. Fatty acids
137. Ketone bodies
138. Glucose

Questions 139–142

(A) Chylomicrons
(B) VLDL
(C) LDL
(D) HDL
(E) Fatty acid-albumin complexes

Match each description below with the appropriate lipid-protein complex.

139. The major donor of cholesterol to peripheral tissues
140. The first lipoprotein to increase in concentration in the blood after ingestion of 400 g of jelly beans (carbohydrate)
141. The site of the LCAT reaction
142. Composed mainly of triacylglycerols synthesized in intestinal epithelial cells

Questions 143–147

(A) Glycogen
(B) Collagen
(C) Dopamine
(D) Valine
(E) A sphingolipid

Each condition below can be caused by a problem with the metabolism of a particular compound. Match each condition with the appropriate compound.

143. Ehlers-Danlos syndrome
144. Parkinson's disease
145. Tay-Sachs disease
146. McArdle's disease
147. Maple syrup urine disease

Questions 148–151

(A) Vitamin C
(B) Niacin
(C) Vitamin D
(D) Biotin
(E) Thiamine

A dietary deficiency of a vitamin can cause each of the conditions below. Match each condition with the appropriate vitamin.

148. Pellagra
149. Scurvy
150. Beriberi
151. Rickets

Answers and Explanations

1–A. Fat contains 9 calories per gram, whereas carbohydrate contains 4 calories per gram. Therefore, when the patient substituted 50 g of fat for 50 g of carbohydrate, he took in more calories per day and gained weight.

2–B. The patient's weight (176 lb × 0.454 lb per kg) is 80 kg. Since the basal metabolic rate (BMR) is approximately 24 kcal/kg/day, her BMR (24 kcal/kg/day × 80 kg) is 1920 kcal/day. She requires 30% more calories for her activity (sedentary) or 1920 × 1.3 = 2500 kcal.

3–E. Although niacin is a vitamin, it can be synthesized to a limited extent from tryptophan.

4–C. Lysine is a strictly ketogenic amino acid; it cannot be used to produce glucose. Glycogen is used within the muscle to produce ATP for muscle contraction. Glycerol from adipose triglycerol stores is a substrate for gluconeogenesis, whereas even-chain fatty acids are not. They produce acetyl CoA, which cannot be used to produce net glucose.

5–D. Galactose is converted to glucose-1-P from which glucose-6-P is formed. Glucose-6-P is cleaved by glucose 6-phosphatase to form blood glucose. Lactate and fructose require fructose 1,6-bisphosphatase to form blood glucose. Muscle glycogen does not produce blood glucose.

6–E. Both fructose and galactose can be converted to blood glucose in the absence of phosphoenolpyruvate carboxykinase, but this enzyme is required for conversion of lactate to blood glucose. Muscle glycogen is not converted to blood glucose.

7–C. The pH and pK are related as follows: $pH = pK + \log([A^-]/[HA])$. Thus, when the concentrations of a weak acid and its base are equal, the pH equals the pK.

8–C. HMG CoA is not formed from glutamic acid, but from acetyl CoA and acetoacetyl CoA. It is also formed by degradation of leucine (but not valine) in muscle. It is cleaved to form acetyl CoA and the ketone body acetoacetate. It is reduced to mevalonic acid in cholesterol biosynthesis.

9–E. According to the Michaelis-Menten equation, the velocity (v) is related to the concentration of substrate, [X], as follows: $v = V_m[X]/(K_m + [X])$. Thus, $4 = (10 \times 2)/(K_m + 2)$. $4 K_m + 8 = 20$. $4 K_m = 20 - 8 = 12$. $K_m = 12/4 = 3 \, \mu M$.

10–D. The Y intercept ($1/V_m$) is the same for the normal enzyme and the patient's enzyme, thus the enzymes have the same V_m. However, the X intercepts ($-1/K_m$) differ. The normal enzyme has a K_m of 1 μM, whereas the patient's enzyme has a K_m of 5 μM. Therefore, more thiamine pyrophosphate is required to saturate the patient's enzyme, and raising the body levels of thiamine should cause more of the patient's enzyme to be in the active complex.

11–A. Acetyl CoA, which contains pantothenic acid as part of its coenzyme A moiety, is a substrate for citrate synthase.

12–D. Red blood cells use glucose (via glycolysis) as their only energy source because they do not have an active tricarboxylic acid (TCA) cycle; they lack mitochondria. The other tissues have mitochondria and can use other fuels.

13–C. Hemoglobin contains two α chains and two β chains, which combine to form the quaternary structure. Each mole of subunit binds 1 mole of heme, which binds 1 mole of O_2. Therefore, 1 mole of HbA binds 4 moles of O_2. In the β chain of HbS, valine replaces glutamate at position 6, thus HbS is more hydrophobic than HbA.

14–B. Hydroxylation of lysine and proline residues requires vitamin C and occurs after these amino acids have been incorporated into the polypeptide chain but before secretion from the cell. Oxidation of hydroxylysine residues results in the formation of cross-links between collagen molecules, causing polymerization.

15–C. After an overnight fast, fatty acids are released from adipose tissue, oxidized by muscle (but not the brain), and converted to ketone bodies in the liver. Glucose is not synthesized from even-chain fatty acids, and ketone bodies are not oxidized by red blood cells because they lack mitochondria.

16–C. A, B, and E occur in prokaryotes, not eukaryotes. 80S ribosomes are utilized in eukaryotes. During synthesis of proteins that are secreted, the ribosomes are attached to the RER. Peptidyl transferase is required.

17–D. hnRNA contains sequences (introns) that are removed to produce mRNA. UAG and UAA are both stop codons. Some genes occur in multiple copies within the genome. Gene sequences may undergo rearrangement in germ cells as they differentiate (e.g., during development of immunoglobulin-producing cells).

18–C. The mutant gene has a four-base insertion (TATC) starting at position 9. Consequently, a frameshift occurs, and the mutant gene encodes a protein with a different amino acid sequence beyond this point. The insertion causes the sequence TGA at position 22 to come into frame. This corresponds with UGA, a termination codon in the mRNA. Therefore, the mutant protein will be shorter than the normal protein. Although AGA is a codon for arginine, another codon for arginine (CGU) is used in this sequence.

19–A. Transcription is catalyzed by RNA polymerase II, which binds to proteins attached to a promoter region that includes a TATA box. The DNA template strand is not covalently bound to histones. The primary transcript (hnRNA) is capped at the 5′ end and polyadenylated at the 3′ end; introns are removed by splicing to form mRNA.

20–B. In the absence of glucose and the presence of lactose, the *lac* repressor will be inactive, cAMP levels will rise, and CAP protein will bind to the *lac* promoter stimulating transcription of the operon. Tryptophan levels in the cell will be low, thus the repressor for the *trp* operon will be inactive and the operon will be transcribed by RNA polymerase. Attenuation of transcription of this operon will decrease.

21–E. In base excision repair, the damaged base is first removed by a glycosylase. Then an endonuclease cleaves the AP site. Nucleotides are removed and replaced by a DNA polymerase, and DNA ligase seals the repaired region to the rest of the DNA strand. Reverse transcriptase uses an RNA template to synthesize DNA. It is not involved in repair.

22–D. The gene sequence is read 5′ to 3′ from the bottom to the top of the gel. The normal and mutant sequences are the same except for a point mutation that converted an A to a T. Thus, the mutant gene contains the sequence 5′-GAATTC-3′, which is cleaved by *Eco* RI, but the normal gene does not. *Kpnl* would not cleave within the sequences shown on the gels. *Kpn1* was used to cleave these two sequences from larger fragments of DNA.

23–D. Okazaki fragments are synthesized on the lagging strand in the 5′ to 3′ direction, moving away from the replication fork and copying the parental DNA strand in the 3′ to 5′ direction. Synthesis starts with an RNA primer to which DNA precursors are attached. The RNA is subsequently removed and replaced with DNA, and the fragments are joined by a ligase. A group of enzymes, not just DNA polymerase, is involved in this process.

24–C. During glycolysis, dihydroxyacetone phosphate (Compound I) is isomerized to glyceraldehyde 3-phosphate, which is oxidized to 1,3-bisphosphoglycerate in a reaction in which inorganic phosphate and NAD^+ are utilized. Then 3-phosphoglycerate (Compound II) is formed as ATP is generated.

25–B. Blood glucose is maintained after about 2 hours of fasting by glycogenolysis, which is subsequently supplemented by gluconeogenesis. However, after about 1 day of fasting, liver glycogen is depleted, so thereafter, gluconeogenesis is solely responsible for maintaining blood glucose.

26–C. After an overnight fast, glycogenolysis and gluconeogenesis act to maintain blood glucose levels in a normal person. Both pathways produce glucose 6-phosphate and require glucose 6-phosphatase to produce free glucose. If the phosphatase is inhibited, blood glucose levels will be lower and liver glycogen stores higher than normal. (When glucose 6-phosphatase is genetically deficient, a similar set of circumstances occurs, and the individual has a glycogen storage disease–von Gierke's disease.)

27–B. Because there are two copies (alleles) of this gene in the genome, two fragments containing this gene are produced from each person. These two restriction fragments have a different number of tandem repeats; one fragment is inherited from the mother and the other from the father. The child received the 9-kb fragment from the mother. An 8.5-kb fragment could only have come from F2; therefore, he is most likely to be the father.

28–D. Almost all fatty acids can undergo β-oxidation, resulting in release of acetyl CoA, which can be converted to ketone bodies (but not glucose) in the liver. The oxidation pathway contains a C2-C3 enoyl intermediate. In most tissues, but not the brain and red blood cells, fatty acids are a major source of energy.

29–A. Pancreatic lipase catalyzes the breakdown of dietary triacylglycerols into free fatty acids and 2-monoacylglycerols, an essential step in the digestion of dietary lipids. Since prostaglandins are produced from linoleate, an essential fatty acid found in the triacylglycerols of dietary plants (or plant oils), a deficiency of pancreatic lipase would eventually cause a prostaglandin deficiency. Bicarbonate from the pancreas raises the intestinal pH, and bile salts aid in micelle formation.

30–A. When oxygen is depleted, the electron transport chain stops; NADH builds up; and the TCA cycle is inhibited. Therefore succinate, an intermediate of the cycle, will not be oxidized. In the absence of oxygen, no ATP is produced.

31–D. For a series of coupled reactions, the individual $\Delta G^{\circ\prime}$ values may be added to give the value of $\Delta G^{\circ\prime}$ for the overall reaction.

32–C. $\Delta G^{\circ\prime} = -2.303\ RT \log K_{eq}$. For the conversion of isocitrate to malate, $\Delta G^{\circ\prime} = +0.9$ and $\log K_{eq}$ is negative. Therefore, K_{eq} is less than 1.

33–B. Pyruvate carboxylase, which converts pyruvate (A) to oxaloacetate (B), is found in brain and liver but not in red blood cells or muscle. It is involved in the synthesis of glucose and fatty acids. It is activated by acetyl CoA and requires biotin and ATP. It is an anaplerotic reaction of the TCA cycle (i.e., it produces a four-carbon intermediate of the cycle).

34–C. A decrease in the concentration of ATP stimulates processes that generate ATP. The proton gradient across the inner mitochondrial membrane decreases; NADH oxidation by the electron transport chain increases; and fuel utilization increases. Palmitate is oxidized, and glycolysis increases because of activation of phosphofructokinase-1 by AMP. As ATP decreases, AMP rises (ATP $\rightarrow$ P_i + ADP. 2ADP $\rightarrow$ ATP + AMP).

35–D. If the cytochromes are inhibited, ATP production, the electrochemical potential, heat production from NADH oxidation, and succinate oxidation all decrease.

36–D. The step in glycolysis catalyzed by pyruvate kinase normally produces ATP and pyruvate. A pyruvate kinase deficiency would slow glycolysis, and less ATP would be produced. The NADH/NAD$^+$ ratio would rise because less pyruvate would be available for conversion to lactate (the reaction in which NADH is converted back to NAD$^+$). Intermediates of glycolysis before the blocked step would accumulate, and glucose 6-phosphate would inhibit hexokinase. Because of a lack of ATP, the lifespan of the cells would decrease. Fatty acids cannot serve as a source of energy because these cells lack mitochondria.

37–E. In the glycogen storage disease caused by a muscle phosphorylase deficiency (McArdle's disease), muscle glycogen could not be oxidized during exercise. Therefore, lactate levels would be low, and the person could not tolerate intense exercise of brief duration and would rely on fuels from the blood (glucose, fatty acids, and ketone bodies) for energy. The person could engage in mild exercise of long duration, using these blood fuels. The liver would not be affected because it contains a different phosphorylase isozyme. Liver could still respond to glucagon by breaking down glycogen.

38–B. Under these conditions, cAMP levels would remain elevated. Phosphorylation of pyruvate kinase causes its inactivation. Phosphorylase kinase and phosphorylase are activated by phosphorylation. Protein kinase A is not regulated by phosphorylation but by dissociation of inhibitory subunits that bind to cAMP.

39–D. A, B, and C would result in decreased glucose production. cAMP via protein kinase A causes inactivation of pyruvate kinase and, thus, promotes glucose production.

40–C. Lactase is a digestive enzyme that cleaves lactose to galactose and glucose. However, galactose is not required in the diet. It can be produced from glucose and would be metabolized normally in this woman. Because of her low intake of dairy products, she might develop a calcium deficiency and would have low levels of galactose 1-phosphate.

41–A. Insulin stimulates activation of pyruvate kinase, pyruvate dehydrogenase, and phosphofructokinase 2 (PFK2). PFK2 then catalyzes formation of fructose 2,6-bisphosphate, which is an activator of PFK1 and an inhibitor of fructose 1,6-bisphosphatase, a gluconeogenic enzyme.

42–D. The glycosaminoglycans (mucopolysaccharides) of proteoglycans contain long chains of repeating disaccharide units that are covalently linked to a protein. Sulfation occurs after the monosaccharides are incorporated into the glycosaminoglycan chain. Proteoglycans are degraded by lysosomal enzymes. Deficiencies of these enzymes result in diseases known as mucopolysaccharidoses.

43–D. The carbohydrates present in glycoproteins are synthesized from UDP-sugars and CMP-NANA. Synthesis occurs in the ER and Golgi complex. Glycoproteins are secreted from cells, targeted to lysosomes, or incorporated into cell membranes (with the carbohydrate portion located on the outer surface). They are degraded by lysosomal enzymes.

44–B. Lactose and sucrose are digested by disaccharidases on the brush border of intestinal epithelial cells. Starch is digested by salivary and pancreatic α-amylase. Therefore, its digestion would be less affected by a lack of pancreatic juice than fat, which is digested mainly by pancreatic lipase. A common finding in cystic fibrosis is steatorrhea (fatty stools).

45–D. In this situation, bile salts could not enter the digestive tract. Therefore, recycling and excretion of bile salts, digestion of fats, and formation of chylomicrons would all decrease. As a consequence, fat in the feces would increase (steatorrhea).

46–B. The acetone on her breath (produced from decarboxylation of acetoacetate) and the ketone bodies in her urine indicate that she is in diabetic ketoacidosis (DKA). Her blood glucose levels would be high because her insulin levels are too low to stimulate glucose transport into muscle and adipose tissue and to stimulate glycogen and triacylglycerol synthesis in the liver. An insulin injection would reduce her blood glucose levels and decrease the release of fatty acids from adipose triacylglycerols. Consequently, ketone body production would decrease. Glucagon administration would make her condition worse by increasing her blood glucose and ketone body levels.

47–C. Fatty acid synthesis is maximal in the fed state when insulin is elevated. Glucose is converted to citrate, which moves from the mitochondrion to the cytosol, where it is cleaved to oxaloacetate and acetyl CoA. The regulatory enzyme acetyl CoA carboxylase requires biotin and converts acetyl CoA to malonyl CoA, which provides the two-carbon units for elongation of the fatty acyl chain by the fatty acid synthase complex. NADPH provides reducing equivalents. The major product is palmitate.

48–C. Citrate transports acetyl units from the mitochondrion to the cytosol. NADPH is provided by the pentose phosphate pathway and the malic enzyme. The liver has glycerol kinase, thus blood glycerol can be used. Phosphatidic acid is an intermediate. 2-Monoacylglycerol is produced only in intestinal cells.

49–E. Adipose cells lack glyceron kinase but have a hormone-sensitive lipase. The glucose transport system of adipose cells (and muscle) is stimulated by insulin. When insulin levels are elevated, liver cells secrete very low density lipoprotein (VLDL) and adipose cells secrete lipoprotein lipase, which cleaves the triacylglycerols of chylomicrons and VLDL.

50–D. Chylomicrons are blood lipoproteins produced from dietary fat. VLDL are produced mainly from dietary carbohydrate. IDL and LDL are produced from VLDL.

51–A. The hormone-sensitive lipase of adipose tissue is activated by glucagon via a cAMP-mediated process. Apoprotein CII is the activator of lipoprotein lipase.

52–C. VLDL levels are elevated because the decreased insulin and increased glucagon cause lipolysis of adipose triacylglycerols. The fatty acids and glycerol are repackaged in VLDL, which are secreted by the liver. Therefore, both triacylglycerols and cholesterol are elevated in the blood. Lipoprotein lipase is decreased because its synthesis and secretion by adipose tissue are stimulated by insulin.

53–A. In the absence of dietary choline, PC can be synthesized de novo from glucose. The last step in this pathway involves methylation of phosphatidylethanolamine by SAM. As dipalmitoylphosphatidylcholine, PC serves as a major component of lung surfactant. PC, also called lecithin, transfers a fatty acyl group in the LCAT reaction that occurs in HDL and produces cholesterol esters.

54–E. Arachidonic acid is cleaved from membrane phospholipids by phospholipase A_2, which is inhibited by glucocorticoids. It requires essential fatty acids for its synthesis. It can be converted to leukotrienes, or it can be oxidized by a cyclooxygenase (which is inhibited by aspirin) and converted to prostaglandins and thromboxanes.

55–C. Reduction of HMG CoA to mevalonic acid is an early step in cholesterol synthesis. Inhibition of this step would lead to an increase in cellular levels of HMG CoA and a decrease in squalene (an intermediate beyond this step) and cholesterol. The decreased cholesterol levels in cells cause ACAT activity to decrease and synthesis of LDL receptors to increase. More receptors cause more LDL to be taken up from the blood. Consequently, blood cholesterol levels decrease, but blood triacylglycerol levels do not decrease much, since LDL does not contain much triacylglycerol.

56–D. Bile salts are synthesized from cholesterol only in the liver. Glycine or taurine is conjugated to the carboxyl group on the side chain. Ionization occurs with a pK of about 4 for the glycoconjugates and 2 for the tauroconjugates. Above the pK, they carry a negative charge and are most effective as detergents. Bile salts are secreted in the bile, participate in lipid digestion, are resorbed in the ileum, and are recycled by the liver.

57–C. In the urea cycle, ammonia provides the nitrogen for synthesis of carbamoyl phosphate, which reacts with ornithine to form citrulline. Aspartate reacts with citrulline to form argininosuccinate, which releases fumarate. The product arginine is cleaved by arginase to form urea and regenerate ornithine. Overall, four high-energy phosphate bonds are cleaved. Carbamoyl phosphate synthetase I is activated by *N*-acetylglutamate.

58–A. If argininosuccinate synthetase activity is low, less citrulline will be converted to argininosuccinate than normal. Citrulline levels will rise, and citrulline will be excreted in the urine. A deficiency of CPSI or OTC would lead to decreased citrulline levels. A deficiency of formininotransferase would lead to increased FIGLU in the urine.

59–A. During fasting, all the carbons of alanine are converted to glucose in the liver, and the nitrogens of alanine are converted to urea. A transamination reaction transfers alanine nitrogen to glutamate. This nitrogen can be transaminated and can appear in aspartate or, via glutamate dehydrogenase, in NH_4^+. BUN rises during fasting.

60–B. Creatine is synthesized from glycine, the guanidinium group of arginine, and the methyl group of methionine.

61–B. Glutamate semialdehyde is transaminated to form ornithine. Glutamate provides the nitrogen and is converted to α-ketoglutarate. The cofactor for transamination is pyridoxal phosphate.

62–B. Homocysteine is produced when *S*-adenosylhomocysteine (SAH) releases adenosine. Homocysteine is used in the synthesis of cystathionine. Homocysteine accepts a methyl group (from FH_4 via vitamin B_{12}) to form methionine. If the enzyme that cleaves adenosine from SAH is deficient, homocysteine levels will decrease. The other deficiencies would lead to increased levels of homocysteine. Elevated levels are associated with atherosclerotic vascular disease.

63–D. Tyrosine is produced by hydroxylation of the essential amino acid phenylalanine. In phenylketonuria, tyrosine cannot be synthesized in adequate amounts and is required in the diet.

64–A. S-Adenosylmethionine (SAM) provides a methyl group for the synthesis of creatine. It is not involved in the other reactions.

65–C. In the synthesis of each of these compounds, a decarboxylation of an amino acid occurs. Amino acid decarboxylation reactions, as well as transaminations, require pyridoxal phosphate.

66–C. In pyrimidine biosynthesis, carbamoyl phosphate, produced from glutamine, CO_2, and ATP, reacts with aspartate to form a base which, after oxidation, reacts with phosphoribosyl pyrophosphate (PRPP) to form a nucleotide. This nucleotide is decarboxylated to form UMP. After reduction of the sugar, dUMP reacts with 5,10-methylenetetrahydrofolate to produce dTMP. In purine biosynthesis, the base is produced on ribose-5-phosphate. Glycine is incorporated into the precursor, and tetrahydrofolate derivatives donate carbons 2 and 8. Glutamine is a nitrogen donor for both purine and pyrimidine biosynthesis.

67–C. Xanthine oxidase is involved in the conversion of the purine bases to uric acid. It catalyzes the oxidation of hypoxanthine to xanthine and of xanthine to uric acid. Allopurinol is used in the treatment of gout, which is caused by the precipitation of uric acid crystals in the joints.

68–C. When red blood cells are destroyed (e.g., by lysis or by phagocytosis), hemoglobin is degraded. Bilirubin is produced from heme at an increased rate. The liver converts bilirubin to the diglucuronide at a rapid rate and excretes it into the bile. In the intestine, bacteria convert bilirubin to stercobilins, which give stool its brown color.

69–C. Iron is normally carried in the blood on transferrin and stored mainly in the liver and spleen as ferritin. If an abnormally large amount of iron is present, hemosiderin is produced. Hemoglobin, which contains iron complexed with heme, is not a storage form of iron.

70–B. Although dietary niacin is the major source of the nicotinamide ring of NAD, it may also be produced from tryptophan.

71–B. Glutamate is produced from α-ketoglutarate by addition of ammonia via glutamate dehydrogenase or by transamination. Histidine produces FIGLU, which forms glutamate. Alanine is produced by transamination of pyruvate; a dehydratase is not required. Vitamin B_{12} is involved in the rearrangement of methylmalonyl CoA to form succinyl CoA.

72–E. ACTH levels were low, thus the elevated cortisol levels were most likely caused by a secretory tumor of the adrenal cortex. The elevated cortisol levels caused the elevation of blood glucose.

73–D. The constant low levels of estrogen provided by use of oral contraceptives prevent the release of FSH (which normally would cause the egg to mature) and of LH (which normally would cause ovulation and maintenance of the corpus luteum). On low levels of estrogen, estradiol does not peak; ovulation does not occur; and a corpus luteum is not produced.

74–C. Thyroxine can be taken orally to compensate for low TSH levels. TSH and ACTH are polypeptide hormones; therefore, they would be digested by pancreatic proteases in the gut. Low vasopressin causes water to be lost in the urine (diabetes insipidus); thus water intake should be increased. Cortisol is required particularly during stress. GnRH, FSH, and LH are required for the production of a mature egg. Estrogen and progesterone, taken alone, will suppress ovulation.

75–A. Thyroid hormone feeds back on the anterior pituitary and inhibits the release of TSH. This patient's TSH levels are elevated, thus her thyroid hormone levels are too low, and her dose should be increased.

76–A. A lack of O_2 causes a slowing of the proton pump, and ATP synthesis decreases. The electron transport chain, the citric acid cycle, and the conversion of glucose to CO_2 all decrease. NADH slows the citric acid cycle, but ADP allosterically activates isocitrate dehydrogenase, stimulating the cycle.

77–A. The hydroxyl group of serine forms hydrogen bonds with water.

78–B. A positively charged amino group (on a cysteine residue) and a negatively charged carboxyl group (on a serine residue) form an electrostatic interaction.

79–C. Two cysteine residues are covalently joined by a disulfide bond.

80–D. In peptides, adjacent amino acids are joined covalently by peptide bonds.

81–A. A person with Type 1 diabetes mellitus (DM) who is not taking insulin behaves metabolically like a person who is fasting, except that glucose levels are elevated. The low insulin levels cause decreased transport of glucose into muscle and adipose cells, decreased conversion of glucose to glycogen and triacylglycerols in liver, and increased production of glucose by the liver via glycogenolysis and glyconeogenesis.

82–A. As insulin decreases, glucagon rises and stimulates glycogenolysis and gluconeogenesis.

83–A. When insulin is low and glucagon is high, the carbon skeletons of amino acids derived from muscle protein are converted to glucose in the liver by gluconeogenesis. The amino acid nitrogen is converted to urea.

84–A. When the insulin:glucagon ratio is low, fatty acids are released from adipose tissue and converted to ketone bodies by the liver.

85–B. A CCA sequence which carries the amino acid, is present at the 3′ end of tRNA.

86–E. DNA is replicated during S phase.

87–A. All species of rRNA are produced in the nucleolus except 5S rRNA, which is produced in the nucleoplasm.

88–E. Approximately 140 base pairs of DNA are wrapped around a core of histones to form a nucleosome.

89–D. hnRNA is produced in the nucleus and converted to mRNA, which migrates to the cytoplasm. DNA is found in the nucleus and in mitochondria.

90–E. A-T pairs are found in DNA. RNA contains A-U base pairs. Both DNA and RNA contain G-C base pairs.

91–B. The deoxyribonucleoside triphosphates dTTP, dATP, dGTP, and dCTP are the precursors for elongation of DNA chains.

92–C. The poly (A) tail of mRNA is produced from ATP.

93–D. GTP is the substrate for the cap of hnRNA (and, therefore, mRNA).

94–B. Elongation factor 2 (EF-2) is required for translocation.

95–A. Eukaryotic initiation factors (e.g., eIF-2) re required for initiation.

96–C. Although initiation factors are required for binding of the methionyl-tRNA that initiates synthesis of a polypeptide chain, internal methionine residues require the elongation factors for their incorporation into growing polypeptide chains. EF-1 is required for binding of aminoacyl-tRNA to the appropriate codon on mRNA.

97–B. Tetracycline prevents aminoacyl-tRNA from binding.

98–A. Streptomycin prevents formation of the initiation complex.

99–D. Erythromycin prevents translocation.

100–D. Galactose and glucose would be lower in a person with a lactase deficiency, because lactose in the milk would not be cleaved to produce galactose and glucose.

101–B. Galactose would be higher, because in classic galactosemia (uridyl transferase deficiency), galactose can be phosphorylated but it cannot be metabolized further. Galactose 1-phosphate and its precursor, galactose, increase.

102–C. Fructose derived from the table sugar (sucrose) would not be converted to fructose 1-phosphate, thus it accumulates in the blood and is excreted in the urine, producing a benign fructosuria.

103–C. An aldolase B deficiency (fructose intolerance) results in a decreased ability to cleave fructose-1-P. This compound increases in liver cells and its precursor, fructose, increases in the blood.

104–B. NAD^+ is required for the conversion of malate to oxaloacetate.

105–A. The transketolase of the pentose phosphate pathway requires thiamine pyrophosphate.

106–C. Glucose 6-phosphate dehydrogenase, the first enzyme in the pentose phosphate pathway, requires $NADP^+$.

107–A. Heme.

108–D. Urea.

109–B. Purines.

110–B. An iron deficiency anemia is characterized by small, pale red blood cells.

111–A. Intrinsic factor is required for the absorption of dietary vitamin B_{12}. Lack of B_{12} (or folate) results in a megaloblastic anemia. In a B_{12} deficiency, irreversible neurologic problems (due to demyelination) also occur. When decreased intrinsic factor causes a B_{12} deficiency, the condition is called pernicious anemia.

112–B. Pyridoxine is required for formation of pyridoxal phosphate, the cofactor for the first reaction in heme formation.

113–A. A B_{12} deficiency results in a megaloblastic anemia plus demyelination of nerves.

114–A. Folate deficiency results in a megaloblastic anemia because of decreased production of purines and the pyrimidine thymine. Thus, lack of folate causes decreased DNA synthesis. In contrast with a B_{12} deficiency, neurologic problems do not occur in a folate deficiency.

115–C. Deficiency of glucose 6-phosphate dehydrogenase results in decreased production of NADPH by the pentose phosphate pathway during oxidative stress. Components of cell membranes are oxidized, and a hemolytic anemia results.

116–B. In the absence of insulin, a person with Type 1 diabetes mellitus (DM) will behave metabolically like a person undergoing prolonged starvation, except that blood glucose levels will be elevated. Lipolysis in adipose tissue will produce fatty acids, which will be converted to ketone bodies in the liver.

117–A. CK is found in large amounts in muscle cells. When a tissue is damaged, cellular enzymes leak into the blood. Heart muscle has more of the MB isozyme of CK than skeletal muscle (which contains mainly the MM isozyme). (Brain has the BB isozyme.)

118–E. Urea is made in the liver. If the liver is infected, less urea will be produced and the blood urea nitrogen will decrease. Consequently, ammonia levels will increase.

119–C. The kidney excretes nitrogenous waste products, including urea, ammonia, creatinine, and uric acid. If the kidneys fail, these waste products will not be excreted into the urine.

Index

Page references in *italics* denote figures; those followed by "t" denote tables

143–B. A defect in the synthesis or processing of collagen causes Ehlers-Danlos syndrome.

144–C. Dopamine levels are low in Parkinson's disease.

145–E. Because a hexosaminidase is deficient in Tay-Sachs disease, partially degraded sphingolipids (gangliosides) accumulate in lysosomes.

146–A. Glycogen accumulates because muscle phosphorylase is deficient in McArdle's disease (a glycogen storage disease).

147–D. In maple syrup urine disease, the α-keto acid dehydrogenase involved in metabolism of the branched chain amino acids (valine, isoleucine, and leucine) is defective.

148–B. A dietary deficiency of niacin causes pellagra.

149–A. Scurvy is caused by lack of vitamin C.

150–E. Lack of thiamine in the diet causes beriberi.

151–C. A dietary deficiency of vitamin D causes rickets.

120–E. Long-term exposure of the liver to alcohol can cause cirrhosis. Because the amount of functional liver tissue decreases, urea production decreases.

121–D. The POMC gene produces a protein that can be cleaved to form ACTH, β-lipotropin, MSH, and endorphins.

122–A. LH binds to plasma membrane receptors on Leydig cells and stimulates the production of testosterone.

123–C. An excess of growth hormone (GH) after epiphyseal closure causes acromegaly, a condition characterized by enlargement of the jaw, nose, hands, feet, and skull.

124–B. Aldosterone causes resorption of sodium ions and, consequently, the resorption of water. Vasopressin (antidiuretic hormone) causes water resorption.

125–D. Prolactin causes synthesis of the milk protein α-lactalbumin, which stimulates lactose synthesis.

126–A. Oxytocin causes uterine contractions during labor and contraction of mammary myoepithelial cells during lactation.

127–B. Low levels of thyroid hormone result in increased production of TSH by the anterior pituitary.

128–D. Somatostatin, produced by the hypothalamus, inhibits growth hormone production and secretion by the anterior pituitary.

129–A. Dopamine is an inhibitor of PRL production and secretion. Thus, if dopamine is low, more PRL will be produced and secreted by the anterior pituitary.

130–E. Low levels of aldosterone (which occurs in Addison's disease) results in low blood pressure.

131–B. Blood glucose is the major fuel for the brain, except when, after 3–5 days of fasting, ketone bodies in the blood reach a concentration at which the brain can use them.

132–B. Red blood cells lack mitochondria and thus are dependent on glucose for energy.

133–C. Fatty acids are the major fuel for the liver during fasting.

134–A. Ketone bodies are used by the brain after 3–5 days of fasting.

135–D. Muscles, particularly those with a preponderance of white fibers, use their glycogen stores when exercising.

136–A. Carnitine is required for the transport of fatty acids into the mitochondria where they undergo β-oxidation. If carnitine is deficient, fatty acids accumulate.

137–B. Ketone bodies are produced in the liver from acetyl CoA generated by fatty acid oxidation. In a carnitine deficiency, fatty acids are not oxidized, thus ketone bodies are not produced.

138–B. More blood glucose will be oxidized for energy because fatty acids cannot be used.

139–C. Cells take up LDL by endocytosis, and cholesterol is released from cholesterol esters by a lysosomal enzyme.

140–B. VLDL is synthesized by the liver from dietary sugar (present in jelly beans).

141–D. HDL removes cholesterol from cell membranes. The lecithin cholesterol acyl transferase (LCAT) reaction, which converts the cholesterol to cholesterol esters, occurs on HDL.

142–A. Chylomicrons contain triacylglycerols synthesized from dietary lipid in intestinal epithelial cells.

Pat Simon

$25

Elyse Shaw

Board Review Series

BIOCHEMISTRY 3rd edition

Dawn B. Marks

- Reflects USMLE changes
- 500 USMLE-type questions with explanations
- Easy-to-follow outline covering all USMLE-tested topics
- Numerous tables and illustrations
- A comprehensive examination

Lippincott Williams & Wilkins